Clinical Companion to The Molecular and Genetic Basis of Neurological Disease

Clinical Companion to The Molecular and Genetic Basis of Neurological Disease Second Edition

Edited by

Roger N. Rosenberg, M.D.

Abe (Brunky), Morris and William Zale Distinguished Chair in Neurology and Professor of Neurology and Physiology, University of Texas Southwestern Medical Center at Dallas; Attending Neurologist, Zale-Lipshy University Hospital, Parkland Hospital, and Children's Medical Center, Dallas

Stanley B. Prusiner, M.D.

Professor of Neurology and Biochemistry, University of California, San Francisco, School of Medicine

Salvatore DiMauro, M.D.

Lucy G. Moses Professor of Neurology, Columbia University College of Physicians and Surgeons, New York

Robert L. Barchi, M.D., Ph.D.

David Mahoney Professor of Neurological Sciences, University of Pennsylvania School of Medicine, Philadelphia; Chairman, Department of Neurology, University of Pennsylvania Medical Center, Philadelphia

Consulting Editor

Gerald M. Fenichel, M.D.

Professor of Neurology and Pediatrics and Chairman, Department of Neurology, Vanderbilt University Medical Center, Nashville, Tennessee

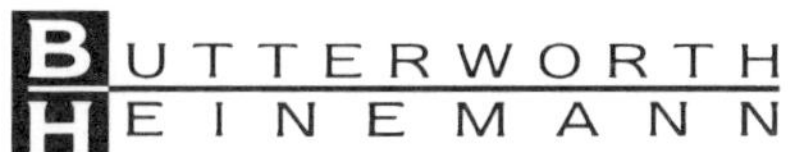

Boston Oxford Johannesburg Melbourne New Delhi Singapore

A member of the Reed Elsevier group

Every effort has been made to ensure that the drug dosage schedules within this text are accurate and conform to standards accepted at time of publication. However, as treatment recommendations vary in the light of continuing research and clinical experience, the reader is advised to verify drug dosage schedules herein with information found on product information sheets. This is especially true in cases of new or infrequently used drugs.

Recognizing the importance of preserving what has been written, Butterworth–Heinemann prints its books on acid-free paper whenever possible.

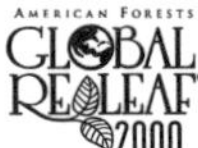

Butterworth–Heinemann supports the efforts of American Forests and the Global ReLeaf program in its campaign for the betterment of trees, forests, and our environment.

ISBN: 0-7506-7043-6

British Library Cataloguing-in-Publication Data
A catalogue record for this book is available from the British Library.

The publisher offers special discounts on bulk orders of this book.

For information, please contact:
Manager of Special Sales
Butterworth–Heinemann
225 Wildwood Avenue
Woburn, MA 01801-2041
Tel: 781-904-2500
Fax: 781-904-2620

For information on all Butterworth–Heinemann publications available, contact our World Wide Web home page at: http://www.bh.com

10 9 8 7 6 5 4 3 2 1

Printed in the United States of America

Contents

Preface

This handbook is designed to serve as a clinical companion to the larger *The Molecular and Genetic Basis of Neurological Disease Second Edition*, which is regarded as the most authoritative book in this area of neuroscience. The book successfully intertwines the clinical and molecular aspects of neurologic disease. To create this companion volume, the editors have extracted from the original book the practical and clinical information that is most useful for neurologists in the diagnosis and treatment of genetic neurologic disease. The text can be used either as a quick reference, stand-alone text, or concise review when the original volume is used as the primary text.

The remarkable achievements in the fields of molecular and cellular neurobiology and molecular neurogenetics have been applied to genetic neurologic disease with equally dramatic results. The study of molecular pathogenesis of neurologic disease is a recent development, and it is fair to say that most of the scientific material presented here was not available even 5 years ago. This surge of molecular data on neurologic disease is a strong testimony to the vitality of investigators in the field. Determination of the molecular pathogenesis of genetic neurologic disease is indispensable to the development of pharmacologic or gene therapy for these disorders. Therapy for proteins is the ultimate goal, and as described herein, such progress is just beginning in several areas such as glycogen storage disease, lipoprotein disorders, lysosomal disorders, Duchenne's muscular dystrophy, genetic forms of epilepsy, and membrane excitability disorders, among others. It is indeed a gratifying and exciting time to be in this rapidly evolving field.

The editors are most grateful to all the contributing authors for their participation in *The Molecular and Genetic Basis of Neurological Disease*. Each author is an authority and scholar in the field and, as such, has greatly enhanced the quality of this work.

The material enclosed herein is of value to clinicians caring for patients with hereditary neurologic disorders and to investigators concerned with the scientific issues that these disorders propose. In addition, we hope that the body of information described will serve to stimulate the next generation of neurologists and neuroscientists to enter this field and move forward aggressively toward a clearer understanding of the molecular and genetic basis of neurologic disease well into the twenty-first century.

The Editors

Clinical Companion to The Molecular and Genetic Basis of Neurological Disease

1

Molecular Genetics and Neurologic Disease: An Introduction

Approximately one-third of recognizable mendelian disease traits show phenotypic expression in the nervous system. Disease gene identification enables presymptomatic and prenatal diagnosis and provides prognostic information.

CLASSIC GENETICS

Gregor Mendel is credited for discovering the laws of inheritance. His first law, the principle of independent segregation, referred to the ability of genes to segregate independently during the formation of gametes, or sex cells. The second law, the principle of independent assortment, postulated that only one "factor" from each pair was independently transmitted to the gamete during sex-cell formation, and any one gamete contains only one type of inherited factor from each gene pair. Genes arising from one parent tend not to stay together except when genes or loci are linked (physically located in close proximity on the chromosome). The closer the link, the more frequently they cosegregate.

The chromosomal theory of heredity emphasizes that the diploid chromosome group consists of two morphologically similar sets for each chromosome, and that during meiosis every gamete receives only one chromosome of each homologous pair. Genes are arranged in linear order on the chromosome, each having a specific position or locus. Two copies exist for each gene at the given locus. The two copies, or alleles, may be identical or homozygous at a specific locus. The genes are passed to the next generation through parental gametes, which contain only one of the two alternative gene copies. Human diploid cells contain 22 chromosome pairs called *autosomes* and one pair of sex chromosomes: two X chromosomes in females and one X matched with one Y chromosome in males. The full complement of chromosomes, or karyotype, is normally 46,XX for females and 46,XY for males.

The major patterns of mendelian inheritance are termed *autosomal dominant, autosomal recessive,* and *X-linked.* Autosomal dominant alleles exert their effect despite the presence of a corresponding normal allele on the homologous chromosome. One-half of individuals in each generation are affected, and an affected individual has a 50% chance of transmitting the disease to each offspring. In autosomal recessive inheritance, both alleles must be abnormal for the disease trait to be expressed. The parents of an affected child are obligate heterozygotes for the mutant allele and are themselves unaffected. Couples who are heterozygous carriers of a recessive mutant allele have a 25% risk of having an affected child with each pregnancy. In X-linked recessive inheritance, a mutation in a gene located on the X chromosome may not express itself in females because of the normal copy on the other X chromosome. All males who inherit the mutant allele, however, will be affected. An important feature of X-linked inheritance is that male-to-male transmission never occurs, but all female offspring of affected males inherit the abnormal gene. X-linked recessive disorders may sometimes be observed in females because of a skewing in the process of lyonization or X inactivation.

VARIABILITY OF EXPRESSION, PENETRANCE, ANTICIPATION, AND IMPRINTING

Establishing a particular mendelian pattern of inheritance enables accurate estimates of recurrence risk but does not address the severity of the disease. *Variability of expression* refers to the differing severity of clinical manifestation found in different patients with a particular disease. *Penetrance* refers to whether a clinical phenotype is expressed when an individual has inherited a mutant gene. Penetrance may be age-dependent or may reflect how the phenotype is measured (i.e., clinical examination or diagnostic studies). *Anticipation* refers to the appearance of a more severe clinical phenotype in successive generations. *Imprinting* refers to variation in phenotype depending on the parent of origin of the mutant allele.

MITOCHONDRIAL INHERITANCE

In addition to the nuclear genome, mitochondria contain DNA that transmits genetic information to subsequent generations. Mitochondrial DNA (mtDNA) encodes several subunits of the mitochondrial respiratory chain and oxidative phosphorylation system. Because sperm contribute no mitochondria to the zygote, the ovum supplies the total complement of mtDNA for the conceptus. Therefore, mtDNA is exclusively maternally transmitted. Disorders resulting from such mutations have great variability in clinical expression. The term *heteroplasmy* is used when different tissues have different percentages of mutant genomes; *homoplasmy* refers to instances in which all the mitochondrial genomes are identical to one another.

CHROMOSOMAL INHERITANCE

Chromosomal disorders may involve several genes. Chromosome abnormalities can involve the entire chromosome or chromosomal segments. *Chromosome aneuploidy* is an abnormal number of chromosomes. *Trisomy* is the presence of three copies of a single chromosome. The frequency of trisomy increases with advanced maternal age. *Monosomy* refers to the absence of one chromosome from the pair. Monosomy usually involves the sex chromosomes. *Uniparental disomy* describes the inheritance of two chromosomes from one parent rather than the usual one chromosome of the homologous pair from each parent. *Heterodisomy* is the inheritance of two different chromosomes for one homologous pair from one parent, whereas *isodisomy* is the inheritance of two copies of one chromosome homologue from one parent. *Segmental aneuploidy* occurs when portions within a chromosome are missing from a deletion or are in excess either because of duplication of a specific region of a chromosome or because of translocation of a portion of one chromosome to another. Translocation carriers have the proper amount of chromosomal material and therefore a normal phenotype but are at a high risk of transmitting a chromosome with missing or excess genetic information and conceiving a child with an unbalanced karyotype.

MUTATION TYPES

Point mutations that occur in the coding region of a gene may have different effects. A *silent mutation* is a base pair change that makes a different triplet codon but still codes for the same amino acid. Such a mutation can cause benign polymorphic changes in DNA. A silent mutation may create a cryptic splice site and alter what is expressed from the gene. *Missense mutations* change a codon so that a different amino acid is substituted at a given position in the protein. *Nonsense mutations* result in a premature translational termination. *Frameshift mutations* result from deletions or additions of one or more base pairs, but not multiples of three. Frameshift mutations usually lead to premature translation termination secondary to encountering a stop codon in a different reading frame.

Deletions refer to the loss of DNA sequence. *Duplications* refer to an additional exact copy of a particular DNA sequence. Either may involve a part of a gene, the entire gene, or a segment of a chromosome with many genes. The phenotypic consequences of duplications may result from gene dosage effects of only one or a small subset of genes.

Transposable genetic elements are discrete segments of DNA that can move or transpose from one region of the genome to another. They usually lead to insertional inactivation of that gene. *Trinucleotide repeat expansions* are unstable mutations that may change in size from generation to generation or even in different tissues in the same individual. They provide a biologic explanation for anticipation, variable penetrance and expressivity, and parental transmission effects.

CLINICAL APPLICATIONS

Even before the isolation of a disease gene, the identification of genetic markers that are closely linked to a disease locus, known as *linked markers*, can be used to identify presymptomatic individuals and for prenatal diagnosis of gene carriers. The estimation of risk for genetic disease using linked markers is an indirect method and has several limitations. The predictive value of a test using a linked marker is a function of the genetic distance between the marker locus and the disease gene. A disadvantage of the linkage approach is that several family members must be available to establish which allele at the marker locus is segregating with the disease gene. This is known as *setting the phase*.

Once a disease gene is isolated and the molecular structure of the normal and mutant forms are delineated, a direct mutation detection test can be designed. The identification of the specific molecular lesion in a patient (1) establishes a secure diagnosis, (2) makes it possible to diagnose or exclude a diagnosis with a simple blood test in other family members in whom there is risk of the disease developing, (3) enables prenatal diagnosis to be offered, and (4) may provide prognostic information.

Table 1.1 shows the chromosomal localization of loci for mutations causing neurologic disease and genes encoding proteins, enzymes, and transmitters involved in normal neurologic functioning as of 1996.

Table 1.1
A neurologic gene map: chromosomes 1–22 and X.

Chromosome/ Region	*Gene/Disease Locus*
1p12	Neurofilament, heavy polypeptide-like
1p13	Beta-nerve growth factor
1p13	*N*-ras oncogene
1p13	Adenosine monophosphate deaminase 1/myopathy
1p21[a]	Glycogen storage disease
1p21–qter	Actin, alpha chains
1p22–p21[a]	Zellweger syndrome type II
1p31	Dihydrolipoyl transacylase/maple syrup urine disease
1p32	Infantile neuronal ceroid lipofuscinoses (Finnish type)
1p34	Alpha-L-fucosidase-1/fucosidosis
1p34	Uroporphyrinogen decarboxylase/porphyria cutanea tarda
1p36–q12	Carnitine palmitoyltransferase/deficiency
1p36.2–p36.1[a]	Neuroblastoma type III
1cen–q32	Muscle phosphofructokinase[b]/glycogenosis type VII
1q21	Glucocerebrosidase/Gaucher's disease
1q21.2–q23[a]	HMSN type I; Po protein mutation
1q21–q23	Nemaline myopathy
1q21–q23	ATPase, Na^+/K^+, $alpha_2$ polypeptide
1q22–q25	ATPase, Na^+/K^+, beta polypeptide
1q31–32	Hypokalemic, periodic paralysis—alpha subunit of the dihydropyridine receptor calcium channel
1q	Usher syndrome type 2
1q	Xeroderma pigmentosum
2p	Carbamoylphosphate synthetase I[b]/carbamoylphosphate synthetase I deficiency
2p[a]	Hereditary spastic paraplegia; autosomal dominant
2p21[a]	Holoprosencephaly type 2
2p24	*N*-myc oncogene
2p23	Proopiomelanocortin
2p12–q11	Neurofilament, light polypeptide-like type 1
2q12–q11	Diazepam-binding inhibitor[b]
2q12–q21	Sodium channel type II, alpha polypeptide[b]
2q21–q32	Muscle nicotinic ACHR, alpha subunit[b]
2q21	Xeroderma pigmentosum
2q31–q32	Nebulin
2q32–qter	Muscle nicotinic ACHR, gamma subunit
2q33–qter	Muscle nicotinic ACHR, delta subunit
2q33–qter	Cerebrotendinous xanthomatosis[b]
2q33–q35[a]	Amyotrophic lateral sclerosis, juvenile
2q	Desmin
2q	Glutamate decarboxylase
3p12–p21.1[a]	Dominant ataxia with retinal dystrophy (ADCA type II)
3pter–3p21	Beta-galactosidase I/GM_1 gangliosidosis
3p14.3[a]	Susceptibility to Wernicke-Korsakoff syndrome

Table 1.1
(continued)

Chromosome/ Region	*Gene/Disease Locus*
3p21	Pyruvate dehydrogenase, E_1 beta subunit/pyruvate dehydrogenase deficiency
3p26–p25	von Hippel-Lindau disease
3q[a]	Usher syndrome type 3
3p24	Retinoic acid receptor, beta
3q23–q25	Ceruloplasmin
3q21–q24[a]	Rhodopsin/retinitis pigmentosa type 4, dominant
3q24–q25	Dandy-Walker anomaly
3q28	Somatostatin[b]
4p16.3[a]	Huntington's disease, CAG repeats
4p16.3[a]	Hurler and Hurler-Scheie syndrome
4p16–q23	ATPase, Na^+/K^+, beta polypeptide-like type 1
4p15.3[a]	Quinoid dihydropteridine reductase/deficiency; phenylketonuria syndrome
4p13–p12	GABA A receptor, $alpha_2$ and $beta_1$ subunits
4q11–q13	Alpha-fetoprotein
4q21–q23[a]	Mucolipidosis types II and III
4q22–q23	Pyruvate dehydrogenase, E_1 alpha peptide-like[b]
4q25	Epidermal growth factor
4q35–qter	Facioscapulohumeral dystrophy
5p11–q13	Arylsulfatase B/Maroteaux-Lamy syndrome
5p13–p12	Growth hormone receptor[b]
5q11.2–q13.3	Acute and chronic childhood spinal muscular atrophy
5q11–q13[a]	Maroteaux-Lamy syndrome
5q11.2–q13.2	Dihydrofolate reductase/deficiency
5q11.2–q13.3	Schizophrenia[b]
5q13	Hexosaminidase B/Sandhoff's disease
5q22–q34	Dominant limb girdle muscular dystrophy
5q23	Diphtheria toxin sensitivity
5q31–q32	Glucocorticoid receptor
5q31–q32	$Beta_2$-adrenergic receptor, surface
5q33–q35	Platelet-derived growth factor receptor, beta chain
5q33–q35[a]	Hereditary hyperekplexia (familial startle syndrome)-dominant glycine receptor
5	GM_2 activator protein[b]/GM_2 gangliosidosis, AB variant
6p21.1–cen[a]	Retinitis pigmentosa, peripherin-related
6p–21.3[a]	Juvenile myoclonic epilepsy
6pter–p21	Tubulin, beta polypeptide
6pter–p23	Mitochondrial malic enzyme 2
6p24–p23[a]	Dominant ataxia (some families); SCA type 1, CAG repeats
6p23–p21.1	Prolactin
6p22–p21	Branch chain ketoacid dehydrogenase E_1/maple syrup urine disease
6p21.3	Major histocompatibility complex

Chromosome/ Region	*Gene/Disease Locus*
6p21.3	Neuraminidase I/possibly sialidosis[b]
6q23	Arginase[b]/argininemia
6q24–q27	Vasoactive intestinal polypeptide
7p13–p12.3[a]	Myopathy due to phosphoglycerate mutase deficiency
7pter–q22	Actin, cytoskeletal[b]
7pter–q22	Neuropeptide Y[b]
7pter–q22	Argininosuccinate lyase/argininosuccinicaciduria
7p21.3	Craniosynostosis (some families)
7p13	Greig's cephalopolysyndactyly syndrome
7p13–p12	Epidermal growth factor receptor
7p15.1–p13[a]	Retinitis pigmentosa type 9
7q[a]	Retinitis pigmentosa type 10
7q[a]	Cavernous malformations of the brain
7cen–q11.2	Myosin, heavy polypeptide 5
7q11.23	Zellweger's syndrome type 1[b]
7q21.2–q22	Beta-glucuronidase/mucopolysaccharidosis type VII
7q31–q35[a]	Myotonia congenita, dominant (Thomsen disease); (*CLCN* 1 gene) (muscle chloride channel protein)
7q36[a]	Holoprosencephaly type 3
8p[a]	Progressive epilepsy with mental retardation, recessive (Finnish type)
8p11–q21	Retinitis pigmentosa type I
8q[a]	Hereditary spastic paraplegia; autosomal recessive
8q13[a]	Friedreich's ataxia, vitamin E deficiency; alpha tocopherol transport protein defect
8q[a]	Benign neonatal seizures
8q13	Corticotropin-releasing hormone
8q23–q24	Proenkephalin[b]
9p13	Galactose-1-phosphate uridyltransferase/galactosemia
9q13–q21.1	Friedreich's ataxia; GAA repeats in first intron; frataxin protein deficiency
9q32–q34.1[a]	Xeroderma pigmentosum, complementation group, type A
9q32–q34[a]	Torsion dystonia (some families)
9q34.1–q34.2	Tuberous sclerosis (some families) type 1[b]
9q33	Sequin/amylin neuropathy (Finnish type)
9q34	Argininosuccinate synthetase/citrullinemia
9q34	Dopamine-beta-hydroxylase
9q34[a]	Porphyria, acute hepatic
9	Coproporphyrin oxidase/coproporphyria
10q[a]	Partial epilepsy
10q23.3–q24.1[a]	Infantile-onset spinocerebellar ataxia of Nikali et al.
10q23–q24	Glutamate dehydrogenase[b]
10q24–q26	Adrenergic alpha$_2$ receptor
10	Glycoprotein neuraminidase[b]/sialidosis
10	Mitochondrial ATPase[b]
11 (centromere)[a]	Dominant ataxia (SCA type 5)
11p	Major affective disorder type l[b]

Table 1.1
(continued)

Chromosome/ Region	*Gene/Disease Locus*
11p[a]	Usher syndrome type 1C
11p15.5	Tyrosine hydroxylase
11p15.4–15.1[a]	Niemann-Pick disease types A and B
11q13–q13.2	Muscle glycogen phosphorylase/McArdle's disease
11q13.5[a]	Usher syndrome type 1B
11q14–q21	Tyrosinase
11q14–q23	Tuberous sclerosis (some families)
11q22–q23	Dopamine D_2 receptor
11q23	Ataxia telangiectasia
11q23[a]	Tuberous sclerosis type 2
11q23–q24	Apolipoprotein Al/amyloid neuropathy, Iowa type
11q23–q24	Neural cell adhesion molecule
11q23.2qter	Porphobilinogen deaminase/acute intermittent porphyria
11q	Pyruvate carboxylase
11q [a]	Usher syndrome type 1C
12p[a]	Dominant episodic ataxia (type 1); K^+ channelopathy
12p13	Gamma neuronal enolase type 2
12p12–ter[a]	Dentato-rubro-pallido-luysian atrophy; CAG repeats
12q22–q24.2	Phenylalanine hydroxylase/phenylketonuria
12q22–q24.1	Tuberous sclerosis (some families)
12q22–qter	Short- and medium-chain acyl CoA dehydrogenase/lipid storage myopathy
12q23–24.1[a]	Dominant ataxia (some families) SCA type 2
13q12–q13[a]	Muscular dystrophy, Duchenne-like, autosomal
13q14.2–q21	Wilson's disease
13q14.2	Retinoblastoma
13q21–q31 or pter–q13	ATPase, Na^+/K^+, alpha polypeptide-like type 1
14	Dominant distal myopathy
14q[a]	Hereditary spastic paraplegia; autosomal dominant
14q[a]	Dopa-responsive dystonia; T_4 biopterin type
14q32[a]	Usher syndrome type 1A
14q32.3	Brain creatine kinase
14q32.33	Immunoglobulin heavy chain gene cluster
14q	Protoporphyrin oxidase/variegate porphyria
14q	Usher syndrome type 1A
14q11.2–q13[a]	Oculopharyngeal muscular dystrophy
14q11.1–q13[a]	Holoprosencephaly type 4
14q12[a]	Central core disease
14q24.3–q32.1[a]	Machado-Joseph disease (SCA type 3) CAG repeats
14q24.3[a]	Early-onset Alzheimer's disease (FAD), dominant
15q[a]	Hereditary spastic paraplegia; autosomal dominant
15q11[a]	Dyslexia (some families)
15q11–q12	Angelman and Prader-Willi syndromes

Chromosome/ Region	*Gene/Disease Locus*
15q15–q22	Recessive limb girdle dystrophy
15q22–qter	Muscle pyruvate kinase
15q23–q24	Hexosaminidase A/Tay-Sachs disease
15	Xeroderma pigmentosum, complementation group F
15	Marfan's syndrome
16p13 [a]	Tuberous sclerosis (some families)
16p12	Batten's disease[b]
16q[a]	Dominant ataxia (SCA type 4)
17pter–p11	Myosin, heavy chain cluster
17p13.3	Miller-Dieker syndrome, lissencephaly
17p13.1	Tumor protein pS3
17p12–p11	Muscle nicotinic ACHR, beta subunit[b]
17p11.2[a]	Neuropathy, recurrent, with pressure palsies (tomaculus type); PMP22 deletion
17p11.2[a]	HMSN type 1 (most families), trisomy; PMP22 protein type
17q11.2[a]	von Recklinghausen's neurofibromatosis (type 1); neurofibrin type
17q22–q24	Growth hormone
17q21–q22[a]	Disinhibition-dementia-Parkinsonism-amyotrophy complex (Lynch-Wilhelmsen type), dominant
17q21–q22	Nerve growth factor receptor
17q23[a]	(Pompe disease) acid alpha-glucosidase/acid maltase deficiency
17q23.1–q25.3[a]	Hyperkalemic periodic paralysis (SCN4 A gene) (muscle sodium channel alpha subunit); paramyotonia congenita
17	Gamma actin
18p[a]	Niemann-Pick disease type C
18pter–q11[a]	Holoprosencephaly type 1
18q11.2–q12.1	Transthyretin/familial amyloid polyneuropathy, several types
18q22.1[a]	? Gilles de la Tourette's syndrome
18q22–qter[a]	Myelin basic protein; multiple sclerosis susceptibility
19p[a]	Mannosidosis
19p[a]	Dominant episodic ataxia type 2, acetazolamide-responsive
19[a]	Hereditary hemiplegic migraine
19[a]	Malignant hyperthermia (muscle ryanodine receptor)
19cen–q13.1	Lysosomal alpha-D-mannosidase B/mannosidosis
19q12[a]	Central arteriopathy with subcortical infarcts and leukoencephalopathy
19q12–13.2	Poliovirus sensitivity
19q12–q13.1	Central core disease
19q12–13.2	Ryanodine receptor/malignant hyperthermia
19q13.1	Myelin-associated glycoprotein
19q13.1–q13.2[a]	Maple syrup urine disease type 1
19q13.3[a]	Myotonic dystrophy; CTG repeats
19q13.2–q13.3	Muscle creatine kinase
19cen–q13.2[a]	Late-onset familial Alzheimer's disease-apolipoprotein E (2,3,4) locus

Table 1.1
(continued)

Chromosome/ Region	*Gene/Disease Locus*
20pter–p12[a]	Prion protein/inherited spongiform encephalopathies CJD and GSS types
20p11.22–p11.21	Cystalin C/Icelandic amyloid angiopathy
20p11.23–qter	Growth hormone–releasing factor
20q13.2–q13.3[a]	Benign neonatal convulsions (EBN type 1) (nicotinic acetylcholine receptor)
20q13.2[a]	Dominant nocturnal epilepsy
20q13.2[a]	Pituitary tumor, growth hormone–secreting
21q22.3	Cystathionine beta-synthase/homocystinuria
21q21.2[a]	Early-onset familial Alzheimer's disease (FAD); amyloid precursor protein gene (codons 670–671, 692, 717)
21q21.2[a]	Dutch hereditary cerebral hemorrhage; amyloid precursor protein gene (codon 693)
21q21.3–q22.05[a]	Schizophrenia, chronic
21q22.1–q22.2[a]	Amyotrophic lateral sclerosis (some families); Cu/Zn superoxide dismutase
21q22.3[a]	Unverricht-Lundborg disease; progressive myoclonus epilepsy
22pter–q11	Alpha-L-iduronidase[b]/Hurler's and Scheie's syndromes
22q11–q13	Thyrotropin-stimulating hormone receptor
22q13.31–qter	Arylsulfatase A/metachromatic leukodystrophy
22q12.2[a]	Bilateral acoustic neurofibromatosis (type 2)
22q12.1–q13.1	Neurofilament, heavy polypeptide
22q12.3–qter	Meningioma
22q13–qter	Neuroaxonal dystrophy
22q13.1–q13.2	Cytochrome P450 IID/debrisoquine sensitivity
22q	Transcobalamin II deficiency
22	Catecholamine-*O*-methyltransferase
Xp22.32	Kallmann syndrome
Xp22.2	X-linked HMSN type 2
Xp22.2–p22.1	Retinoschisis
Xp22.1	Pyruvate dehydrogenase E_1 alpha polypeptide[b]/pyruvate dehydrogenase
Xp22.1–p21.2	Glycine receptor[b]
Xp22	Aicardi's syndrome[b]
Xp22	Ocular albinism; two types
Xp21.3–p21.2	Retinitis pigmentosa 6
Xp21.2	Duchenne's and Becker's muscular dystrophies
Xp21.1	Kell blood group precursor/McLeod's syndrome
Xp21.1	Ornithine transcarbamylase/deficiency
Xp21.1–p11.4	Retinitis pigmentosa type 3
Xp11.4–p11.2	Retinitis pigmentosa type 2
Xp11.4–11.3	Norrie's disease
Xp11.3–p11.23	Monoamine oxidase A

Chromosome/ Region	*Gene/Disease Locus*
Xp11.3–p11.23	Monoamine oxidase B
Xp11.21–cen	Incontinentia pigmenti type 1
Xp11–q13	X-linked mental retardation without dysmorphic features
Xq11–q13	X-linked HMSN type 1, dominant
Xq12–q13[a]	Menkes' disease
Xq12–q22	X-linked spastic paraplegia[b]
Xq12cen–q22[a]	Bulbospinal neuronopathy of Kennedy; androgen receptor; CAG repeats
Xq21	Dystonia/parkinsonism (Filipino type)
Xp21[a]	Mental retardation of the Snyder-Robinson type
Xq21.1–q21.2	Choroideremia
Xq21.3–q22	Alpha-galactosidase A/Fabry's disease
Xq21.3–q22	Myelin proteolipid protein/Pelizaeus-Merzbacher disease
Xq22[a]	Hereditary spastic paraplegia
Xq22.2[a]	X-linked HMSN type 3, connexin 32 protein type; recessive
Xq25–q26.1	Lowe's oculocerebral syndrome
Xq26	Hypoxanthine-guanine phosphoribosyltransferase/Lesch-Nyhan syndrome
Xq27	Paraneoplastic cerebellar degeneration–related protein
Xq27–q28	Incontinentia pigmenti type 2
Xq27–q28	Centronuclear myopathy[b]
Xq27–q28	Rud's syndrome
Xq27–q28	Major affective disorder type 2
Xq27.3[a]	Fragile X mental retardation syndrome; CGG repeats
Xq27.3–q28	Iduronate-2-sulfatase/Hunter's syndrome
Xq27.3–q28[a]	Emery-Dreifuss muscular dystrophy (emerin type)
Xq28[a]	Fragile X type E; GCC repeats
Xq28	Adrenoleukodystrophy, adrenoleukomyeloneuropathy
Xq28[a]	Myotubular myopathy
Xq28	Deutan and protan color blindness
Xq28	γ-Amino butyric acid (GABA) A receptor $alpha_3$ subunit
Xq28[a]	Hydrocephalus aqueductal stenosis type
Xq	Ataxia and dementia syndrome

ADCA = autosomal dominant cerebellar ataxia; CJD = Creutzfeldt-Jakob disease; GSS = Gerstmann-Sträussler-Scheinker disease; CLCN = chloride channel gene; FAD = familial Alzheimer's disease; HMSN = hereditary motor and sensory neuropathy; SCA = spinocerebellar ataxia; SCN = sodium channel(opathy); p = short arm; q = long arm; ter = end of short or long arm; cen = centromere (e.g., 6q23 = band 23 on the long arm of chromosome 6 [band numbers increase moving in either direction away from the centromere], 3p21–cen = between band 21 on the short arm of chromosome 3 and the centromere, and 5 implies localized to chromosome 5, but not to any specific region).

Note: Numerous X-linked mental retardation syndromes have been mapped to the X chromosome (1).

[a]Added with the second edition of *The Molecular and Genetic Basis of Neurological Disease*.

[b]Provisional assignment only.

For a more detailed discussion, see Lupski JR, Zoghbi HY. Molecular Genetics and Neurologic Disease: An Introduction (Chapter 1; pp. 3–22); Harding AE, Rosenberg RN. A Neurologic Gene Map (Chapter 2; pp. 23–28); Merette C, Ott J. Finding and Excluding Gene Locations by Linkage Analysis (Chapter 3; pp. 29–32); Moore RC, Melton DW, Gene Targeting (Chapter 4; pp. 33–48), in RN Rosenberg, SB Prusiner, S DiMauro, RL Barchi (eds), **The Molecular and Genetic Basis of Neurological Disease** *(2nd ed). Boston: Butterworth–Heinemann, 1997.*

2

Chromosome Disorders

DOWN SYNDROME

Down syndrome (DS) is the prototype of all chromosome abnormality syndromes.

Clinical Neurology of Down Syndrome

Hypotonia

Hypotonia is the most characteristic feature of DS in newborns and infants. It is even more pronounced in infants with moderate to severe congenital heart disease. Tone improves but remains decreased as compared to normals throughout childhood. Strength is decreased in direct relation to the severity of hypotonia. Tendon reflexes, a reflection of tone, are less smooth and brisk. The hypotonia is assumed to be central in origin. Proposals that tone results from a decrease in the concentration of 5-hydroxytryptamine (serotonin) in the peripheral blood and that it can be improved by administration of 5-hydroxytryptophan have not been confirmed by subsequent investigation. Indeed, administration of 5-hydroxytryptophan may induce infantile spasms. Similarly, vitamin B_6 administration, which also elevates blood serotonin, had no beneficial effects on tone or development.

Mental Retardation

With the exception of the profound hypotonia, the behavior of infants with DS is generally normal at birth. Developmental retardation usually becomes obvious during the first several months of life, and the mean age at which developmental landmarks are attained becomes increasingly more delayed as time goes on. The developmental quotient during infancy is usually 50% of normal. During childhood, development continues to progress but at a slower rate, finally plateaus between 5 and 10 years of age, and ultimately declines. Cardiac status influences motor development but not mental development. Both appear to correlate with muscle tone. The decline in developmental rate may not be entirely biological; decreased active participation in the learning process as a consequence of poor or inadequate motivation may also play a role.

The mental retardation associated with DS may have some features that are characteristic but not specific. These include lexical and grammatical impairments, a selective inattention to detail in visuospatial constructions, and greater difficulty in recalling sequences of verbal information presented auditorially. Anomalous dominance (lateralization) of language has been observed in young adults with DS.

In rare instances, children with DS without known mosaicism have attained IQs above 80 and have performed in the low average range. These cases illustrate the variability of the syndrome and raise the question about what factors could influence mental development. One possible factor is intrinsic genetic differences among individuals and another is the different environments in which they are raised. Studies of both factors have provided contradictory results. The long-term effects of early intervention programs remain unproved.

Other Neurologic Abnormalities

Atlantoaxial/atlanto-occipital instability is a risk in 15–20% of children with DS, but only a few with instability become symptomatic. Seizures occur in less than 10% of children with DS. Infantile spasms and tonic-clonic seizures with myoclonus are the more common seizure types during infancy, whereas tonic-clonic, partial simple, or partial complex seizures are more common later on. The prevalence of seizures increases with age, reaching 46% after age 50. Seizures beginning after age 35 indicate the development of dementia.

Dementia and Cognitive Decline

The brains of older people with DS show the senile plaques and neurofibrillary tangles characteristic of Alzheimer's disease (AD). Although these changes are reliable semiquantitative markers for AD, it is not known if they cause dementia. A significant number of adults with DS do not have dementia; some who are thought to be demented are suffering instead from severe depression.

Table 2.1
Physical characteristics of Down syndrome.

Feature	*Frequency (%)**
Oblique (upslanting) palpebral fissures	82
Loose skin on nape of neck	81
Narrow palate	76
Brachycephaly	75
Hyperflexibility	73
Flat nasal bridge	68
Gap between first and second toes	68
Short, broad hands	64
Short neck	61
Abnormal teeth	61
Epicanthic folds	59
Short fifth finger	58
Open mouth	58
Incurved fifth finger	57
Brushfield spots	56
Furrowed tongue	55
Transverse palmar crease	53
Folded or dysplastic ear	50
Protruding tongue	47

*Means of frequencies in Table 1 of SM Pueschel et al. Biomedical Aspects in Down Syndrome. In SM Pueschel, JE Rynders (eds), Down Syndrome. Advances in Biomedicine and the Behavioral Sciences. Cambridge, MA: Ware, 1982;169.
Source: Adapted from CJ Epstein. The Consequences of Chromosome Imbalance: Principles, Mechanisms, and Models. New York: Cambridge University Press, 1986.

Physical Features of Down Syndrome

The most immediately apparent manifestations of DS are the minor dysmorphic features that collectively constitute its distinctive physical phenotype. A list of these features is presented in Table 2.1. Although any individual with DS will have many of the characteristic features and be easily recognized as having the syndrome, none of these features is present in all affected individuals.

Neuropathology

During infancy and childhood, brain weight is in the low normal range, and the size of the cerebellum and brain stem may be reduced to an even greater extent. The fronto-occipital diameter of the forebrain is foreshortened and the superior temporal gyrus is narrowed. Among the nonspecific findings in DS are nerve cell heterotopias in the white layers of the cerebellum and vermis and delayed myelination. The main pathologic changes seen in adults are those of AD. The pathologic changes found in adult DS brains may differ quantitatively in some areas from those found in AD; in DS, the density of amyloid deposition is greater and the distribution more widespread.

Therapy for Down Syndrome

Therapy for DS is presently symptomatic and is addressed to the treatment of the various medical and surgical conditions that may be associated with the syndrome. No specific form of pharmacologic or other therapy is known to have beneficial effects on neurologic and cognitive functioning in DS.

Mode of Inheritance and Epidemiology

Chromosome Abnormalities

DS is the phenotypic manifestation of trisomy 21. It occurs when an extra copy of chromosome 21 is present in the genome, whether as a free whole chromosome (93–96% of the time), as part of a robertsonian fusion chromosome carrying the long arm of chromosome 21 in combination with the long arm of another acrocentric chromosome (2–5%), or in rare instances as part of a reciprocal translocation (<1%). All cells of the body are trisomic except for those in the 24% of cases in which mosaicism exists. In the latter, two populations of cells, one diploid and one trisomic, are present, with the number and distribution of trisomic cells being sufficient to cause the DS phenotype. Because the frequency of 47, + 21 is a function of maternal age, whereas the other forms of aneuploidy producing DS do not appear to be, its proportion and that of 47, + 21/46 mosaicism rise progressively with maternal age, whereas that of the robertsonian fusions decreases. When these factors are considered together with the age dependence of nontranslocation/nonfusion trisomy 21, the likelihood that a person with DS has an unbalanced translocation of familial origin falls from 2.2% at maternal age 20 years to 1% at age 30, 0.4% at age 35, and 0.1% at age 40.

Mosaicism

Trisomy 21 mosaicism is generally recognized in one of three ways: during the cytogenetic investigation of typical cases of DS; during the evaluation of so-called mild or possible cases of DS, or of mildly retarded or dysmorphic children without any obvious diagnosis; and in the course of studies on parents who have had more than one child with trisomy

21. Parental mosaicism, as defined by the detection of at least two trisomic cells, is present in about 3% of women having one child with trisomy 21. The proportion of trisomic cells present in either peripheral blood lymphocytes or fibroblasts does not correlate with mental development. The physical phenotype can be quite variable, ranging from typical DS to only mental retardation and subtle dysmorphic features. Congenital heart disease appears to occur infrequently, if at all.

Maternal Age and Parental Origin

The risk of having a child with DS increases with maternal age and the distribution of maternal age in the population of women having children is the primary determinant of the overall incidence of DS. The incidence of DS in the newborn population is estimated at 1 per 1,000. The rate of DS increases gradually in a linear fashion, about 0.05 per 1,000 per year, until approximately age 30 years, then abruptly shifts to more of an exponential pattern of increase. Approximately 88% of full trisomy 21 are maternal in origin, 9% are paternal, and 3% occur at mitosis after fertilization.

Molecular Neurobiology

Structure of Chromosome 21

Chromosome 21 is the smallest of the human autosomes, constituting approximately 1.7% of the length of the haploid genome. The long arm (21q), which constitutes the major part of chromosome 21, has a characteristic banding pattern consisting of three or four bands at low resolution and as many as 11 dark and light bands resolvable by prometaphase banding. Only this arm of chromosome 21 is essential for normal development and function.

Down Syndrome Region: Genotype-Phenotype Correlations

Cases in which only part of chromosome 21 is duplicated have been intensively studied to arrive at a phenotypic map that will permit a correlation of particular phenotypic features of DS with specific regions or loci of the chromosome. The consensus of the earlier studies carried out before molecular markers became available is that the full DS phenotype, as manifested by mental retardation, congenital heart disease, characteristic facial appearance, hand anomalies, and dermatoglyphic changes, appears when band 21q22 is duplicated, and, of this, subbands 21q22.1 and probably 21q22.2 are required. This region is estimated to carry 50–100 genes. Many of the components of the DS phenotype, including the facies, short stature, hypotonia, abnormal dermatoglyphics, and mental retardation, however, may be influenced by genes outside of 21q22.

General Principles of the Effects of Aneuploidy

The problem of defining how an extra copy of all or part of chromosome 21 results in the phenotype of DS is a specialized case of the general problem of explaining how chromosome imbalance involving any part of the genome produces abnormalities of function and development. Aneuploid phenotypes, although frequently overlapping, are differentiable from one another. Thus, although the same dysmorphic features or congenital malformations may be part of the phenotype of two or more different aneuploid states, the patterns of individual aneuploid states are specific enough to permit them to be distinguished from one another clinically. Although there may be a significant degree of variability in the expression of the phenotype of a given type of chromosome imbalance, no single phenotypic feature, with the possible exceptions of mental retardation and hypotonia, is always present in DS.

Variability in phenotypic expression stems from three sources: genetic, stochastic, and extrinsic. Stochastic factors refer to the inherent variability normally present in any developmental process such that, all else being equal, more than one outcome is possible. Extrinsic factors include all nongenetic influences except for those randomly generated developmental events that are referred to as stochastic. The genetic factors are of two kinds: differences in the precise genetic constitution of the chromosomes or chromosome segments that are unbalanced and, conversely, differences in the balanced remainder of the genome. Imbalance of one part of the genome does not operate in a vacuum; it is superimposed on the overall genetic constitution of the organism, a genetic constitution that, except in identical twins, necessarily differs from individual to individual.

Pathogenesis of Down Syndrome

The immediate consequence of an aneuploid state is a *gene dosage effect* for each of the loci present on the unbalanced chromosome or chromosome segment. With the exception of the amyloid precursor protein, the measured increases in activities or concentrations in trisomic cells in brains of fetuses with DS were close to the theoretically expected values of 1.5. Taken in the aggregate, these results confirm the existence of quite precise dosage effects in cells aneuploid for chromosome 21. Proposals to explain the development of AD in adults with DS can be summarized in two principal categories. The first category is that the genetic imbalance present in trisomy 21 indirectly causes AD either by causing the nervous system to be intrinsically defective from early in life, thereby enhancing the susceptibility of the brain to exogenous agents that cause AD, or by causing premature aging. The second category is that the genetic imbalance in trisomy 21 directly causes AD because the increased dosage of one or more chromosome 21 loci results in increased activities or concentrations of one or more gene products, which, in turn, produce injury to the brain. One candidate for the responsible gene product has been CuZn-superoxide dismutase.

FRAGILE X SYNDROME

X-linked inheritance of mental retardation has long been recognized. A fragile site was noted on the X chromosome in cases of X-linked mental retardation and the site became known as FRAXA. Other fragile sites were later discovered on the X chromosome and were designated FRAXB through FRAXF. Of these, only FRAXE is also associated with a mental retardation syndrome. The routine diagnosis of fragile X syndrome was made possible by the discovery that folic acid deficiency is a factor in the in vitro cytogenetic expression of fragile X. Fragile X syndrome is the second most common genetic form of mental retardation after DS. The prevalence is estimated at 0.2–0.6 per 1,000 females and 0.4–0.9 per 1,000 males.

The inheritance and penetrance of fragile X syndrome are unlike those of any other X-linked disorder. Males with the gene can be clinically normal but transmit the disorder through all their daughters, who are also normal, to affected grandchildren. The unaffected male carrier of fragile X is called the *transmitting male* (TM). Some unusual observations in fragile X syndrome are (1) the penetrance rate of affected females (33%) is much higher than in other X-linked disorders; (2) TMs have fewer daughters with mental retardation than do unaffected carrier females; and (3) mentally retarded females have more retarded offspring than do unaffected carrier females.

The molecular basis of fragile X syndrome is an expansion of a repetitive trinucleotide sequence, CGG. In fragile X families, the region lengthens through a series of intergenerational steps from premutations, which are silent, to full mutations, which affect the transcription of an adjacent gene. That gene, *FMR1*, normally produces a previously unknown but apparently important protein known as FMRP or FMR1 protein.

Clinical Aspects

Physical Phenotype

The fully expressed, characteristic physical phenotype of affected fragile X males includes a long, oblong face with a large mandible; large ears, prominent ears, or both; and macro-orchidism. These signs are often absent or subtle in prepubertal males and are not always present in postpubertal affected males. The craniofacial traits are less frequent in affected black males. Mild macrocephaly and above-average height may be noted in childhood, but adult fragile X males tend to be shorter than average. TMs are phenotypically normal.

Females, both children and adults, who carry a full mutation on one X chromosome, regardless of IQ, usually show physical features of fragile X syndrome, including a long face, prominent ears, and hyperextensible finger joints. As with those of affected males, the characteristic facial features of females are less common in childhood. Typical craniofacial features, especially prominent ears, are more frequent in females with a premutation than in control females, although to a milder degree than in females with a full mutation. Women who carry a premutation may enter menopause at a significantly earlier age than normal and have a higher rate of dizygotic twinning. This suggests that the *FMR1* gene has some role in female gonadal function. Surprisingly, these trends are not seen in women with full mutations.

Cognitive and Behavioral Phenotype

Prepubertal males may function at a mildly retarded level, although psychomotor delay is evident from birth. Most adults are moderately mentally retarded, and 30% are severely or profoundly retarded. The IQ appears to decrease with age in fragile X males. The number of CGG repeats does not correlate with IQ. Fragile X males with a mosaic DNA pattern (some premutation-size repeats in addition to a full mutation) or with incomplete methylation of the mutant *FMR1* gene have higher IQs than those who have a nonmosaic DNA pattern or a fully methylated *FMR1* gene. Such males may have a low normal or normal IQ but have learning disabilities.

Affected males usually show weaknesses in quantitative skills, short-term memory for abstract stimuli, spatial visualization, and visuomotor coordination and integration; relative strengths appear in short-term memory for meaningful stimuli, vocabulary, verbal expressive skills, and comprehension. Despite relative cognitive strengths in verbal areas, fragile X males have delayed speech and language development and frequently exhibit perseveration, cluttering, staccato speech, and litany speech. Boys tend to have low-pitched voices with a hoarse or harsh quality. The typical behavioral phenotype that begins in childhood includes hyperactivity, social avoidance and anxiety, and stereotypic behaviors such as hand-flapping, hand-biting, gaze aversion, and tactile defensiveness.

TMs, although of normal intelligence, score significantly lower than their male relatives with a normal *FMR1* gene on psychometric tests and show more behavioral and psychiatric disorders than control males, suggesting that some males with a premutation may be mildly affected.

At least 35% of females with cytogenetic fragile X expression are mentally impaired or retarded and at least 50% have learning disabilities. The wide range of phenotypic variation in full-mutation females is unexplained. As a group, females with a full mutation have a significantly lower mean IQ than premutation carriers, but their individual IQs may range from less than 40 to greater than 115. It remains impossible to predict whether a female with a full mutation will be mentally retarded or normal. In general, the patterns of strength and weakness on formal psychometric testing in affected females are similar in kind to those of fragile X males. IQ scores in young fragile X females tend to decrease over time, although they may remain stable in women older than 18 years. The behavioral phenotype of the full mutation is similar in females and males.

Females with the premutation have IQs above 85, appear to have a normal cognitive profile, and are not different from control women on measures of neuropsychological function, in psychiatric diagnoses or symptoms, or on self-rated personality profiles.

Neurologic Findings

Clumsy gait and impaired coordination are always present, and hypotonia and oculomotor dysfunction (strabismus or ptosis) are common. Seizures occur in up to 25% of affected males. Seizures are typically infrequent and generalized and have their onset during childhood. They respond to anticonvulsants and disappear after adolescence. Some affected males have benign centrotemporal epilepsy of childhood.

Molecular and Biochemical Aspects

Triplet Repeat Diseases

Fragile X syndrome is one of the class of hereditary diseases caused by DNA expansions at areas of repeated trinucleotide (triplet) sequences. In each triplet repeat disease, the effect of the triplet repeat varies, depending on its sequence, location within the gene, and the length to which it expands. In fragile X syndrome, three basic states of expansion can occur: (1) normal, in which intelligence is normal and the length is stable from generation to generation; (2) premutations, in which intelligence is normal but intergenerational changes of increasing magnitude are possible; and (3) full mutations, which are the massive, somatically unstable changes found in affected individuals.

The number of triplets is less than 50 for normal, 50–200 for premutation, and more than 200 for full mutation. For diagnostic or genetic counseling, it is not necessary to determine precisely the number of CGG repeats. It is more appropriate to describe the expansion in terms of "additional kilobases," or Δkb. In these terms, every premutation has a discrete Δkb between 0.1 and 0.6, and every full mutation is a collection of molecules with a Δkb between 0.6 and approximately 5.0. A likely mechanism for the expansion of the number of repeats is that repetitive DNA sequences have a tendency to slip out of alignment during replication and incorporate more, or fewer, units of the repeat. Those that become longer are more prone to slippage in the future, leading to the incorporation of successively larger numbers of additional repeats.

Fragile Sites

A unique property associated with expanded triplet repeats of 100% CGG composition is the formation of rare folate-sensitive fragile sites. In general, fragile sites are chromosome locations identified in vitro as areas of nonstaining gaps or areas prone to chromosome breakage. There are more than 100 identified fragile sites in the human chromosome map, with more than 75% classified as common. The remainder are considered rare, and, of these, most are folate sensitive. FRAXA and four other folate-sensitive fragile sites, FRAXE, FRAXF, FRA11B (from chromosome 11), and FRA16A (from chromosome 16) have been sequenced.

The FMR1 Gene

Gene Organization. The involved gene, *FMR1*, is composed of 17 exons. The first exon, containing the untranslated CGG region, is unusually long even in the normal state, as well as unusually distant from the next exon. *FMR1* normally produces an RNA-binding protein active in brain and other tissues. In fragile X syndrome, transcription of the *FMR1* gene is prevented by a large expansion in a nearby region of CGG repeats. A preliminary expansion of moderate length accounts for the silent carrier state. DNA testing can now detect expansions of all sizes. In the past, diagnosis depended on the fact that the fully expanded CGG region forms a characteristic cytogenetic fragile site at chromosome band Xq27.3.

LOCATIONS OF GENE EXPRESSION. The sites and timing of *FMR1* expression have been studied in human tissues. High levels of mRNA are found in brain and testes and have strong expression in placenta, lung, and kidney but very little expression in liver or pancreas. In human fetuses of 8–9 weeks' gestation, mRNA was detected in proliferating and migrating cells of the brain, spinal cord ganglia, and neural retina, as well as in all cartilaginous structures, the cephalic mesenchyme, and the liver. In 25-week-old human fetuses, expression was detected in nearly all differentiated structures of the brain, with the highest levels in cholinergic neurons of the nucleus basalis magnocellularis and in pyramidal neurons of the hippocampus. Significant expression is also seen in thalamic and subthalamic nuclei and in the cerebral cortex and the cerebellum, especially in Purkinje cells.

ROLE IN REPRODUCTION. Men with full mutations or mosaicism for premutations and full mutations produce only sperm (or daughters) with premutations. This suggests that a requirement for internal *FMR1* expression selects against sperm bearing full mutations. However, a family has been reported in which a man, apparently a mosaic, appears to have fathered four daughters who inherited an X chromosome from him with a deletion in *FMR1*. An alternative explanation for the preservation of premutation-bearing sperm in males with full mutations is that the expansion to a full mutation in the embryo takes place in somatic cells only.

FMRP Deficiency

FAILURE OF *FMR1* TRANSCRIPTION IN FULL MUTATIONS. The direct cause of fragile X syndrome, brought about by full-length expansion at the CGG repeat, is the absence of FMRP protein. This is primarily due to the suppression of transcription. If any mRNA molecules containing more than 200 CGG repeats are transcribed, they are inefficiently translated. Transcription of mRNA from premutation alleles is indistinguishable from normal levels. The suppression of transcription is mediated by DNA methylation rather than the length of the CGG region alone.

Confirmation of the Role of FMRP from Rare Deletion and Missense Patients. Like any other gene, *FMR1* can undergo direct mutations such as deletions and point mutations. Although such patients are extremely rare, they prove that deficiency of FMRP is sufficient to cause the phenotypic features of the syndrome. These patients do not have CGG expansions or chromosome fragility at Xq27.3, although their deletions may in some cases be the result of erroneous removal of an expansion. Deletions and point mutations would be inherited in a straightforward X-linked manner, without the phenomenon of normal TMs.

Inheritance Aspects

Rules of Inheritance

With the advent of DNA analysis for fragile X syndrome, the stages of expansion of the triplet repeat could be traced through families. The old mysteries of inheritance and penetrance were explained by the discovery of the apparently silent premutation state. The rules of fragile X syndrome inheritance as they are now understood are:

1. Every affected child has a carrier mother. New mutations never occur directly from normal to full mutation. Mothers of affected children always have expansions. Males with expansions never pass on full mutations.
2. Carrier mothers may carry premutations or full mutations. Mothers who have fragile X–related mental impairment have full mutations. Unaffected mothers can have nonpenetrant full mutations or premutations. If the mother has a full mutation, the maternal grandmother is an obligate carrier, but if the mother has a premutation, the source could be either maternal grandparent.
3. The probability of a female carrier having a child with a full mutation is proportional to the size of the expansion she carries. Small maternal premutations (fewer than approximately 90 total repeats or approximately 0.2 Δkb) do not always become full length on passage to offspring. Passage of premutations greater than approximately 90 repeats almost always results in full mutations.
4. Premutations are inherited silently for many years. No intergenerational transition from a stable, average-length allele to a premutation has ever been documented. Therefore, widely separated branches of an extended family are at risk.

Mosaicism

The two types of mosaicisms are methylation mosaicism, in which a fraction of full mutation molecules escapes methylation, and premutation/full mutation mosaicism. Both are thought to be favorable findings.

Diagnosis of Fragile X Syndrome

Clinical Diagnosis

More than 100 X-linked disorders with mental retardation exist. In developmentally delayed young children, the characteristic behavioral phenotype, together with a family history of X-linked mental retardation, may more readily suggest the fragile X syndrome than will the child's physical appearance.

DNA-Based Diagnosis

All methods of DNA-based diagnosis for fragile X syndrome have one goal: to identify a fragment of DNA containing the CGG region and determine its length by electrophoresis, such that it can be classified as normal, as a premutation, or as a full mutation. Detection of a full mutation of any size in a known developmentally delayed individual is considered confirmation of fragile X syndrome. If a full mutation is detected in a female before clinical diagnosis—for example, by prenatal analysis—it is not certain that she will be affected, or how severely.

A premutation detected in a developmentally delayed individual in the absence of mosaicism for a full mutation does not establish a diagnosis of fragile X syndrome, but it does mean that the patient and relatives are carriers. A normal result found in a developmentally delayed individual, in the absence of mosaicism for a full mutation, provides a definitive exclusion of fragile X syndrome.

FRAXE Syndrome

FRAXE is so close to FRAXA that they cannot be distinguished cytogenetically. The gene that is presumably affected by proximity to FRAXE has not yet been identified. It is a mistake to trivialize the misidentification of the site. This would be a particular risk if other members of the family have carrier testing with the FRAXA DNA tests and are mistakenly tested at the wrong gene. The confirmed cases have relatively mild mental retardation and no characteristic physical features. Other differences between FRAXE and FRAXA are that, in

FRAXE syndrome, males with large expansions are not always affected, and affected fathers can have affected daughters.

Carrier Detection and Prenatal Diagnosis

The mothers of affected children are inevitably carriers. Other male or female relatives who could share one of her X chromosomes should have genetic counseling and consider carrier testing. Prenatal DNA testing is indicated primarily if not exclusively in families in which the mother is a known carrier of a proven CGG expansion of significant size. There is no indication for testing fetuses, the mothers of which are not carriers. Offspring of carrier fathers (TMs) need not be tested because no sons are expected to inherit the father's X, whereas all daughters must inherit the involved X and be carriers. No male with a premutation or full mutation has ever been reported to have a daughter with a full mutation.

TREATMENT

No cure exists for the fragile X syndrome. The attention deficit disorder and hyperactivity may be ameliorated by central nervous system stimulants such as methylphenidate, dextroamphetamine, and pemoline. Low doses appear to be most effective because higher doses tend to increase the frequency of tantrums, mood swings, and motor and vocal tics. Some adult fragile X males with intermittent violent outbursts have been most commonly treated with thioridazine. Seizures are easily controlled by drugs such as carbamazepine. Awareness of the frequency of other medical problems in the fragile X syndrome, such as floppy mitral valve, scoliosis, and strabismus, will lead to early recognition and appropriate management.

For a more detailed discussion, see Epstein CJ. Down Syndrome (Chapter 5; pp. 51–79); Maddalena A, Schneider NR, Howard-Peebles PN. Fragile X Syndrome (Chapter 6; pp. 81–99), in RN Rosenberg, SB Prusiner, S DiMauro, RL Barchi (eds),* The Molecular and Genetic Basis of Neurological Disease *(2nd ed). Boston: Butterworth–Heinemann, 1997.

3

Prions

BIOLOGY OF PRIONS

Prions cause a group of human and animal neurodegenerative diseases that are now classified together because their etiology and pathogenesis involve modification of the prion protein. The normal prion protein (PrP) gene product, a protein of 33–35 kd, designated *PrP^C*, is protease-sensitive and soluble in nondenaturing detergents. PrP^C differs from all other known infectious pathogens in three respects: (1) it does not contain a nucleic acid genome that codes for its progeny; (2) its only known component is a modified protein that is encoded by a cellular gene; and (3) the major, and possibly only, component of the disease-causing prion is the scrapie isoform (PrP^{Sc}), which is a pathogenic conformer of the cellular isoform PrP^C. The fundamental event in prion diseases is a conformational change that occurs during the conversion of PrP^C into PrP^{Sc}. PrP^C is anchored to the external surface of cells by a glycolipid moiety, and its function is unknown. A posttranslational chemical modification that distinguishes PrP^{Sc} from PrP^C has not been identified. PrP^C contains approximately 45% α-helix and is virtually devoid of β-sheet. Conversion to PrP^{Sc} creates a protein that contains approximately 30% α-helix and 45% β-sheet. The mechanism of conversion is unknown, but PrP^C appears to bind to PrP^{Sc} to form an intermediate complex during the formation of nascent PrP^{Sc}. PrP^{Sc} in the inoculum interacts preferentially with homotypic PrP^C during the propagation of prions.

The human prion diseases are kuru, Creutzfeldt-Jakob disease (CJD), Gerstmann-Sträussler-Scheinker (GSS) disease, and fatal familial insomnia (FFI) (Table 3.1); animal prion diseases are scrapie of sheep and goats and bovine spongiform encephalopathy (BSE). The discovery that prion diseases in humans are uniquely both genetic and infectious has greatly strengthened and extended the prion concept. Nineteen different mutations in the human PrP gene, all resulting in

Table 3.1
Human prion diseases.

Disease	*Etiology*
Kuru	Infection
Creutzfeldt-Jakob disease	
Iatrogenic	Infection
Sporadic	Unknown
Familial	PrP mutation
Gerstmann-Sträussler-Scheinker disease	PrP mutation
Fatal familial insomnia	PrP mutation
Progressive subcortical gliosis	Unknown

Animal prion diseases.

Disease	*Host*
Scrapie	Sheep and goats
Bovine spongiform encephalopathy	Cattle
Transmissible mink encephalopathy	Mink
Chronic wasting disease	Mule deer and elk
Feline spongiform encephalopathy	Domestic and great cats
Exotic ungulate encephalopathy	Nyala and greater kudu

nonconservative substitutions, have been found either to be linked genetically to or segregate with the inherited prion diseases. Yet, the transmissible prion particle is composed largely, if not entirely, of the abnormal isoform PrP^{Sc}. These findings suggest that prion diseases should be considered pseudoinfections, in that the particles transmitting disease appear to be devoid of a foreign nucleic acid and therefore differ from all known micro-organisms as well as viruses and viroids.

MOLECULAR NEUROPATHOLOGY OF PRION DISEASES

The neuropathologic features common to all prion diseases are spongiform (vacuolar) degeneration of neurons and their processes, neuronal loss, and reactive astrocytic gliosis. Amyloid plaques containing PrP are a variable feature, but when present, they are usually found within gray matter and are diagnostic. PrP amyloid plaques are not usually surrounded by a halo of dystrophic neurites, except in GSS, which presents with neurofibrillary tangles. Prion diseases do not show inflammation or viral inclusion bodies. The etiology and pathogenesis of prion diseases appear to be related solely to abnormalities of PrP. Because scrapie is such an accurate animal model of the human illnesses, more is known about the etiology and pathogenesis of CJD and related diseases than any of the human neurodegenerative disorders.

The first evidence that PrP^{Sc} participates in the pathogenesis of prion diseases was the finding that the amyloid plaques in human and animal prion diseases react specifically with PrP antibodies. However, amyloid plaques are not a constant feature of prion diseases. The amyloidogenic potential of PrP^{Sc} is probably inherent in its high content of β-sheet in that all amyloids are composed of proteins with a β-pleated sheet conformation.

The evidence that accumulation of PrP^{Sc} in the gray matter causes spongiform degeneration and nerve cell loss is as follows: (1) PrP^{CJD} and PrP^{Sc} are found only in human and animal prion diseases, respectively; (2) a temporal relationship exists between the accumulation of PrP^{Sc} in scrapie and the development of spongiform degeneration and reactive astrocytic gliosis; and (3) PrP^{Sc} accumulation, spongiform degeneration, and reactive astrocytic gliosis co-localize in the brains of mice and Syrian hamsters in scrapie.

Human prion diseases are the only known neurodegenerative disorders that present as sporadic, genetic, and infectious variants. There are two key elements of the disease mechanism: (1) PrP can exist in two or more structurally stable states in a cell. One of these, PrP^{C}, performs an as yet unknown normal cellular function, and the other, PrP^{Sc}, is pathogenic. (2) In the pathogenesis of these disorders, a normal cellular metabolic pathway converts PrP^{C} into PrP^{Sc} when PrP^{Sc} is presented to the cell either as exogenously or endogenously derived prion particles. Once begun, the process becomes self-perpetuating, and the conversion of PrP^{C} into PrP^{Sc} in the presence of preexisting PrP^{Sc} spreads from one susceptible neuron population to another. Although prion diseases are relatively uncommon, it may be that a variant of their pathogenic mechanisms plays key roles in the pathogenesis of other diseases.

ANIMAL PRION DISEASES

Scrapie

Scrapie is the most common natural prion disease of animals. It is unique among the prion diseases in that it seems to be readily communicable within flocks, but the mechanism of natural spread is not understood. In Iceland, scrapied flocks of sheep were destroyed and the pastures left vacant for several years; however, reintroduction of sheep from flocks known to be free of scrapie eventually resulted in scrapie in the new flock. The source of the scrapie prions that attacked the sheep from flocks without a history of scrapie is unknown.

Bovine Spongiform Encephalopathy

Beginning in 1986, an epidemic of a previously unknown disease appeared in cattle in Great Britain. It was initially named *bovine spongiform encephalopathy* (BSE), but it is frequently called *mad cow disease*. BSE was shown to be a prion disease by identifying protease-resistant PrP in the brains of ill cattle. The offal of scrapied sheep in Great Britain is thought to be responsible for the current epidemic of BSE. Prions in the offal from scrapie-infected sheep were contained in the meat and bone meal fed to cattle as a nutritional supplement.

HUMAN PRION DISEASES

Infectious forms of prion diseases result from the horizontal transmission of infectious prions, as occurs in iatrogenic CJD and kuru. Transmission of prions from animals to humans has not been established despite repeated attempts to implicate scrapie prions from sheep as a cause of CJD. Whether BSE poses any risk to humans is unknown, but three teenagers and eight young adults in Britain and France died of atypical CJD in 1995 and 1996.

Inherited forms, notably GSS, familial CJD, and FFI, constitute 10–15% of all cases of prion disease. A mutation in the open reading frame (ORF) or protein-coding region of the PrP gene has been found in all reported kindreds with inherited human prion disease.

Sporadic forms of prion disease produce most cases of CJD and possibly some cases of GSS. How prions arise in patients with sporadic forms is unknown; hypotheses include horizontal transmission from humans or animals, somatic mutation of the PrP gene, and spontaneous conversion of PrP^{C} into PrP^{Sc}. An infectious link between sporadic CJD and a pre-existing prion disease in animals or humans is not established.

Diagnosis of Human Prion Diseases

Human prion disease should be considered in any patient who develops a progressive subacute or chronic decline in cognitive or motor function. Most affected individuals are between 40 and 75 years of age. The symptom complex in each disease is often sufficiently characteristic to suggest the diagnosis. A specific diagnostic test for prion disease in the cerebrospinal fluid is not available. Definitive diagnosis of human prion diseases, which are invariably fatal, can often be made from the examination of brain tissue. Molecular genetic diagnosis of inherited prion diseases has been possible in living patients by using peripheral tissues. The common feature to all prion diseases, whether sporadic, dominantly inherited, or acquired by infection, is the aberrant metabolism of the prion protein. A definitive diagnosis of human prion disease can be accomplished if PrP^{Sc} can be detected immunologically.

Kuru

For many decades, kuru devastated the lives of the Fore Highlanders of Papua New Guinea. Contamination during ritualistic cannibalism appears to have been the mode by which kuru spread among the Fore people. Cannibalism ceased by 1960 in the Fore region; individuals now developing kuru presumably were exposed to the kuru agent more than three decades ago. In many of the new cases, a history of cannibalism of a near relative who had died of kuru can be obtained. The ability of the kuru prions to remain quiescent in these patients for a period of two decades is supported by incubation periods of more than 7.5 years in some monkeys inoculated with kuru agent.

The clinical features of kuru are uniform. The prodromal symptoms are headache and joint pain. These are followed 6–12 weeks later by difficulty walking, and death usually occurs within 12 months and no later than 2 years after onset. Signs of cerebellar dysfunction always dominate the clinical picture. Patients remain ambulatory with the aid of a stick for more than half of the clinical phase of their illness.

No individual born in the south Fore region after cannibalism ceased has developed kuru. Kuru has progressively disappeared, first among children and thereafter among adolescents. Each year the youngest new patients are older than those of the previous year. Of several hundred kuru orphans born since 1957 to mothers who later died of kuru, none has yet developed the disease. Therefore, the many children with kuru seen in the 1950s were not infected prenatally, perinatally, or neonatally by their mothers. Attempts to demonstrate consistent transmission of prion disease from mother to offspring in experimental animals have been unsuccessful. The regular disappearance of kuru is inconsistent with the existence of any natural reservoirs for kuru besides humans. Patients dying of kuru over the past decade seem to have incubation periods exceeding two or even three decades. It has been suggested that kuru began at the turn of the century as a spontaneous case of CJD that was propagated by ritualistic cannibalism.

Creutzfeldt-Jakob Disease

Epidemiology

CJD is worldwide in distribution, and the overall incidence is less than 1 case per million per year. In Libyan Jews living in Israel, the annual incidence is 31.3 per million. The high incidence in specific populations is most often the result of familial (inherited) disease associated with PrP gene mutations. The incubation period is estimated to range from less than 10 years to more than 30 years.

Iatrogenic Transmission

Accidental transmission of CJD to humans has occurred by corneal transplantation, contaminated electroencephalographic (EEG) electrode implantation, and surgical operations using contaminated instruments or equipment. Since 1985, at least 61 cases of CJD after implantation of dura mater grafts have been recorded. All of the grafts were thought to have been acquired from a single manufacturer whose preparative procedures were inadequate to inactivate human prions. The possibility of transmission of CJD from contaminated human growth hormone (HGH) preparations derived from human pituitaries has been raised by the occurrence of fatal cerebellar disorders with dementia in more than 90 patients ranging in age from 10 to 41 years who received injections of HGH every 2–4 days for 4–12 years. CJD in patients younger than 40 years of age is very rare. The clinical course resembles kuru more than ataxic CJD.

Clinical Features

The clinical tetrad of CJD is a subacute progressive dementia, myoclonus, periodic complexes on the EEG, and normal cerebrospinal fluid. One-fourth of patients show prodromal symptoms of asthenia, altered sleep patterns and appetite (bulimia and anorexia), weight loss, and loss of libido. Once the dementia is established, patients complain of problems with concentration, memory, and problem solving; family members report apathy, paranoia, self-neglect, irresponsibility, and inappropriate behavior. Less frequent disturbances are episodes of disorientation, hallucinations, and emotional lability. In most, deterioration occurs over weeks or months but may also occur over days. Ataxia at onset is a feature in one-third of patients and will ultimately occur in 70%. Seizures are uncommon.

Gerstmann-Sträussler-Scheinker Syndrome

GSS is caused by a mutation in the protein-coding region of the PrP gene. Onset is in the third or fourth decades, and a protracted clinical course over several years is common. Cerebellar dysfunction occurs before dementia. Presenting signs are clumsiness, unsteadiness, difficulty with walking, or incoordination. Ataxia, dysarthria, and nystagmus develop with increasing severity. In some families, extrapyramidal or parkinsonian features predominate; others show gaze palsies, deafness, and blindness. Examination frequently reveals loss of deep tendon reflexes in the legs with extensor plantar responses. Myoclonus is rarely seen.

Fatal Familial Insomnia

FFI is an autosomal dominant disorder that presents with intractable, progressive insomnia and autonomic systemic disturbances caused by sympathetic overactivity such as hypertension, hyperthermia, hyperhidrosis, and tachycardia. Motor system abnormalities include tremor, ataxia, hyperreflexia, and spontaneous and induced myoclonus. Dementia does not develop, but the patients may show attention and memory deficits, disorientation, confusion, and complex hallucinations. Endocrine abnormalities consist of loss of circadian rhythm for the secretion of melatonin, prolactin, and growth hormone. Secretion of adrenocorticotropic hormone is decreased, whereas secretion of cortisol is increased.

For a more detailed discussion, see Prusiner SB. Biology of Prions (Chapter 7; pp. 103–143); DeArmond SJ, Prusiner SB. Molecular Neuropathy of Prion Diseases (Chapter 8; pp. 145–163); Prusiner SB. The Prion Diseases of Humans and Animals (Chapter 9; pp. 165–186), in RN Rosenberg, SB Prusiner, S DiMauro, RL Barchi (eds),* The Molecular and Genetic Basis of Neurological Disease *(2nd ed). Boston: Butterworth–Heinemann, 1997.

4

Mitochondrial Disorders

THE MITOCHONDRIAL GENOME

Mitochondria are organelles located in the cytoplasm of almost all mammalian cells. Several important biochemical functions take place in mitochondria, such as the citric acid cycle, amino acid biosynthesis, fatty acid oxidation, and oxidative phosphorylation (Figure 4.1).

GENOME ORGANIZATION

The human mitochondrial genome is a double-stranded circle of DNA containing 37 genes. Only 13 genes specify polypeptides, and all are components of the respiratory chain/oxidative phosphorylation system. This system is a set of five biochemically related complexes located in the mitochondrial inner membrane. Complexes I, III, IV, and V are composed of polypeptides encoded by both nuclear DNA (nDNA) and mitochondrial DNA (mtDNA). The nDNA-encoded genes are imported into mitochondria and are co-assembled with the mtDNA-encoded genes into the respective enzyme complexes in the mitochondrial inner membrane. Complex II, unlike the other four complexes, contains no mtDNA-encoded subunits.

mtDNA has several unique features: (1) its genetic code is different from nDNA, (2) it is tightly packed with information because it contains no introns, (3) spontaneous mutations occur at a higher rate than nDNA, (4) it has less efficient repair mechanisms than nDNA, (5) it is present in hundreds or thousands of copies in each cell, and (6) it is transmitted by maternal inheritance.

MITOCHONDRIAL INHERITANCE

Mammalian mitochondria are maternally inherited. A mother transmits mitochondria to all of her children, both boys and girls, but only

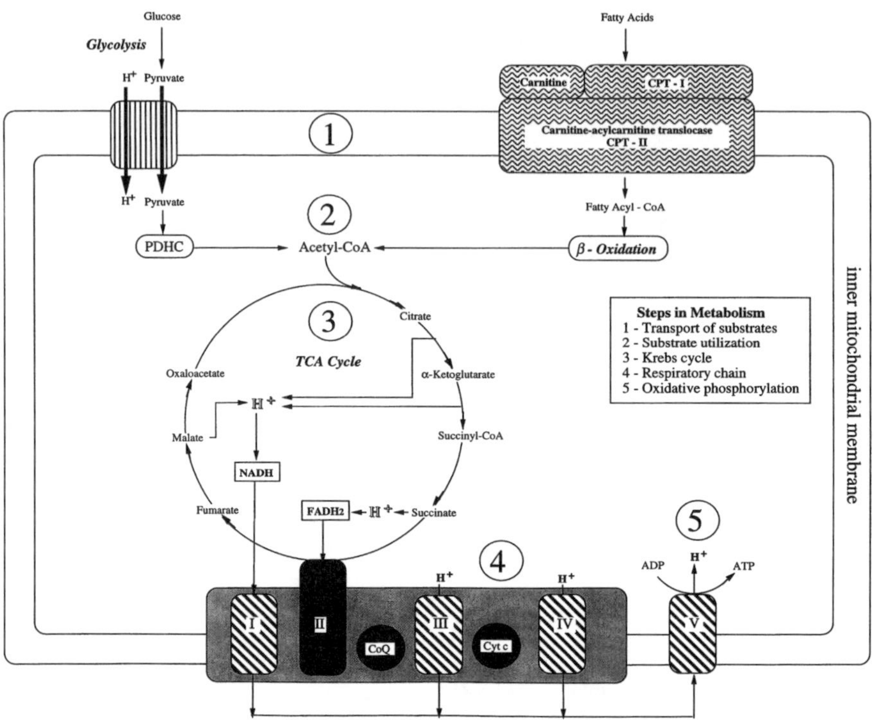

Figure 4.1 Schematic representation of mitochondrial metabolism. For details, see text. Respiratory chain complexes or components encoded exclusively by the nuclear genome are stippled; complexes containing some subunits encoded by the nuclear genome and others encoded by mtDNA are crosshatched. (CPT = carnitine palmitoyltransferase; PDHC = pyruvate dehydrogenase complex; CoA = coenzyme A; TCA = tricarboxylic acid; NADH = nicotinamide adenine dinucleotide, reduced; $FADH_2$ = flavin adenine dinucleotide, reduced; I, II, III, IV, V = complexes of the respiratory chain; CoQ = coenzyme Q; Cyt c = cytochrome *c*; ADP = adenosine diphosphate; ATP = adenosine triphosphate.) (Reprinted with permission from S DiMauro, M Hirano, E Bonilla, DC DeVivo. The Mitochondrial Disorders. In O Berg [ed], Principles of Child Neurology. New York: McGraw-Hill, 1996;1201.)

her daughters will transmit their mitochondria to their children. Because the respiratory chain complexes are derived from both mitochondrial and nuclear genes, mitochondrial respiratory-chain disorders can be transmitted by either mendelian or maternal inheritance. An important feature of mitochondrial inheritance is that the number of mitochondria in a cell depends on its energy requirements. Because the timing of mtDNA replication is unrelated to the cell cycle, the numbers of mitochondria present in a cell vary among cells and tissues and during development and aging. A mutation affecting some mtDNA in the ovum or in the zygote is passed on randomly to subsequent generations of cells. Some cells receive no mutant genomes (normal or wild-type homoplasmy), others receive exclusively mutant genomes (mutant homoplasmy), and still others receive a mixed population of mutant and wild-type mtDNA (heteroplasmy).

The concepts of maternal inheritance and heteroplasmy have four implications for disease. (1) Inheritance of the disease is maternal as in X-linked traits, but both sexes are equally affected. (2) The phenotypic expression of an mtDNA mutation depends on the relative proportions of mutant and wild-type genomes; a minimum critical number of mutant genomes is required for expression (threshold effect). (3) At cell division, the proportion of mutant and normal genomes may shift in daughter cells (mitotic segregation), and the phenotype may change accordingly. (4) All children of an affected mother would be affected were it not for the threshold effect. The threshold effect is relative because the critical number of mutant mtDNAs needed to cause cell dysfunction varies from tissue to tissue depending on its vulnerability to impairments of oxidative metabolism and may vary in the same tissue with time.

mtDNA mutations arise in single molecules spontaneously, probably during DNA replication. Once a mutation is fixed, the cell is now considered to be *heteroplasmic* (coexistence of different mtDNA genotypes). If the mutation arises in the female germline, it can be transmitted to the next generation. The number of mtDNAs transmitted from mother to child is small, however—as few as five maternal mtDNAs actually repopulate the mtDNA in the next generation—so that even if the germline is heteroplasmic, reversion to homoplasmy can occur within a few generations.

MITOCHONDRIAL ENCEPHALOMYOPATHIES

Clinical Considerations

Mitochondrial diseases are clinically heterogeneous (Table 4.1). Pure myopathies vary in age at onset from birth to adult life, in rapidity of course from progressive to static, or even reversible, and in distribution of weakness from generalized with respiratory failure to progressive external ophthalmoplegia. Other possible features are exercise intolerance or hypermetabolism. Multisystem disorders show considerable over-

Table 4.1
Clinical and laboratory features and inheritance of disorders caused by mtDNA mutations.

		Δ-mtDNA		*tRNA*		*ATPase*	
Tissue	*Symptoms and Signs*	*KSS*	*Pearson*	*MERRF*	*MELAS*	*NARP*	*MILS*
Central nervous system	Seizures	–	–	+	+	–	+
	Ataxia	+	–	+	+	+	±
	Myoclonus	–	–	+	±	–	–
	Psychomotor retardation	–	–	–	–	–	+
	Psychomotor regression	+	–	±	+	–	–
	Hemiparesis/hemianopia	–	–	–	+	–	–
	Cortical blindness	–	–	–	+	–	–
	Migraine-like headaches	–	–	–	+	–	–
	Dystonia	–	–	–	+	–	+
Peripheral nervous system	Peripheral neuropathy	±	–	±	±	+	–
Muscle	Weakness	+	–	+	+	+	+
	Ophthalmoplegia	+	±	–	–	–	–
	Ptosis	+	–	–	–	–	–
Eye	Pigmentary retinopathy	+	–	–	–	+	±
	Optic atrophy	–	–	–	–	±	±
	Cataracts	–	–	–	–	–	–
Blood	Sideroblastic anemia	±	+	–	–	–	–
Endocrine	Diabetes mellitus	±	–	–	±	–	–
	Short stature	+	–	+	+	–	–
	Hypoparathyroidism	±	–	–	–	–	–
Heart	Conduction block	+	–	–	±	–	–
	Cardiomyopathy	±	–	–	±	–	±
Gastrointestinal tract	Exocrine pancreatic dysfunction	±	+	–	–	–	–
	Intestinal pseudo-obstruction	–	–	–	–	–	–

Ears, nose, and throat	Sensorineural hearing loss	–	–	+	+	±	–
Kidney	Fanconi syndrome	±	±	–	±	–	–
Laboratory	Lactic acidosis	+	+	+	+	–	±
	Muscle biopsy: RRFs	+	±	+	+	–	–
Inheritance	Maternal	–	–	+	+	+	+
	Sporadic	+	+	–	–	–	–

Note: Boxes highlight the typical clinical features of different syndromes, except for maternally inherited Leigh syndrome, which is defined by neuroradiologic or neuropathologic techniques.

Δ-mtDNA = deleted mtDNA; ATPase = adenosine triphosphatase; KSS = Kearns-Sayre syndrome; MELAS = mitochondrial encephalomyopathy with lactic acidosis and strokelike episodes; MERFF = myoclonic epilepsy with ragged-red fibers; MILS = maternally inherited Leigh syndrome; NARP = neurogenic atrophy, ataxia, retinitis pigmentosa; RRFs = ragged-red fibers.

Source: Adapted from S DiMauro, M Hirano, E Bonilla, DC DeVivo. The Mitochondrial Disorders. In O Berg (ed), Principles of Child Neurology. New York: McGraw-Hill, 1996;1201.

lap in clinical features. Distinct mutations underlie different syndromes. A single syndrome can be associated with different mutations, however, and different syndromes can be associated with the same mutation.

Biochemical Classification

Mitochondrial encephalomyopathies may be classified according to the area of mitochondrial metabolism specifically affected (Table 4.2).

1. *Substrate transport.* Because the inner mitochondrial membrane is impermeable to anions and neutral metabolites, these are transported across the membranes by a set of carriers or translocases. Pyruvate is transported into the matrix with hydrogen ions flowing inward down their electrochemical gradient (symport system). Long-chain fatty acids are transported through a system involving carnitine palmitoyltransferase I (CPT I) and CPT II, a carrier molecule, l-carnitine, and a translocase that shuttles fatty acyl-carnitine esters into the matrix and free carnitine out (see Figure 4.1).

2. *Substrate transport utilization.* In the matrix, pyruvate is oxidized by the pyruvate dehydrogenase complex and fatty acids by the β-oxidation pathway.

3. *Krebs cycle.* The common product of intramitochondrial oxidation, acetyl-CoA, is oxidized in the Krebs cycle. Oxaloacetate is regenerated, two molecules of carbon dioxide are formed, and high-energy electrons are extracted in the form of NADH and $FADH_2$.

4. *Electron transport chain.* The reducing equivalents produced by the oxidation of acetyl-CoA are passed along the respiratory chain through a series of oxidation/reduction reactions in which the final hydrogen acceptor is molecular oxygen and the final product is water.

5. *Oxidative phosphorylation coupling.* The energy released is harnessed to pump protons from the matrix side of the inner membrane to the space between the inner and outer mitochondrial membranes. The resulting electrochemical proton gradient is used to synthesize adenosine triphosphate (ATP) through the action of a large protein complex (complex V or ATP synthetase). This process is known as *oxidation/phosphorylation coupling.*

Genetic Classification

The genetic defects are classified as defects in nDNA, mtDNA, and the communication between nuclear and mitochondrial genomes.

1. *Mutations of nuclear genes.* Mutations of nDNA-encoding mitochondrial proteins are mainly transmitted as autosomal recessive traits;

Table 4.2
Biochemical classification of mitochondrial diseases.

1. Defects of *substrate transport*
   CPT deficiency
   Carnitine deficiency
2. Defects of *substrate utilization*
   PDHC deficiency
   Defects of β-oxidation
3. Defects of the *Krebs cycle*
   Fumarase deficiency
   Aconitase deficiency
   α-Ketoglutarate dehydrogenase deficiency
4. Defects of the *electron transport chain*
   Complex I deficiency
   Complex II deficiency
   Complex III deficiency
   Complex IV (COX) deficiency
   Combined defects of complexes I, III, and IV
5. Defects of *oxidation/phosphorylation coupling*
   Loose coupling of muscle mitochondria (Luft's disease)
   Defects of complex V (ATP synthetase)

CPT = carnitine palmitoyltransferase; PDHC = pyruvate dehydrogenase complex; COX = cytochrome *c* oxidase; ATP = adenosine triphosphate.

a few are X-linked recessive. Nuclear defects involving genes encoding tissue-specific proteins cause diseases confined to one or a few tissues. Those involving encoding proteins common to all tissues cause multi-system disease.

2. *Defects of the mitochondrial genome*. Defects consist of point mutations, deletions, and duplications. As of 1995, more than 50 point mutations were reported in association with neurologic and non-neurologic syndromes (Table 4.3).

3. *Defects of communication between nuclear and mitochondrial genomes*. The nuclear and mitochondrial genomes work coordinately under the control of the nuclear genome. nDNA-encoded factors are required for mtDNA transcription, translation, and replication. Two groups of human disorders are caused by faulty communications between nuclear and mitochondrial genomes. One includes autosomal dominant or recessive disorders dominated by progressive external ophthalmoplegia (PEO) and characterized by multiple deletions of mtDNA; the other includes autosomal recessive disorders affecting muscle or liver and characterized by depletion of mtDNA.

Table 4.3
Pathogenic mtDNA point mutations.

Nucleotide	*Mutation**	*Gene Location*	*Phenotype*
1555	A→G	12s rRNA	Aminoglycoside-induced deafness
3243	A→G	tRNA-Leu(UUR)	MELAS/PEO/diabetes/hearing loss
3250	T→C	tRNA-Leu(UUR)	Myopathy
3251	A→G	tRNA-Leu(UUR)	Multisystem
3252	A→G	tRNA-Leu(UUR)	Multisystem
3256	C→T	tRNA-Leu(UUR)	Multisystem/PEO/MELAS
3260	A→G	tRNA-Leu(UUR)	MICM/myopathy
3271	T→C	tRNA-Leu(UUR)	MELAS
3271	Del T	tRNA-Leu(UUR)	MELAS
3291	T→C	tRNA-Leu(UUR)	MELAS
3302	A→G	tRNA-Leu(UUR)	Myopathy
3303	C→T	tRNA-Leu(UUR)	MICM
3394	T→C	ND1	LHON
3460	G→A	ND1	LHON
4136	A→G	ND1	LHON
4160	T→C	ND1	LHON
4216	T→C	ND1	LHON
4269	A→G	tRNA-Ile	MICM/multisystem
4300	A→G	tRNA-Ile	MICM
4917	A→G	ND2	LHON
5244	G→A	ND2	LHON
5549	G→A	tRNA-Trp	Chorea, dementia
5692	T→C	tRNA-Asn	PEO
5703	C→T	tRNA-Asn	PEO
5814	T→C	tRNA-Cys	MELAS-like
5877	G→A	tRNA-Tyr	PEO
7444	G→A	COX I	LHON
7445	T→C	tRNA-Ser(UCN)	Deafness
7471	Ins C	tRNA-Ser(UCN)	Deafness, ataxia, myoclonus
8344	A→G	tRNA-Lys	MERRF
8356	T→C	tRNA-Lys	MERRF/MELAS
8363	G→A	tRNA-Lys	MICM/PEO/ataxia/deafness
8851	T→C	ATPase 6	FBSN
8993	T→G	ATPase 6	NARP/MILS
8993	T→C	ATPase 6	NARP/MILS
9101	T→C	ATPase 6	LHON
9176	T→C	ATPase 6	FBSN
9438	G→A	COX III	LHON
9804	G→A	COX III	LHON
9957	T→C	COX III	MELAS
9997	T→C	tRNA-Gly	MICM
11778	G→A	ND4	LHON
13708	G→A	ND5	LHON
14459	G→A	ND6	LHON/dystonia
14484	T→C	ND6	LHON

Nucleotide	Mutation*	Gene Location	Phenotype
14709	T→C	ND6	Myopathy/diabetes
15257	G→A	Cyt b	LHON
15812	G→A	Cyt b	LHON
15923	A→G	tRNA-Thr	Infantile respiratory deficiency
15990	C→T	tRNA-Pro	Myopathy

MELAS = mitochondrial encephalomyopathy with lactic acidosis and strokelike episodes; PEO = progressive external ophthalmoplegia; LHON = Leber's hereditary optic neuropathy; MICM = maternally inherited cardiomyopathy; FSBN = familial bilateral striatal necrosis; MERRF = myoclonus epilepsy with ragged-red fibers; NARP = neurogenic atrophy, ataxia, retinitis pigmentosa.
*L-strand sequence.

MITOCHONDRIAL DISEASES

In describing individual mitochondrial disease, the genetic classification is primary and the biochemical classification is secondary.

Diseases Caused by Defects of Nuclear DNA

Defects of Substrate Transport

The main defects of mitochondrial substrate transport affect lipid metabolism and are caused by deficiency of CPT or carnitine (see Chapter 13).

Defects of Substrate Oxidation

Enzyme defects in the β-oxidation pathway are described in Chapter 13. Defects of the pyruvate dehydrogenase complex (PDHC) can affect each of its three catalytic components, E_1 (pyruvate decarboxylase), E_2 (dihydrolipoyl transacetylase), or E_3 (dihydrolipoyl dehydrogenase), and both regulatory components, PDH-kinase, which inactivates the enzyme, and PDH-phosphatase, which activates it.

The E_1 unit is most commonly involved. It is composed of two α and two β subunits. The α subunit is encoded by a gene on the X chromosome and the β subunit by a gene on chromosome 3. Three syndromes are identified with disturbances of the E_1 unit:

1. The neonatal form is characterized by hypotonia, episodic apnea and lethargy, seizures, failure to thrive, and severe lactic acidosis. Dysmorphic features and agenesis of the corpus callosum are often asso-

ciated. Males predominate, suggesting involvement of the X-linked $E_1\alpha$ subunit in many patients.

2. The infantile form has its onset before 6 months and consists of psychomotor delay, hypotonia, seizures, episodic apnea, lethargy, ataxia, ophthalmoplegia, optic atrophy, and mild to moderate lactic acidosis. Death usually occurs before 3 years of age. Postmortem findings in most patients shows the symmetric necrotic lesions in the basal ganglia and brain stem characteristic of Leigh syndrome. There is a slight predominance of affected males, and the most common defects are in $E_1\alpha$ and $E_1\beta$.

3. The benign form occurs in males. The features are mild lactic acidosis, usually normal psychomotor development, and intermittent ataxia or exercise intolerance, which is responsive to thiamine administration. The clinical severity correlates with residual enzyme activity. The disorder can be caused by several mutations in the α-subunit gene.

The E_2 subunit deficiency was described in a child with hyperammonemia and severe lactic acidosis at 2 weeks of age who later showed severe psychomotor retardation.

The E_3 unit is a homodimer whose subunit is shared by two other α-ketoacid dehydrogenases, α-ketoglutarate dehydrogenase and branched-chain ketoacid dehydrogenase. Defects of E_3 are never isolated and result in blood accumulation (and urinary excretion) of pyruvate, lactate, α-ketoglutarate, and branched-chain α-ketoacids. Patients with E_3 deficiency show demyelination and cavitation of the basal ganglia, thalamus, and brain stem, sparing the cortex.

PDH-phosphatase deficiency causes the clinical and neuropathologic features of Leigh syndrome.

Defects of pyruvate carboxylase, the first enzyme in gluconeogenesis, usually causes a severe syndrome characterized by psychomotor retardation and death during infancy. A benign variant causes recurrent vomiting, dehydration, and metabolic acidosis and is compatible with normal development.

Defects of the Krebs Cycle

The known defects of the Krebs cycle involve α-ketoglutarate dehydrogenase, fumarase, and aconitase. α-Ketoglutarate dehydrogenase deficiency is described above as part of the PDH-E_3 subunit deficiency state.

Fumarase deficiency is a devastating encephalomyopathy of infancy characterized by poor feeding, failure to thrive, persistent vomiting, developmental delay, microcephaly, lethargy alternating with irritability, impaired vision, hypotonia, and hyporeflexia. Laboratory examinations show lactic acidosis, hyperammonemia, and a distinctive organic aciduria with excessive excretion of succinic and fumaric acid. Postmortem examination shows abnormalities of neuronal migration in the brain. Aspartate administration should benefit these patients by increasing oxaloacetate concentrations, except that it does not enter the brain freely.

Aconitase deficiency has been described in association with succinate dehydrogenase deficiency in a patient with exercise intolerance and myoglobinuria, but the enzyme defect appears to be secondary to a more generalized abnormality of iron-sulfur cluster metabolism (see later).

Defects of the Respiratory Chain

This section deals only with clinical entities presumed to be caused by defects of nDNA.

COMPLEX I DEFICIENCY (NADH-COQ REDUCTASE). Complex I is the largest complex of the respiratory chain. Deficiencies fall into three broad categories:

1. Fatal infantile multisystem disorders are characterized by severe congenital lactic acidosis, psychomotor delay, diffuse hypotonia and weakness, cardiopathy, and cardiorespiratory failure causing death in the neonatal period. Therapeutic trials with thiamine, biotin, carnitine, and ketogenic diet have been unsuccessful.
2. Myopathy with exercise intolerance followed by fixed weakness can start in childhood or in adult life. It is usually accompanied by lactic acidosis at rest, which is exaggerated by exercise.
3. Mitochondrial encephalomyopathy (excluding mitochondrial encephalomyopathy, lactic acidosis, and strokelike episodes [MELAS]), with onset in childhood or adult life, occurs in variable combination with ophthalmoplegia, seizures, dementia, ataxia, neurosensory hearing loss, pigmentary retinopathy, sensory neuropathy, and involuntary movements. This heterogeneous group is likely to include some patients with nDNA defects and others with mtDNA defects.

COMPLEX II DEFICIENCY. Biochemical documentation of complex II deficiency has been incomplete and largely based on more or less severe defects of succinate-cytochrome *c* reductase activity in five patients with encephalomyopathy. Onset was in infancy or childhood and symptoms included failure to thrive, developmental delay, hypotonia, weakness, lethargy, respiratory insufficiency, ataxia, and myoclonus. Three died in infancy. Partial complex II deficiency was documented in two sisters with clinical and neuroradiologic evidence of Leigh syndrome, in whom a molecular defect was documented in the riboflavin subunit of the complex.

Coenzyme Q_{10} Deficiency. Coenzyme Q_{10} (CoQ_{10}) deficiency affects both muscle and brain. The myopathic features are exercise intolerance, myoglobinuria, and progressive weakness. Blood concentrations of creatine kinase are elevated and muscle histology may show excessive accumulation of lipid droplets and mitochondria in type 1 fibers and ragged-red fibers (RRF). The cerebral features are learning disabilities, seizures, and ataxia. Marked improvement of brain and muscle symptoms occurs when CoQ_{10} is replaced.

Complex III Deficiency. Complex III is composed of 11 subunits. The clinical features of complex III deficiency are heterogeneous, but patients can be divided into two major groups: those with multisystem disease (encephalomyopathy) and those with tissue-specific defects such as myopathy or cardiopathy. The encephalomyopathies include a fatal infantile form with severe lactic acidosis and hypotonia with onset a few hours after birth, accompanied by generalized amino aciduria and terminally by dystonic posturing, seizures, and coma, and later-onset forms (childhood to adult life) characterized by various combinations of weakness, short stature, dementia, ataxia, sensorineural deafness, pigmentary retinopathy, sensory neuropathy, and pyramidal signs.

Myopathy is characterized by exercise intolerance with premature fatigue and hyperpnea, often followed by fixed weakness. Complex III deficiency has been described in one patient with facioscapulohumeral (FSH) muscular dystrophy and suspected in a large family with FSH who showed an abnormal accumulation of lipid droplets and mitochondria in muscle. Biochemical studies of isolated muscle mitochondria showed impaired respiratory control. The administration of menadione (vitamin K_3) and ascorbate (vitamin C), in an attempt to bypass the block in the electron transport chain, provided clinical relief in some patients but not others.

Complex IV Deficiency. Clinical phenotypes associated with complex IV (COX) deficiency are of two types: one characterized by myopathy, the other involving multiple tissues but dominated by encephalopathy. Two forms of myopathy are described, both presenting soon after birth with severe diffuse weakness, respiratory distress, and lactic acidosis but with very different outcomes. Fatal infantile myopathy causes respiratory insufficiency and death before 1 year of age. Although heart, liver, and brain are clinically spared, many patients have renal disease with de Toni-Fanconi syndrome. The benign infantile myopathy starts the same way, but spontaneous improvement occurs and affected infants are usually normal by 2 or 3 years of age. This disorder is life-threatening in the neonate and requires life-sustaining measures. The spontaneous recovery in children with the benign infantile myopathy corresponds to a gradual return to normal COX activity in muscle. Other myopathic phenotypes are characterized by recurrent myoglobinuria, progressive myopathy, and exercise intolerance.

Among the encephalomyopathies, the most important is Leigh syndrome (subacute necrotizing encephalomyelopathy). COX deficiency is the most common known biochemical cause of Leigh syndrome. Leigh syndrome is a devastating encephalopathy of infancy or childhood, characterized by psychomotor regression, ataxia, optic atrophy, ophthalmoplegia, nystagmus, dystonia, tremor, pyramidal signs, and respiratory abnormalities. The pathologic hallmark consists of focal, symmetric areas of necrosis in the thalamus and brain stem that can be seen on magnetic resonance images of the brain.

Complex V (ATP Synthase) Deficiency. Two patients with different phenotypes are described. One was a 37-year-old woman with a congenital, slowly progressive myopathy. Muscle histology showed RRFs and a profusion of paracrystalline inclusions in virtually all mitochondria. The other was a 17-year-old boy with a multisystem disorder characterized by weakness, ataxia, retinopathy, dementia, and peripheral neuropathy. Although the family history was uninformative in both cases, the clinical picture in the second patient is reminiscent of maternally inherited NARP (neuropathy, ataxia, retinitis pigmentosa), associated with a mutation in subunit 6 of complex V (see the section on Neuropathy, Ataxia, Retinitis Pigmentosa, and Maternally Inherited Leigh Syndrome, below).

Defects of Oxidation/Phosphorylation Coupling. Nonthyroidal hypermetabolism (Luft's disease) has been reported only in two women, both sporadic. Onset is in adolescence, with fever, heat intolerance, profuse perspiration, polyphagia, polydipsia, and resting tachycardia. Exercise intolerance is present, but weakness is only mild to moderate. Muscle histology shows numerous RRFs and abundant capillaries. Electron microscopy shows greatly enlarged mitochondria, many of which contained osmiophilic inclusions. Biochemical analyses in both patients showed that muscle mitochondria had lost the physiologic control exerted by ATP on the rate of respiration (i.e., oxidation and phosphorylation were "loosely coupled"). Both women died in middle-age.

DEFECTS OF MITOCHONDRIAL PROTEIN TRANSPORT. Errors in protein transport cause a variant of methylmalonic acidemia and may cause a congenital myopathy and adult-onset exercise intolerance and myoglobinuria.

Diseases Caused by Defects of Mitochondrial DNA

Deletions

Three major syndromes can be identified: Kearns-Sayre syndrome, sporadic PEO with RRFs, and Pearson marrow/pancreas syndrome. Although the genetic defect and pathogenesis are common, the distribution of deletions among tissues differentiates these syndromes rather precisely.

KEARNS-SAYRE SYNDROME. The invariant clinical triad of Kearns-Sayre syndrome (KSS) is (1) onset before age 20 years, (2) PEO, and (3) pigmentary retinopathy plus at least one of the following: heart block, cerebellar syndrome, or a cerebrospinal fluid protein level above 100 mg/dl. Other common but nonspecific features include dementia, neurosensory hearing loss, and endocrine abnormalities (short stature, diabetes, hypoparathyroidism). Muscle biopsy shows RRFs and a variable number of COX-negative fibers. Most patients die in the third or fourth decade, even after placement of a pacemaker. Almost all patients with the clinical features of KSS have mtDNA deletions. Some patients have PEO plus a few but not all of the features required for the diagnosis of KSS. These cases of incomplete KSS may develop the full syndrome later in life. The presence of mtDNA deletions in most of these patients underlines the identity with KSS.

SPORADIC PROGRESSIVE EXTERNAL OPHTHALMOPLEGIA WITH RAGGED-RED FIBERS. Sporadic PEO with RRFs is a condition characterized by ophthalmoplegia, ptosis, and proximal limb weakness. Onset is usually in adolescence or young adult years, and the course is slowly progressive and compatible with a relatively normal life. Muscle biopsy specimens show RRFs and COX-negative fibers. Half of patients with PEO have mtDNA deletions. Other family members are not affected, and this helps in the differential diagnosis from other forms of PEO with RRFs, such as autosomal dominant PEO with multiple mtDNA deletions or maternally inherited PEO with various mtDNA point mutations (see the section on Diseases Caused by Defects of Communication Between Nuclear and Mitochondrial Genome).

PEARSON MARROW/PANCREAS SYNDROME. Pearson marrow/pancreas syndrome is a non-neurologic disease of childhood characterized by refractory sideroblastic anemia, vacuolization of marrow precursors, and exocrine pancreatic dysfunction. Death usually occurs in early childhood as a result of sepsis secondary to bone marrow failure. A few patients with Pearson marrow/pancreas syndrome may survive into adolescence only to develop symptoms and signs of KSS.

Duplications

Duplications of mtDNA were initially reported in two patients with KSS. Maternally inherited duplications were associated with deletions in two sisters with a syndrome including cerebellar ataxia, proximal tubular nephrosis, and diabetes mellitus. A similar association of maternally inherited duplications and deletions was described in other patients and may be the underlying cause of all maternally transmitted single deletions of mtDNA, including the very large deletion (approximately 10 kb) observed in a family with diabetes mellitus and deafness. That duplications can be pathogenic was indicated by two patients with adult-onset, slowly progressive mitochondrial myopathy without PEO, whose muscle biopsy specimens showed no mtDNA deletions but contained relatively high levels of mtDNA-harboring duplications.

Point Mutations

Point mutations in mtDNA were first associated with Leber's hereditary optic neuropathy (LHON). As of 1995, more than 50 distinct point mutations had been described (see Table 4.3). The clinical presentations are diverse and can affect all body tissues. Only the most common syndromes of neurologic interest are listed below.

LEBER'S HEREDITARY OPTIC NEUROPATHY. LHON is characterized by acute or subacute loss of vision because of severe bilateral optic atrophy. Onset is usually between 18 and 30 years and has marked predominance in men. Typical ophthalmoscopic features are circumpapillary telangiectatic microangiopathy and pseudoedema of the optic disc. Associated features may include hyper-reflexia, cerebellar ataxia, peripheral neuropathy, or cardiac conduction abnormalities (pre-excitation syndrome). One unusual form of LHON is associated with progressive generalized dystonia and striatal degeneration.

Several distinct mutations, all in structural genes and most in genes encoding complex I subunits, have been described. Of these, some (primary mutations) are found exclusively in LHON families and appear to cause the disease even when present in isolation; others (secondary mutations) are found both in LHON families and in controls and may become pathogenic only when they coexist with another mtDNA mutation.

Myoclonic Epilepsy with Ragged-Red Fibers. In its full clinical expression, myoclonic epilepsy with ragged-red fibers (MERRF) is characterized by myoclonus, seizures, mitochondrial myopathy, and cerebellar ataxia. Less common features are dementia, hearing loss, optic atrophy, peripheral neuropathy, pigmentary retinopathy, ophthalmoparesis, and multiple lipomatosis. Evidence of maternal inheritance is another important feature that distinguishes MERRF from four other neurologic syndromes dominated by progressive myoclonic epilepsy: Unverricht-Lundborg disease (Baltic myoclonus), Lafora-body disease, sialidosis, and neuronal ceroid-lipofuscinosis. Recognition of a highly specific, although not exclusive, point mutation at nt 8344 (A8344G) in the $tRNA^{Lys}$ gene of mtDNA allows the identification of patients independent of the severity of their clinical phenotype.

Onset can be in childhood or in adult life, and the course can be slowly or rapidly progressive. A hierarchy of vulnerability of different organs exists, parallel to their dependence on oxidation/phosphorylation, in which the brain suffers first, followed by muscle and heart. No specific therapy is available, but coenzyme Q_{10} administration appeared to benefit a mother and daughter with the MERRF mutation.

Mitochondrial Encephalomyopathy, Lactic Acidosis, and Strokelike Episodes. MELAS is characterized by the strokelike episodes and in their absence may be difficult to diagnose clinically. As with MERRF, the identification of a highly specific, although not exclusive, point mutation at nt 3243 (A3243G) in the $tRNA^{Leu(UUR)}$ gene of mtDNA has provided a valuable diagnostic tool. This point mutation is found in about 80% of patients defined on the basis of (1) strokelike episodes (with CT or MRI evidence of focal brain abnormalities); (2) lactic acidosis, RRFs, or both; and (3) at least two of the following: focal or generalized seizures, dementia, recurrent headache, or vomiting. The mutation is always present in oligosymptomatic maternal relatives and most asymptomatic maternal relatives. Therefore, the MELAS mutation should be looked for in patients with nonspecific symptoms, signs of mitochondrial encephalomyopathy, and evidence of maternal inheritance. Other mutations, both in tRNA genes and in structural genes, have been associated with typical MELAS.

The onset of symptoms is usually before age 15 years. Hemianopia and cortical blindness are the most common initial features, and the first strokelike episode occurs before age 40 years in almost all patients.

Seizures and lactic acidosis are almost invariable. A substantial number of patients with the A3243G mutations have a distinct phenotype, which is dominated by PEO but often is associated with various combinations of other symptoms, including hearing loss, endocrinopathy, heart block, cerebellar ataxia, and pigmentary retinopathy. Although the A3243G mutation is by far the most common cause of maternally inherited PEO, ptosis and ophthalmoparesis have also been reported in a few patients with different mtDNA point mutations. A distinctive feature of the muscle histology in most patients with typical MELAS (but not in those with PEO) is RRFs that are COX-positive. Biochemical studies of muscle had shown complex I deficiency in many patients.

Patients with the full syndrome have a poor prognosis. Therapeutic trials have included corticosteroids and CoQ_{10}. In patients with severe lactic acidosis, simply lowering the blood level of lactic acid may cause marked clinical improvement.

NEUROPATHY, ATAXIA, RETINITIS PIGMENTOSA, AND MATERNALLY INHERITED LEIGH SYNDROME. NARP is a maternally inherited multisystem disorder associated with a heteroplasmic point mutation (T8993G) in the ATPase 6 gene of mtDNA. The clinical features include developmental delay, retinitis pigmentosa, dementia, seizures, ataxia, proximal weakness, and sensory neuropathy. Muscle histology does not show RRFs. The disease severity correlates with the abundance of mutant genomes. Infants with at least 90% of mutant mtDNA develop a severe encephalomyopathy with the neuroradiologic and neuropathologic features of Leigh syndrome. The A8993G mutation is, together with PDHC and COX deficiencies, one of the most important causes of Leigh syndrome.

Onset of maternally inherited Leigh syndrome is in early infancy with developmental delay, hypotonia, seizures, pyramidal signs, ataxia, retinitis pigmentosa, and ophthalmoparesis. Retinitis pigmentosa is not seen in patients with PDHC or COX deficiency and, when present, represents a useful diagnostic clue. The coexistence of patients with NARP and Leigh syndrome in the maternal lineage is another clue to the correct diagnosis. The results of biochemical analyses of the electron transport chain in muscle may be normal or may show multiple partial defects, but studies in mitochondria containing high levels of the T8993G mutation consistently show marked decreases in ATP synthesis caused by structural instability and altered assembly of the ATP synthase complex. A different mutation in the very same nucleotide (T8993C) causes a milder and more variable clinical phenotype and a less severe defect of ATP synthesis. Two additional mutations in the ATPase 6 gene (T8851C and T9176C) have been reported in children with bilateral striatal necrosis, suggesting that this gene may represent a hotspot for mutations associated with

Leigh-like syndromes, just as the $tRNA^{Leu(UUR)}$ gene is a hotspot for mutations causing MELAS.

Diseases Caused by Defects of Communication between Nuclear and Mitochondrial Genomes

Multiple mtDNA Deletions

PEO is the constant feature in this group of disorders.

Autosomal Dominant Progressive External Ophthalmoplegia. Autosomal dominant progressive external ophthalmoplegia is characterized by exercise intolerance, weakness of proximal limb and respiratory muscles, cataracts, hearing loss, and early death. Analysis of muscle mtDNA shows multiple bands representing species of mtDNA molecules harboring deletions of different sizes. Clinical features vary in different families and may include tremor, ataxia, peripheral neuropathy, mental retardation, hypoparathyroidism, and psychiatric disorders. Lactic acidosis, RRFs, and low-density areas in the basal ganglia, centrum ovale, and brain peduncle may be associated. Biochemical studies of muscle show combined defects of the respiratory chain of varying severity. The autosomal dominant mode of transmission in these families suggests that the alteration of an nDNA-encoded transacting factor (or factors) either facilitates an intrinsic propensity of mtDNA to undergo rearrangements or leads to a failure to recognize and eliminate spontaneously occurring rearrangements.

Autosomal Recessive Progressive External Ophthalmoplegia. In two families, PEO was associated with proximal weakness and severe hypertrophic cardiomyopathy causing cardiac insufficiency and death at an early age. A distinctive autosomal recessive PEO multisystem disorder with PEO and gastrointestinal involvement often associated with multiple mtDNA deletions is the myoneurogastrointestinal disorder and encephalopathy (MNGIE) syndrome. MNGIE syndrome consists of short stature, PEO, limb weakness, peripheral neuropathy, gastroenteropathy, lactic acidosis, RRFs, and decreased COX activity in muscle and liver.

Other Conditions with Multiple mtDNA Deletions. Multiple mtDNA deletions in muscle have been described in several other conditions, including sporadic inclusion body myositis, late-onset mitochondrial myopathy, and an assortment of individual cases with diverse clinical features. The pathogenic role of multiple deletions in these conditions is questionable, because they may be a consequence of normal aging.

Depletion of mtDNA

Depletion of mtDNA has been described in several patients, and two main clinical pictures have emerged: a congenital and rapidly fatal condition characterized by myopathy or hepatopathy and a progressive infantile myopathy causing death from respiratory failure within a few years. The first syndrome is sometimes associated with glycosuria, phosphaturia, and generalized aminoaciduria (de Toni-Fanconi-Debre syndrome) and has a decreased amount of mtDNA in the kidneys. The later onset and slower course in children with the infantile myopathy may be because the mtDNA depletion affects some but not all muscle fibers. Biochemical studies showed combined defects of respiratory chain complexes containing mtDNA-encoded subunits, such as complexes I, III, and IV, that were more marked in patients with severe mtDNA depletion than in those with partial mtDNA depletion.

Transmission appears to be autosomal recessive for both the congenital and the infantile forms of mtDNA depletion, suggesting that the genetic defect (or defects) may involve a nuclear gene (or genes) controlling mtDNA replication. The clinical spectrum of mtDNA depletion may be wider than described. A less severe, secondary form of mtDNA depletion is probably the cause of the mitochondrial myopathy described in patients with acquired immunodeficiency syndrome after prolonged therapy with zidovudine (AZT).

For a more detailed discussion, see Schon EA. The Mitochondrial Genome (Chapter 10; pp. 189–200); DiMauro S, Bonilla E, Mitochondrial Encephalomyopathies (Chapter 11; pp. 201–235), in RN Rosenberg, SB Prusiner, S DiMauro, RL Barchi (eds),* The Molecular and Genetic Basis of Neurological Disease *(2nd ed). Boston: Butterworth–Heinemann, 1997.

5

Peroxisomal Disorders

PEROXISOMES

Morphology

Peroxisomes appear as round or oval cellular organelles, bounded by a single membrane with an average diameter of 500 nm. They lie in close apposition to other organelles such as the mitochondrion, endoplasmic reticulum, and the Golgi apparatus but do not interconnect with them. Except for mature erythrocytes, peroxisomes are probably present in all tissues and organs. They are prominent in liver, kidney, the intestinal epithelium, the adrenal cortex of pregnant rats, and in tissues that synthesize lipids, such as the sebaceous gland. Nervous system peroxisomes are smaller and fewer than those in the liver. They are most prominent in oligodendrocytes during the period of myelination, probably because peroxisomes are required for the synthesis of plasmalogens, a group of lipids that includes the myelin constituent phosphatidylethanolamine.

Peroxisomes contain a series of membrane proteins (PMPs) that are organelle-specific. The basic defect in the disorders of peroxisome assembly involves the import of proteins into the peroxisome, a process that must involve the PMP.

Biochemical Reactions

Table 5.1 lists the biochemical reactions that take place mainly or even exclusively in peroxisomes, and these reactions are defective in disorders of peroxisome assembly. Other peroxisomal processes, such as fatty acid oxidation and cholesterol biosynthesis, also occur in other organelles, and the physiologic role and the alterations that occur in disease states are not yet fully understood. This section provides a brief overview of biochemical reactions that have been localized to the peroxisomes, with emphasis on those that are relevant to peroxisomal diseases.

Table 5.1
Diagnostically significant abnormalities in Zellweger syndrome.

1. Peroxisomes absent or reduced in number
2. Catalase in cytosol
3. Deficient synthesis and reduced tissue levels of plasmalogens
4. Defective oxidation and abnormal accumulation of very long-chain fatty acids
5. Deficient oxidation and age-dependent accumulation of phytanic acid
6. Defects in certain steps of bile acid formation and accumulation of bile acid intermediates
7. Defect in oxidation and accumulation of L-pipecolic acid
8. Increased urinary excretion of dicarboxylic acids

Hydrogen Peroxide–Based Respiration

Peroxisomes contain several oxidases that reduce oxygen to hydrogen peroxide. The substrates of these oxidases include D- and L-amino acids, pipecolic acid, L-α-hydroxy acids, glutaryl-coenzyme A (CoA), oxalate, very long-chain fatty acids (VLCFAs), and branched-chain fatty acids. Catalase, the enzyme that decomposes hydrogen peroxide, has been localized to the peroxisomes.

Fatty Acid β-Oxidation

Peroxisomes play an active role in many aspects of fatty acid oxidation. In contrast to mitochondrial β-oxidation, peroxisomal fatty acid oxidation is not dependent on carnitine, and it is not inhibited by cyanide. The peroxisomal fatty acid oxidation system shows maximum catalytic activity toward saturated acyl-CoAs with chain length C12–16 and long-chain unsaturated fatty acids. The main role of peroxisomal β-oxidation is to supply acetyl-CoA for anabolic reactions when the cells are well supplied with energy. Such anabolic reactions include cholesterol, phospholipid, and bile acid synthesis. Peroxisomes are not able to oxidize short-chain fatty acids. VLCFAs, those with a carbon chain length of 24 or greater, are oxidized mainly, and perhaps exclusively, in the peroxisomes. Increased levels of VLCFA are the hallmark of peroxisomal disorders.

All enzymes of peroxisomal β-oxidation have been purified and defects are associated with human disease states. Three separate CoA ligases are identified. A defect in the VLCFA CoA ligase is the primary defect in X-linked adrenoleukodystrophy. Peroxisomes are also involved in the oxidation of monounsaturated and polyunsaturated fatty acids and in the chain shortening of prostaglandins. The prostaglandin chain shortening reactions are analogous to fatty acid β-oxidation and are part of the processes that inactivate them.

Bile Acid Synthesis

The formation of bile acids from cholesterol involves a series of microsomal and mitochondrial hydroxylation, dehydration, and oxidation steps that lead to the formation of 3α,7α,12α-trihydroxybetacholestanoic acid (THCA) and 3α,7α-dihydrobetacholestanoic acid (DHCA). The CoA derivatives of these compounds are converted to cholic and chenodeoxycholic acid, respectively, by the action of one chain shortening cycle. These reactions take place in peroxisomes, and THCA and DHCA accumulate in many peroxisomal disorders.

Cholesterol Biosynthesis

Peroxisomes synthesize cholesterol, and patients with disorders of peroxisome assembly have abnormally low levels of plasma cholesterol.

Plasmalogen Synthesis

Plasmalogens belong to the class of ether lipids. They constitute 5–20% of the phospholipids in most cell membranes and are particularly abundant in nervous tissue. One-third of myelin phospholipids are plasmalogens. The initial two steps in plasmologen synthesis take place in the peroxisomes, the third step in both peroxisomes and microsomes, and all subsequent steps are microsomal.

Amino Acid Metabolism

The subcellular localization of alanine-glyoxalate aminotransferase (AGT) in humans is peroxisomal. AGT catalyzes the transamination of glyoxylate to glycine, with alanine serving as the amino group donor. L-Pipecolic acid oxidase is a peroxisomal enzyme. Pipecolic acid is an intermediate in the lysine degradation pathway that serves as the main route of lysine degradation in brain.

CLASSIFICATION OF PEROXISOMAL DISORDERS

Table 5.2 lists the current classification of peroxisomal disorders. The two main categories are (1) disorders of peroxisome assembly and (2) defects of single peroxisomal proteins. In the disorders of peroxisome assem-

Table 5.2
Genetically determined peroxisomal disorders.

Assembly Deficiencies	*Single Peroxisomal Enzyme Deficiencies*
Zellweger syndrome*	X-linked adrenoleukodystrophy*
Neonatal adrenoleukodystrophy*	Acyl-coenzyme A oxidase deficiency*
Infantile Refsum disease*	Bifunctional enzyme deficiency*
Hyperpipecolatemia*	Peroxisomal thiolase deficiency*
Rhizomelic chondrodysplasia punctata*	DHAP alkyl transferase deficiency*
	Alkyl DHAP synthase deficiency*
	Glutaric aciduria type III*?
	Classic Refsum disease*
	Hyperoxaluria type 1
	Acatalasemia

DHAP = dihydroxyacetone phosphate.
*Disorders associated with mental retardation or neurologic deficits.

bly, the organelle fails to form normally, and multiple peroxisomal functions are defective. In defects of single peroxisomal proteins, peroxisome structure is intact. Among disorders of peroxisome assembly, four conditions have a Zellweger phenotype: Zellweger syndrome, neonatal adrenoleukodystrophy, infantile Refsum disease, and hyperpipecolic acidemia. These will be discussed together, with rhizomelic chondrodysplasia punctata considered separately. Disorders with defects of single peroxisomal proteins with phenotypes that resemble the disorders of peroxisome assembly are discussed together, and X-linked adrenoleukodystrophy and hyperoxaluria type 1 are discussed separately. In addition, a brief summary of acatalasemia and of recently described peroxisomal disorders is provided.

DISORDERS OF PEROXISOME ASSEMBLY WITH THE ZELLWEGER PHENOTYPE

The Zellweger syndrome, neonatal adrenoleukodystrophy (NALD), infantile Refsum disease (IRD), and hyperpipecolic acidemia (HA) all share a panel of morphologic and biochemical abnormalities (see Table 5.1). The Zellweger cerebrohepatorenal syndrome was the first disorder shown to be caused by the absence of peroxisomes. The recognition and naming of the three other disorders followed the demonstration of a single biochemical abnormality for each. The first patient with hyperpipecolic acidemia represented the first time that pipecolic acid accumulation was noted in any human disease state. It was later noted to be a feature of the Zellweger syndrome. It is now clear that all four disorders share the abnormalities listed in Table 5.1 and that they differ only in disease severity. Zellweger syndrome is the most severe, infantile Refsum disease the least severe (although still severely disabling), and neonatal ALD intermediate in severity.

Clinical Features

Newborns with Zellweger syndrome have characteristic abnormalities (Table 5.3). Of central importance are the typical face (high forehead, hypoplastic supraorbital ridges, epicanthal folds, midface hypoplasia), severe weakness and hypotonia, eye abnormalities (cataracts, glaucoma, corneal clouding, Brushfield spots, pigmentary retinopathy, optic nerve dysplasia), and neonatal seizures. Infants with Zellweger syndrome rarely live beyond the first year, and most show no signs of psychomotor development.

Newborns with neonatal ALD are severely ill at birth with seizures, mild to moderate dysmorphic features, hypotonia, and poor feeding. Pigmentary degeneration of the retina and an enlarged liver with micronodular cirrhosis develop in the first months. Some children make minimal maturational gains, such as evidence of ocular pursuit, some degree of head control, and the ability to sit with support; others show no psychomotor development.

Children with infantile Refsum disease show mild dysmorphic features (high arched palate, epicanthal folds, anteverted nostrils, midface hypoplasia) and have an enlarged liver and pigmentary degeneration of the retina. Hypotonia is present but not as severe as in the Zellweger syndrome. These patients differ from those with Zellweger syndrome and neonatal ALD in that early motor development does occur. Most patients are able to stand, albeit with an ataxic component. Speech is usually not attained, and affected children function in the profoundly retarded range. Seizures are not part of the syndrome.

Laboratory Features

The main laboratory abnormalities are listed in Table 5.1. The concentrations of saturated and unsaturated VLCFA are increased in tissues and body fluids. Pipecolic acid concentrations are elevated in plasma and urine. Plasma concentrations of phytanic acid increases with age, whereas plasmalogen concentrations in red blood cells decrease. Abnormally high plasma concentrations of THCA and DHCA are a consistent feature. Studies with cultured skin fibroblasts show increased

Table 5.3
Main clinical abnormalities in Zellweger syndrome.

	Cases in Which Information About the Feature Was Available		*Cases in Which the Feature Was Present*	
Abnormal Feature	*Number*	*Percent*	*Number*	*Percent*
High forehead	60	53	58	97
Flat occiput	16	14	13	81
Large fontanelle(s)	57	50	55	96
Shallow orbital ridges	33	29	33	100
Low/broad nasal bridge	23	20	23	100
Epicanthus	36	32	33	92
High arched palate	37	32	35	95
External ear deformity	40	35	39	97
Micrognathia	18	16	18	100
Redundant skin folds of neck	13	11	13	100
Brushfield spots	6	5	5	83
Cataract/cloudy cornea	35	31	30	86
Glaucoma	12	11	7	58
Abnormal retinal pigmentation	15	13	6	40
Optic disk pallor	23	20	17	74
Severe hypotonia	95	83	94	99
Abnormal Moro response	26	23	26	100
Hyporeflexia or areflexia	57	50	56	98
Poor sucking	77	68	74	96
Gavage feeding	26	23	26	100
Epileptic seizures	61	54	56	92
Psychomotor retardation	45	39	45	100
Impaired hearing	21	18	9	40
Nystagmus	37	32	30	81

Source: From a survey of 114 patients with Zellweger syndrome reported in the literature by HSA Heymans. Cerebro-hepato-renal (Zellweger) syndrome: clinical and biochemical consequences of peroxisomal dysfunction. Thesis, University of Amsterdam, 1984.

quantities of VLCFA, deficient activity of acyl:CoA dihydroxyacetone phosphate acyl transferase and of the peroxisomal steps of plasmalogen synthesis, and impaired oxidation of phytanic acid. Liver biopsy shows the lack of catalase-containing peroxisomes.

Mode of Inheritance

An autosomal recessive mode of inheritance is likely for all of the disorders of peroxisome assembly.

Neuropathology

The brain of patients with Zellweger syndrome shows striking and characteristic abnormalities of neuronal migration: heterotopia, microgyria, and pachygyria. Leukodystrophy may also be present.

Diagnosis

Disorders of peroxisome assembly should be suspected in newborns with the combination of hypotonia, weakness, seizures, dysmorphic features, enlarged liver, renal cysts, chondrodysplasia punctata, glaucoma, and cataracts. Dysmorphic features associated with classic Zellweger syndrome need not be present. Tests for these disorders should be conducted in neonates with unexplained failure to thrive, particularly when this is associated with hypotonia, seizures, dysmorphic features, and an enlarged liver. In older children or young adults, the most important diagnostic leads are severe or profound mental retardation, mild or moderate dysmorphic features, pigmentary degeneration of the retina and optic nerve atrophy, hearing loss, enlarged liver, and impaired liver function.

The initial laboratory test should be the measurement of plasma concentrations of VLCFA, pipecolic acid, phytanic acid, and bile acid intermediates and plasmalogen concentrations in red blood cells. In those cases in which the proband is known to have increased levels of bile acid intermediates, prenatal diagnosis can be achieved by showing increased levels of THCA and DHCA in amniotic fluid.

All of the biochemical abnormalities are secondary to the peroxisomal defects, but the primary defect in all disorders of peroxisome assembly is unknown. The lack of definition of the primary defect accounts for the fact that no tests for the carrier state are available.

Therapy

The severe multiple malformations present at birth limit the possibilities of postnatal therapy. For patients with classic Zellweger syndrome, therapy is confined to supportive care, with addition of vitamin K when prothrombin deficiency exists in association with liver disease. More active therapy may be considered for children with the somewhat milder phenotypes, and gratifying, albeit limited, progress has been achieved with multidisciplinary habilitative approaches, including hearing aids and communication training, ophthalmologic treatment, and physical and occupational therapy. It is possible to normalize, at least in part, some of the biochemical abnormalities, and several of the more mildly affected children have been placed on special diets. The regimens that are being used include oral ether lipid therapy and the dietary restriction of VLCFA and phytanic acid.

RHIZOMELIC CHONDRODYSPLASIA PUNCTATA

The term *chondrodysplasia punctata* is applied to infants with punctate epiphyseal and extraepiphyseal calcifications on radiographs. It is a nonspecific finding that can be caused by toxins, but most cases are genetically determined. The modes of inheritance may be autosomal dominant or recessive and X-linked dominant or recessive. Two forms are distinguished. The mild form (Conradi-Hünermann type) is transmitted as an autosomal dominant trait; intelligence is normal, cataracts are uncommon, and survival to adulthood is expected. The severe form is transmitted as an autosomal recessive trait; the limbs are severely shortened, psychomotor retardation is severe, and death occurs during infancy. The severe form is called *rhizomelic chondrodysplasia punctata* (RCDP).

Clinical Features

The clinical features of classical RCDP are short stature with disproportionate shortening of the proximal parts of the extremities, microcephaly, abnormal facial appearance, severe mental retardation, cataracts, and ichthyosis. Radiologic features include severe shortening, metaphyseal cupping, splaying, and disturbed ossification of the humeri and femora; a coronal cleft of the vertebral bodies; and stippling of the epiphyses at the knee, hip, elbow, and shoulder. Stippling in the vertebral column is uncommon in RCDP but is prominent in the Conradi-Hünermann syndrome.

Diagnosis

RCDP must be differentiated from other genetic and acquired causes of chondrodysplasia punctata. All infants with RCDP have three biochemical defects: (1) marked reduction of plasmalogen levels secondary to an impairment of plasmalogen synthesis; (2) increased plasma levels of phytanic acid secondary to impaired capacity of phytanic acid oxidation; and (3) the presence of 3-oxoacyl-CoA thiolase in the immature form. This biochemical profile is seen only in RCDP. The most readily available tests are measures of erythrocyte plasmalogen concentrations and plasma phytanic acid concentrations. Prenatal diagnosis uses the same assays in cultured amniocytes or chorionic villus samples.

Pathophysiology

RCDP differs from the disorders of peroxisome assembly in that peroxisomes are present and differs from the single enzyme defects in that the activities of at least two unrelated enzymes are deficient, namely acyl-CoA:dihydroxyacetone phosphate acyltransferase and the enzyme for phytanic acid oxidation. In addition, the enzyme 3-oxoacyl-CoA thiolase is present in its unprocessed form. In disorders of peroxisome assembly, both pristanic and phytanic acid accumulate, whereas in classic Refsum disease and in RCDP, only phytanic acid accumulates. This suggests that the metabolic block in RCDP, as in classic Refsum disease, involves the phytanic acid α-oxidation step. The basic defect of phytanic acid oxidation, however, is different in the two disorders. The presence of the immature form of peroxisomal thiolase is also found in patients with Zellweger syndrome and in neonatal ALD.

Molecular Neurobiology

RCDP is associated with a defect for the receptor for peroxisome targeting sequence 2. This sequence is located at the amino terminal of peroxisomal 3-oxoacyl-CoA thiolase. The impaired import of this enzyme into the peroxisome accounts for the inability of RCDP patients to process the precursor form of this enzyme. Mutations have not been identified in any of the RCDP patients.

Therapy

Therapeutic options are limited because the abnormalities are severe at birth. In addition to habilitative therapy, consideration may also be given to dietary measures that may correct at least in part the plasmalogen deficiency and the phytanic acid accumulation (see the section on Disorders of Peroxisome Assembly with the Zellweger Phenotype).

SINGLE PEROXISOMAL ENZYME DEFICIENCIES

X-Linked Adrenoleukodystrophy

Clinical Features

X-linked adrenoleukodystrophy (X-ALD) has several different phenotypes (Table 5.4). The childhood cerebral form is the most severe phenotype. Boys develop normally until age 4 to 8 years, when they become hyper-

Table 5.4
X-Linked adrenoleukodystrophy phenotype distributions (%) at the Kennedy Krieger Institute (KKI), United States; the Academic Medical Center, the Netherlands; and Hôpital de la Salpetriere, France.

Phenotype	*KKI Total up to 1995 (N = 2,088)*	*KKI United States and Canada (N = 1,416)*	*KKI 54 Most Informative U.S. and Canadian Families (N = 252)*	*France 1993 (N = 116)*	*Netherlands 1994 (N = 77)*
Childhood cerebral	40.5	38.4	34.5	43.1	31.0
Adolescent cerebral	4.9	4.8	4.4	16.3	
Adult cerebral	2.7	2.8	1.2	2.6	1.0
Adrenomyeloneuropathy	25.2	26.4	27.0	15.5	46.0
Addison's only	9.6	9.6	10.3	7.8	14.0
Asymptomatic	7.9	8.6	10.3	Not included	8.0
Insufficient information	9.2	9.4	12.3	14.7	Not included

Note: Estimate of the relative frequencies of X-linked adrenoleukodystrophy phenotypes. The first two columns show the overall experience at the Kennedy Krieger Institute. Although they include a large number of patients, it is likely that mildly involved or neurologically asymptomatic patients are underrepresented, because until recently it was not possible to diagnose them. Columns 3 and 5 provide the most reliable data. Column 3 shows the distribution in 54 U.S. and Canadian families studied at the Kennedy Krieger Institute for whom we have the most complete information. The data in column 5 were derived from 30 kindreds in the Netherlands in whom extensive family data were available. Comparison of columns 3 and 5 indicates that the proportion of patients with the childhood cerebral phenotype is smaller (31.0–34.5%) than suggested from the earlier series (columns 1 and 2). The proportion of adrenomyeloneuropathy patients in the Netherlands series is higher than it is in the United States. This discrepancy is in need of further investigation. Some of it may be resolved by definition of the phenotype of the 12.7% (column 3) of the U.S. and Canadian patients for whom clinical information is still incomplete.

active, withdrawn, or emotionally labile. School performance drops off. Impaired auditory discrimination is a common early symptom that causes difficulty in understanding speech in a noisy room. Other early features are visual impairment (field cuts, impaired visual acuity, and cortical blindness) and seizures. Both occur in one-third of patients. The course is rapidly progressive and characterized by spastic paresis; dysphagia; and loss of speech, vision, and hearing, leading to a vegetative state within 2 years from the onset of the initial neurologic symptoms. Neurologic manifestations precede adrenal insufficiency in most patients, but impaired cortisol response to ACTH stimulation usually coexists at the time of neurologic disease. The initial features of adrenal insufficiency are unexplained vomiting, dehydration, weakness, and hyperpigmentation.

The term *adolescent cerebral ALD* is applied when the onset of symptoms that resemble the childhood cerebral form is between the ages of 10 and 21 years. The adult cerebral form is characterized by the onset of behavioral disturbances, dementia, or seizures after age 21 years. The illness may be misdiagnosed as schizophrenia, brain tumor, or multiple sclerosis.

Adrenomyeloneuropathy (AMN) contrasts with the childhood cerebral form of ALD because of its later age of onset, rate of progression, and site of main neurologic involvement. Unlike the cerebral forms of ALD, AMN involves mainly the spinal cord. The mean age of onset is 27.6 ± 8.7 years, and the progression is over decades rather than years. The main neurologic deficits are spasticity, weakness of the legs, and impaired vibration sense that is most severe in the feet. Bladder function is almost always impaired. Adrenal insufficiency is present in two-thirds of cases. One-half of AMN patients also have some degree of cerebral involvement.

The *Addison's only* category includes patients who have Addison's disease in the absence of neurologic signs or symptoms. Half of males with Addison's disease have the ALD biochemical defect. Most develop signs of AMN later in life. Correct diagnosis is important for genetic counseling.

Symptomatic Heterozygotes

Women who are heterozygous for ALD may develop progressive spastic paraparesis, impaired vibration sense in the feet, and sphincter disturbances. The clinical syndrome resembles AMN in males but is milder and occurs later (mean age of onset: 37.8 ± 14.6 years). Some symptomatic women have dementia or visual disturbances. Exacerbations and remissions may occur, suggesting multiple sclerosis. Adrenal insufficiency is rare among heterozygotes.

Laboratory Diagnosis

Diagnosis is established by showing increased concentrations of saturated VLCFA in plasma, erythrocyte membranes, leukocytes, or cultured skin fibroblasts. MRI studies show striking white matter lesions in the parieto-occipital region, with accumulation of contrast material at the advancing edges of the lesions. These lesions are characteristic and occur early in the course of the disease so that abnormal findings on MRI often provide the first clue to the diagnosis.

Pathogenesis

It is likely that the pathogenesis of X-ALD is related in some way to the accumulation of VLCFA secondary to a defect that involves peroxisomal lignoceroyl-CoA ligase. Although considerable evidence indicates that excess VLCFA impairs adrenal function in a dose-related fashion, plasma VLCFA concentrations do not correlate with the severity of neurologic disease. The plasma VLCFA concentration in boys with the rapidly progressive childhood cerebral form does not differ from that in men with AMN or in those adolescents or adults who are neurologically intact. It is suspected that inflammatory or immunopathogenetic mechanisms are involved in the rapidly progressive white matter lesions of the childhood cerebral form of ALD. The hypothesis that the accumulation of saturated VLCFA triggers a cytokine-mediated myelinolytic cascade has led to clinical trials of new therapeutic approaches.

Molecular Neurobiological Features

A putative X-ALD gene localizes to Xq28, in proximity to the red-green color vision genes. Abnormalities in this gene have been demonstrated in all X-ALD families studied so far and not in controls. Large deletions have been identified throughout the genome but do not correlate with phenotype.

Therapy

Two forms of therapy are under active consideration: dietary therapy and bone marrow transplantation. Dietary restriction of VLCFA does not lower VLCFA plasma concentrations and has no effect on clinical course.When glyceryl trioleate and glyceryl trierucate (Lorenzo's oil) are added, however, the plasma concentration of C26:0 and the microviscosity of erythrocytes normalize. Red cell membrane microviscosity is increased in untreated ALD patients and may be of pathogenetic significance. This regimen does not alter the course of disease in boys who are already symptomatic with cerebral ALD or AMN, but preliminary data suggest that severe disability may be prevented when the diet is started before the onset of neurologic abnormality.

Bone marrow transplantation was beneficial in one 8-year-old boy with mild neurologic disability and changes evident on MRI. The transplant came from an unaffected twin. Four years after transplant, the neurologic disability and MRI abnormalities had cleared, and cognitive function was the same as that of his twin. Transplants in boys with advanced disease have caused worsening of neurologic status in the period immediately after transplantation and are contraindicated. Further experience with bone marrow transplantation continues to indicate a favorable response in mildly affected patients when a matched donor is available. Boys with moderately advanced disease or with the rapidly progressive childhood form are not candidates. Therapy is not recommended for asymptomatic heterozygotes.

Disorders That Resemble the Zellweger–Neonatal Adrenoleukodystrophy–Infantile Refsum Disease Phenotype

Three disorders involve defects of a single peroxisomal fatty acid oxidation enzyme that catalyzes sequential reactions in the peroxisomal fatty acid β-oxidation pathway: acyl-CoA oxidase deficiency (oxidase deficiency), bifunctional enzyme deficiency, and 3-oxo-acyl-CoA thiolase deficiency (thiolase deficiency). They have a similar phenotype that more closely resembles the Zellweger phenotype than X-linked ALD, which also involves an enzyme in the β-oxidation pathway. Thiolase deficiency is also called *pseudo–Zellweger syndrome*, and oxidase deficiency is called *pseudo–neonatal ALD*.

Clinical Features

All three syndromes are characterized by neonatal hypotonia and seizures. Thiolase deficiency is also associated with slight dysmorphic features and hepatomegaly. Infants with thiolase deficiency and the bifunctional enzyme deficiency show no psychomotor development and die during infancy. Children with oxidase deficiency make slight psychomotor gains but then regress and become totally disabled. Death occurs during childhood.

Laboratory Diagnosis

The plasma VLCFA concentrations are increased to the same extent as in disorders of peroxisome assembly. Bile acid intermediate (THCA and DHCA) concentrations are increased in the bifunctional enzyme and thiolase deficiency, but not in oxidase deficiency. All other peroxisomal functions are normal, and peroxisome structure is intact.

Neuropathology

Postmortem examination reveals a combination of cerebral maldevelopment, as in disorders of peroxisome assembly, and demyelination, with an inflammatory response that resembles neonatal adrenoleukodystrophy.

Diagnosis

In these disorders, unlike disorders of peroxisome assembly, the biochemical abnormality is confined to VLCFA and, depending on the nature of the defect, to bile acid intermediates. The plasma concentrations of THCA and DHCA are increased in the thiolase and bifunctional enzyme defects but are normal in the oxidase deficiency. Peroxisome structure is intact; catalase is sedimentable; and pipecolic acid, plasmalogen, phytanic acid levels, and metabolism are normal.

Molecular Biology

In oxidase deficiency, siblings of both sexes are affected and are often the product of a consanguineous marriage, suggesting autosomal recessive inheritance. The gene for peroxisomal acyl-CoA oxidase has been cloned and a large deletion accounts for the deficiency state. The gene for human peroxisomal bifunctional enzyme has been cloned and mapped to 3q26.3–3q28.

Disorders That Resemble the Rhizomelic Chondrodysplasia Punctata Phenotype

Isolated deficiencies of dihydroxyacetonephosphate acyltransferase or of alkyldihydroxyacetone phosphate synthase, two peroxisomal enzymes required for the synthesis of plasmalogens, produce clinical features indistinguishable from RCDP. The biochemical abnormalities are confined to defects in plasmalogen synthesis. Phytanic acid metabolism and the processing of peroxisomal thiolase are unimpaired. Therefore, defects in plasmalogen synthesis alone can cause the full spectrum of clinical abnormalities in RCDP. Therapeutic options are limited because of the malformations present at birth.

SUMMARIES OF OTHER PEROXISOMAL DISORDERS

Acatalasemia

Most cases of acatalasemia are asymptomatic. The most severe Japanese variant may be associated with oral ulcerations thought to be caused by infection by peroxide-generating bacteria. These patients have greatly reduced catalase activity, but the electrophoretic mobility of the small amount of enzyme is normal.

Hyperoxaluria Type 1

Hyperoxaluria type 1 presents as progressive renal failure associated with urolithiasis. Neurologic function is intact. It is inherited as an autosomal recessive trait. Diagnosis depends on showing abnormally high urine concentrations of oxalate and glycolate. Therapeutic success is achieved with combined liver and kidney transplants.

Peroxisomal Glutaryl CoA Oxidase Deficiency

Peroxisomal glutaryl CoA oxidase deficiency was first described in an infant with failure to thrive and postprandial vomiting. The urine glutaric acid level was 500 mmol per mole of creatinine compared with the normal value of less than 2. She also was homozygous for β-thalassemia. The glutaric aciduria was responsive to riboflavin, 200 mg twice daily, and at 5 years her development was normal. It is not known whether the normal development is attributable to the vitamin therapy. Detailed metabolic investigations ruled out glutaric aciduria types 1 and 2. The peroxisomal hydrogen-peroxide producing oxidases in cultured skin fibroblasts were measured. The activity of glutaryl-CoA oxidase was reduced to less than 10% of the control value, whereas lauroyl-CoA and dodecanedoyl-CoA oxidase activities were normal. Loading studies suggested that the glutaric acid was derived from lysine, presumably via the pathway in which pipecolic acid is an intermediate, and not from leucine.

This disorder is a third cause of glutaric aciduria in addition to the mitochondrial disorders glutaric aciduria types 1 and 2. Because mitochondrial metabolism of glutaric acid was normal, the data suggest little interchange between the mitochondrial and peroxisomal glutaric acid pools. Because the activities of the other peroxisomal oxidases were normal, it appears likely that the peroxisomal glutaryl-CoA oxidase is a separate enzyme.

PEROXISOMAL DISORDERS THAT ARE STILL INCOMPLETELY CHARACTERIZED

Zellweger-like Syndrome with Detectable Peroxisomes

Liver peroxisomes were present in a male infant with the Zellweger phenotype. His disease differed from the pseudo–Zellweger syndrome (thiolase deficiency) because multiple peroxisomal functions were deficient, including plasmalogen synthesis.

Congenital Syndrome Associated with Calcific Epiphyseal Stippling and Peroxisomal Dysfunction

In a child with a congenital syndrome of calcific epiphyseal stippling and peroxisomal dysfunction, phytanic acid levels in serum were greatly increased and plasma VLCFA concentrations were mildly elevated. Plasmalogen synthesis was mildly impaired.

Ataxia and Peripheral Neuropathy: A Benign Variant of Peroxisome Assembly

A single patient presented with calcium oxalate renal stones, ataxia, and peripheral neuropathy, but normal intellect. VLCFA and pipecolic acid levels were increased greatly, and catalase in cultured skin fibroblasts was in the cytosolic fraction.

Di- and Trihydroxycholestanaemia without Other Evidence of Peroxisomal Dysfunction

Four patients showed elevated plasma concentrations of THCA and DHCA but normal levels of VLCFA and no other evidence of peroxisomal dysfunction. The phenotype varied from severe psychomotor retardation, hypotonia, and dysmorphic features, to fatal progressive liver failure, to a relatively mild disability. An isolated defect of peroxisomal THCA-CoA β-oxidation was considered and found to be normal. The biochemical basis for the THCA and BHCA accumulation remains unexplained.

REFSUM DISEASE

Refsum disease (*heredopathia atactica polyneuritiformis*) is a rare familial neurologic disorder characterized by elevated plasma and tissue concentrations of phytanic acid. Although an increased plasma phytanic acid concentration distinguishes Refsum disease from other neurologic disorders, this finding is not pathognomonic, because elevated levels are also found in several peroxisomal disorders.

Clinical Features

A diagnostic tetrad of clinical findings includes retinitis pigmentosa, peripheral polyneuropathy, cerebellar ataxia, and a high protein concentration in the cerebrospinal fluid (CSF) without pleocytosis. In addition, nerve deafness and cardiac involvement are present in most cases. Features of the disorder that are less commonly found include anosmia, pupillary abnormalities, cataracts, ichthyosis, and skeletal abnormalities.

Onset is usually in the second or third decade. Night blindness is the first symptom. It is followed by a progressive neuropathy that eventually leads to wasting and distal paralysis. Ataxia, particularly unsteadiness of gait, and other cerebellar signs are also early features. If untreated, the disease is slowly progressive with respiratory failure as the cause of death.

Pathophysiology

The only source of phytanic acid is dietary. Its principal food sources are dairy products and ruminant meats and fats. Phytanic acid accumulates in Refsum disease because of a defect in its oxidation pathway. Phytanic acid cannot be degraded by β-oxidation unless it is first shortened by one carbon in an α-oxidation process. In α-oxidation, hydroxylation of the 2-carbon precedes decarboxylation, yielding pristanic acid, which can be catabolized by β-oxidation. The metabolic defect in Refsum disease appears to be at the α-hydroxylation step.

Molecular Biology

Refsum disease is transmitted as an autosomal recessive trait, and a single gene defect is believed responsible. Although the gene coding for the enzyme (α-hydroxylase) is suspected to be defective, it has not been purified, cloned, or sequenced.

Treatment

Increased levels of phytanic acid are directly or indirectly responsible for the clinical disease, although the precise role of phytanic acid in the pathophysiology of Refsum disease has not been identified. Dietary restriction of foods containing phytanic acid results in a reduction of the plasma phytanic acid concentration and the mobilization of tissue stores. Gradual clinical improvement in the polyneuropathy, ataxia, and cardiac and CSF abnormalities occurs during diet therapy, but retinitis pigmentosa and symptoms of cranial nerve involvement are not reversed. Plasma exchange has been successfully used as an adjuvant to dietary therapy.

For a more detailed discussion, see Moser HW. Peroxisomal Disorders (Chapter 13; pp. 273–314); Watkins PA, Mihalik SJ. Refsum Disease (Chapter 14; pp. 315–330), in RN Rosenberg, SB Prusiner, S DiMauro, RL Barchi (eds), **The Molecular and Genetic Basis of Neurological Disease** ***(2nd ed). Boston: Butterworth–Heinemann, 1997.***

6

Lysosomal Disorders

THE MUCOPOLYSACCHARIDOSES

The mucopolysaccharidoses are a group of inherited disorders caused by specific enzyme defects in the degradation of the glycosaminoglycans (mucopolysaccharides) (Table 6.1). The enzyme deficiencies result in the accumulation of glycosaminoglycans in lysosomes of several tissues and in the excessive excretion of partially degraded glycosaminoglycans in urine (Table 6.2). For each enzyme deficiency, there is a spectrum of clinical manifestations. The mucopolysaccharidoses are inherited as autosomal recessive diseases with the exception of Hunter's syndrome, which is transmitted as an X-linked recessive trait. Carrier detection and prenatal diagnosis are available.

Hurler's Syndrome (Mucopolysaccharidosis Type I)

Hurler's syndrome is the prototype of all the mucopolysaccharidoses. It is the most severe form of α-L-iduronidase deficiency. Milder forms are the Hurler-Scheie and Scheie syndromes. The deficiency of α-L-iduronidase leads to the accumulation of dermatan sulfate and heparan sulfate and to the urinary excretion of these glycosaminoglycans. In patients with Hurler's syndrome, vacuolated cells containing lysosomes engorged with glycosaminoglycans are seen in many tissues.

Clinical Features

Infants with Hurler's syndrome appear normal at birth but develop a coarse facial appearance after 6 months. Other features are dysostosis multiplex (see the section on Radiographic Findings), organomegaly, umbilical and inguinal hernias, and chronic rhinorrhea. Recurrent upper airway infection, otitis media, and hypertrophy of the tonsils and adenoids may persist beyond early childhood. Mild kyphosis is first

Table 6.1
Enzyme defects of the mucopolysaccharidoses.

Disease	*Enzyme Defect*	*Inheritance*
Hurler's syndrome	α-L-Iduronidase	Autosomal recessive
Hurler-Scheie syndrome	α-L-Iduronidase	Autosomal recessive
Scheie's syndrome	α-L-Iduronidase	Autosomal recessive
Hunter's syndrome (types A and B)	Iduronosulfate sulfatase	X-linked recessive
Sanfilippo's syndrome type A	Sulfamidase	Autosomal recessive
Sanfilippo's syndrome type B	α-*N*-Acetyl-glucosaminidase	Autosomal recessive
Sanfilippo's syndrome type C	Acetyl-CoA: α-glucosaminide *N*-acetyltransferase	Autosomal recessive
Sanfilippo's syndrome type D	*N*-Acetylglucosamine-6-sulfate sulfatase	Autosomal recessive
Morquio syndrome type A	*N*-Acetylgalactosamine-6-sulfate sulfatase	Autosomal recessive
Morquio syndrome type B	β-Galactosidase	Autosomal recessive
Maroteaux-Lamy syndrome	*N*-Acetylgalactosamine-4-sulfate sulfatase	Autosomal recessive
β-Glucuronidase deficiency	β-Glucuronidase	Autosomal recessive

Table 6.2
Major glycosaminoglycan stored and excreted in urine in the mucopolysaccharidoses.

Disease	*Glycosaminoglycan*
Hurler's syndrome	Dermatan sulfate and heparan sulfate
Hurler-Scheie syndrome	Dermatan sulfate
Scheie's syndrome	Dermatan sulfate
Hunter's syndrome (types A and B)	Dermatan sulfate and heparan sulfate
Sanfilippo's syndrome (types A, B, C, and D)	Heparan sulfate
Morquio syndrome type A	Keratan sulfate, chondroitin-6-sulfate
Morquio syndrome type B	Keratan sulfate
Maroteaux-Lamy syndrome	Dermatan sulfate
β-Glucuronidase deficiency	Chondroitin-4/6-sulfate, dermatan sulfate, and heparan sulfate

seen on attempted sitting and progresses to gibbus later on. Vision is impaired because of clouding of the corneas. Developmental milestones are attained in the first year and then lost. Developmental regression progresses to severe mental retardation and a vegetative state.

Children with Hurler-Scheie syndrome have severe joint involvement, short stature, small thorax, organomegaly, coarse facial features, and corneal clouding but normal or near-normal mentality. In Scheie syndrome, normal height is usually attained and organomegaly is mild. Affected children are not retarded and do not have coarse features.

Biochemical and Molecular Features

It is difficult to differentiate clinically or enzymatically among the α-iduronidase deficiency syndromes during infancy. This has implications for experimental therapy because the milder forms of α-L-iduronidase defects may not require treatment. α-L-Iduronidase is required for the hydrolysis of α-L-iduronic acid from the terminal ends of dermatan and heparan sulfates. In patients with Hurler's syndrome, the excretion of dermatan and heparan sulfate is increased, whereas only dermatan sulfate is excreted in the milder forms. Human α-L-iduronidase has been purified and the cDNA and gene isolated. The gene is located on chromosome 4p16.3 in proximity to the Huntington's disease region. The isolation of the cDNA should make it possible to investigate and explain phenotypic variants of iduronidase deficiency. Studies of genomic DNA do not reveal any gross alterations in the iduronidase gene suggesting point mutations or small insertions or deletions.

Hunter's Syndrome (Mucopolysaccharidosis Type II)

Clinical Features

Hunter's syndrome is the only X-linked recessive disease among the mucopolysaccharidoses. Two phenotypes exist, one with and one without mental retardation. Both forms have similar facial features, with slightly less coarseness in the mild form. In general, the Hunter phenotype is similar to the Hurler phenotype except the corneas are not involved, hearing deteriorates rapidly, and gibbus formation is delayed until the second decade. A macular skin rash over the arms, shoulders, and thighs is characteristic. With time, individuals with the mild variant develop severe hearing problems, carpal tunnel syndrome, and progressive upper airway obstruction. Death may occur from upper airway obstruction and heart failure. Some have survived beyond the fifth or sixth decade.

Biochemical and Molecular Features

Patients with Hunter's syndrome excrete dermatan and heparan sulfate similar to Hurler's syndrome, but no difference exists in the glycosaminoglycan excretion between the severe and mild forms. The gene for iduronosulfatase has been cloned and localized to the Xq28 region. Deletions in the iduronosulfatase gene are a common finding. Complete deletions, partial deletions, or gross rearrangements of the gene are all associated with the severe phenotype. The gross deletion in some patients with Hunter's syndrome suggests that some features in severely affected patients may be caused by the deletion of neighboring genes.

Sanfilippo's Syndrome (Mucopolysaccharidosis Type III)

Sanfilippo's syndrome has four types with different enzyme defects. The enzyme deficiencies can be assayed in white blood cells and cultured skin fibroblasts. The urine contains increased concentrations of heparan sulfate but not dermatan sulfate.

Clinical Features

All forms have some degree of dysostosis multiplex, coarse facial features, and organomegaly. With time, the liver and spleen may resume normal size. Sanfilippo's type A syndrome is the most common form. The enzyme defect is sulfamidase. Hyperactivity, speech delay, and frank mental retardation are initial symptoms. Rapid neurologic deterioration occurs by age 10 years leading to profound disability and death in adolescence. Sanfilippo's type B is second in frequency and has a similar phenotype to type A. The enzyme deficiency is α-*N*-acetylhexosaminidase. Sanfilippo's type C is the mildest type in terms of mental retardation, dysostosis multiplex, and coarse features. Affected children show symptoms of hyperactivity and mental retardation as they get older. Joint stiffness is not a prominent feature. The enzyme defect is acetylCoA:α-glucosamide *N*-acetyltransferase. Sanfilippo's type D syndrome is the least common. The phenotype is usually mild. One child had only speech delay. Children with Sanfilippo's type D excrete not only heparan sulfate but also *N*-acetylglucosamine-6-sulfate. This is caused by the action of hexosaminidase A, which also cleaves sulfated glucosamine.

Biochemical and Molecular Features

Sulfamidase is required for the hydrolysis of *N*-acetylglucosamine residues from heparan sulfate. Heparan sulfate accumulates in all types of Sanfilippo's syndrome, in Hunter's syndrome, and in Hurler's syndrome. The gene for this enzyme has not been cloned. *N*-Acetyl-glucosamine-6-sulfatase hydrolyzes the sulfate on position 6 of the glucosamine of heparan sulfate. The enzyme has been purified and its cDNA cloned. The gene for *N*-acetyl-glucosamine-6-sulfatase has been localized to chromosome 12q14.

Morquio Syndrome (Mucopolysaccharidosis Type IV)

Clinical Features

Morquio's syndrome is characterized by severe skeletal dysplasia and keratan sulfaturia. Mental development is normal. Skeletal abnormalities include shortened vertebrae causing short stature, short neck, pectus carinatum, genu valgum, pes planus, and lax joints. The odontoid process is underdeveloped and may cause atlantoaxial subluxation. Corneal clouding is present in 50% of cases. Midfacial hypoplasia and protrusion of the mandible gives the appearance of a permanent grin. Tooth enamel is very thin. Hepatomegaly may be present but is not prominent. Patients with Morquio syndrome usually survive until middle age.

Variability in phenotypic expression is considerable, and sometimes Morquio syndrome is only distinguishable from other skeletal dysplasias by keratan sulfaturia.

Biochemical and Molecular Features

Two types of Morquio syndrome are differentiated by their enzyme defect. Type A is caused by deficiency of *N*-acetylgalactosamine-6-sulfate sulfatase, and type B by deficiency of β-galactosidase. Type B usually lacks enamel hypoplasia. The enzyme defect in both conditions can be assayed in white blood cells and cultured skin fibroblasts. Galactosamine-6-sulfate sulfatase, the enzyme that hydrolyzes sulfate from galactose-6-sulfate and *N*-acetylgalactosamine-6-sulfate, has been purified and found to be specific for the galactose configuration. Deficiency leads to accumulation in tissues and excretion in urine of keratan sulfate. Chondroitin also accumulates in tissues. The cDNA and gene for *N*-acetylgalactosamine-6-sulfatase has been cloned and the gene has been localized to chromosome 16q24.3. Three different mutations in the coding sequence have been reported in Morquio type A. β-Galactosidase is also required for the sequential degradation of keratan sulfate. Deficiency of this enzyme leads to Morquio type B syndrome (see the section on Beta-Galactosidase Deficiency).

Maroteaux-Lamy Syndrome (Mucopolysaccharidosis Type VI)

Clinical Features

Maroteaux-Lamy syndrome resembles Hurler's syndrome but lacks the mental retardation. The phenotype includes coarse facial features, corneal clouding, organomegaly, and dysostosis multiplex. Urinary mucopolysaccharides show increased excretion of dermatan sulfate, which is caused by the deficiency of *N*-acetylgalactosamine-4-sulfate sulfatase (arylsulfatase B). Maroteaux-Lamy syndrome has a spectrum of severity, and children with the severe form die from a constricted chest and upper airway obstruction.

Biochemical and Molecular Features

Arylsulfatase B is synthesized as a precursor and then converted into an active enzyme form. Both the precursor and active form have enzyme activity. The cDNA clone for human arylsulfatase B has been isolated and the gene localized to chromosome 5q13–14. Mutations causing the severe, moderate, and mild forms have been identified.

Sly Syndrome (Mucopolysaccharidosis Type VII)

Clinical Features

Sly syndrome (β-glucuronidase deficiency) has mild and severe forms. The severe forms cannot be distinguished from Hurler's syndrome, although the coarse facial features are usually milder, and the gibbus is not pronounced. The mucopolysacchariduria consists mostly of chondroitin-4/6-sulfate. The enzyme defect of β-glucuronidase can be documented using white blood cells and cultured skin fibroblasts.

Biochemical and Molecular Features

Glucuronic acid, found in heparan sulfate, dermatan sulfate, and chondroitin 4/6 sulfate, is hydrolyzed by β-glucuronidase. The enzyme has been purified and the gene cloned. The gene for human β-glucuronidase has been localized to 7q21.11. The severe phenotype has been reported with three point mutations leading to two missense and one nonsense change. Two mutations result in hydrops fetalis.

Radiographic Findings

The mucopolysaccharidoses have specific skeletal changes referred to as *dysostosis multiplex*. Dysostosis multiplex can also be seen in glycoprotein storage diseases such as mannosidosis, aspartylglucosaminuria, and GM_1 gangliosidosis. The skull is usually dolichocephalic and the calvarium is thickened with hyperostosis of the cranium. The sella turcica is large and boot shaped. The clavicles are thickened, especially in the middle third. The vertebral bodies are ovoid with beaklike projections on their anterior lower margins. T12 is hypoplastic, which may result in a gibbus formation. The ribs widen distally. The iliac bones are flared with shallow acetabula. The hips are deformed, and the head of the femur has changes that resemble aseptic necrosis. The hands show tapering of the terminal phalanges and tapering of the proximal ends of the metacarpals. The long bones show areas of cortical thinning and irregular widening associated with expansion of the medullary cavity. The radius curves toward the ulna at the distal end, forming a V deformity. The humerus is angulated, and the glenoid fossa is shallow.

Diagnosis

Diagnosis of the mucopolysaccharidoses is suggested clinically by coarse features, developmental delay, enlarged spleen and liver, and radiographic findings of dysostosis multiplex. Increased urinary excretion of glycosaminoglycans will be an added feature confirming a mucopolysaccharide disorder. Qualitative and quantitative determination of the glycosaminoglycans in the urine may be helpful in suggesting a specific disease. Table 6.2 summarizes the typical glycosaminoglycans observed in the various mucopolysaccharidoses. The final confirmatory diagnosis depends on the determination of a specific enzyme defect.

Treatment

Effective treatment of the mucopolysaccharidoses is not available. In general, when the disease does not affect the brain, bone marrow transplantation has been effective in reversing upper airway disease and organomegaly, ameliorating the coarse facial features, clearing the corneas, and diminishing the mucopolysacchariduria. Long-term follow-up is needed to determine the optimal age for bone marrow transplantation and its efficacy for reversing the somatic and neurologic involvement. Symptomatic treatment of the mucopolysaccharidoses for congestive heart failure, removal of tonsils and adenoids, shunting of hydrocephalus, and surgical correction of hernias and carpal tunnel syndrome are important in improving the overall quality of life.

THE MUCOLIPIDOSES

The mucolipidoses were once incorrectly considered to be part of the mucopolysaccharidoses. Lipids and polysaccharides are stored within tissues, and mucopolysacchariduria does not occur.

Sialidosis (Mucolipidosis I)

Clinical Features

Sialidosis type I results from a neuraminidase deficiency. The usual age of onset is the second decade. The main clinical features are progressive visual impairment (cherry-red spot), myoclonic seizures, and gait disturbances. Neuraminidase deficiency can be detected in cultured skin fibroblasts. Sialidosis type II is associated with β-galactosidase deficiency in addition to neuraminidase deficiency. The onset is early, and newborns may have hydrops fetalis. Affected children have coarse facies and dysostosis multiplex. Organomegaly may be present at birth. Foam cells and vacuolated lymphocytes are found in aspirated bone marrow. The storage material is oligosaccharide with *N*-acetylneuraminic acid at the nonreducing end. These compounds are excreted in the urine.

Biochemical and Molecular Features

Neuraminidase and β-galactosidase exists in vivo as a protein complex in association with a protective protein. The deficiency of the protective protein is genetically distinct from GM_1 gangliosidosis and sialidosis and leads to the combined deficiencies of β-galactosidase and neuraminidase. This is referred to as *galactosialidosis* or severe form of mucolipidosis I. The cDNA for the protective protein has been cloned. Its expression restores the biologic activity of β-galactosidase and neuraminidase in galactosialidosis cells.

I-Cell Disease (Mucolipidosis II)

Clinical Features

I-cell disease is characterized by coarse features, severe mental retardation, and dysostosis multiplex. These features are seen earlier than in Hurler's syndrome. The thorax is usually small, joint movement is restricted, the tongue is large, and there is gingival hyperplasia. Corneal haziness is common. Cardiac involvement includes cardiomegaly and aortic insufficiency. Usually these children die in the first decade of life of cardiopulmonary insufficiency.

Biochemical and Molecular Features

In I-cell disease, the lysosomal enzymes are synthesized normally but are excreted because they lack mannose-6-phosphate, a recognition marker that targets the enzymes to lysosomes. The mannose-6-phosphate is added to lysosomal enzymes by UDP-*N*-acetylglucosamine: *N*-acetylglucosaminyl-1-phosphotransferase. Two mucolipidoses are associated with this enzyme deficiency: mucolipidosis II (I-cell disease), which is the more severe, and mucolipidosis III.

Mucolipidosis III

Clinical Features

Mucolipidosis III (pseudo-Hurler polydystrophy) is a milder form of mucolipidosis II, with onset between 2 and 4 years of age. Patients may live to adulthood, and some are not retarded. Linear growth is severely affected, and some have joint stiffness, claw hand deformities, and aortic regurgitation. Coarseness of the face is minimal. Corneal clouding may be associated. Radiologic examination shows moderate dysostosis multiplex.

Biochemical and Molecular Features

The defects in I-cell disease and mucolipidosis III are identical except that the amount of residual enzyme activity is greater in mucolipidosis III.

Mucolipidosis IV

Clinical Features

Children with mucolipidosis IV share some phenotypic resemblance to other patients with storage diseases. They have corneal clouding and psychomotor retardation but lack facial dysmorphism, dysostosis multiplex, and organomegaly. Conjunctival biopsy specimens show storage material within lysosomes, with a lamellar configuration similar to those seen in Tay-Sachs disease. Most are of Ashkenazi Jewish extraction. Mucopolysacchariduria does not occur.

Biochemical and Molecular Features

The storage material in fibroblasts is similar to that observed in I-cell disease. The enzyme defect has not been characterized. Suggestions that a specific neuraminidase deficiency causes this disease are not confirmed, and the diagnosis relies primarily on the use of conjunctival biopsy.

DISORDERS OF GLYCOPROTEIN DEGRADATION

Sialidosis

The true sialidoses are genetic disorders in which damage to the gene for glycoprotein sialidase (α-L-*N*-acetylneuraminidase) results in decreased activity of the enzyme. Sialidase alone is deficient. The true sialidoses have been divided into two groups: the nondysmorphic group (sialidosis type 1, also known as the *cherry-red spot–myoclonus syndrome*) and the dysmorphic group (sialidosis type 2, which includes mucolipidosis I).

Clinical Features

In sialidosis type I, the onset of myoclonus or decreasing visual acuity is between ages 8 and 15 years. Action myoclonus begins in the limbs and becomes increasingly debilitating. Patients may become unable to walk or stand and become bedridden. Cherry-red spots are seen on funduscopy. Corneas are clear, but punctate lens opacities or lamellar cataracts may be seen. Other features sometimes present are generalized tonic-clonic seizures, cerebellar ataxia, hyperactive tendon reflexes, and burning pain in the limbs, which is worse in hot weather. Intelligence is usually normal and the Hurler phenotype is not present. Renal impairment is not a feature of this disorder, but severe renal involvement has occurred in two siblings with otherwise typical cherry-red spot–myoclonus syndrome. The cherry-red spot may disappear with time. Although the underlying disorder is not treatable, 5-hydroxytryptophan may improve the action myoclonus.

Patients with sialidosis type II have deficiency of glycoprotein sialidase, without deficiency of β-galactosidase, and show clinical features of somatic dysmorphism (facial dysmorphism, skeletal dysmorphism, and organ enlargement). The onset may be at birth, in childhood, or later.

Congenital sialidosis is the most severe form. Affected neonates are born prematurely and have the clinical appearance of hydrops fetalis. They may be stillborn or survive 3 months and perhaps longer. At birth, they are plethoric, hypotonic, and depressed, with generalized skin edema, ascites, organomegaly, puffy face and eyelids, and a prominent telangiectatic skin rash. Seizures may occur, and neurologic development is arrested.

Patients with severe infantile sialidosis show many similarities to patients with congenital sialidosis, but they survive into the second year. They have congenital ascites, progressive organomegaly, slow neurologic development, and progressive renal disease in the second year. It is not clear whether severe infantile sialidosis and congenital sialidosis are different manifestations of the same phenotype or different phenotypes.

Nephrosialidosis was defined in studies that focused on the renal component of this disorder. They have a milder phenotype than congenital sialidosis or severe infantile sialidosis. Infants come to medical attention at ages 4–6 months because of hernias, organomegaly, facial dysmorphism, and psychomotor retardation. Late in the course, severe progressive renal disease with proteinuria, a cherry-red spot, and fine corneal opacities develop. The term *mucolipidosis I* is used for the forms of sialidosis that may be noted in infancy but are more slowly progressive and are usually diagnosed in childhood. The term is now appropriately applied only to those patients with the characteristic phenotype and sialidase deficiency without β-galactosidase deficiency. Development is normal for the first 6 months, then slows. Somatic abnormalities appear in the second or third year but are milder than those in Hurler's syndrome. Impaired hearing, corneal opacity, and macular cherry-red spots are usually seen, and growth disturbance is common. Neurologic findings include slowly progressive gait ataxia, tremor, cerebellar signs, myoclonic jerks, hypotonia, muscle wasting, peripheral neuropathy, and seizures.

Diagnosis

Diagnosis requires a compatible clinical picture, the presence of abnormal sialo-oligosaccharides in the urine, and the demonstration of sialidase deficiency in cultured skin fibroblasts or other tissues. Rectal biopsy is a useful confirmatory test because the stored material is visible on ultrastructure of rectal ganglion cells. Radiographs show mild to moderate dysostosis multiplex. Kyphoscoliosis and hypoplasia of the odontoid may occur.

Biochemical and Molecular Features

Sialic acid content is increased in all tissues. Ganglioside accumulation in the sialidoses is a secondary event, perhaps induced by inhibition of a ganglioside sialidase by substances stored because of the primary sialidase deficiency. Lysosomal sialidase is markedly deficient in both type 1 and type 2 sialidoses. Carrier detection and prenatal diagnosis are available. The isolated sialidase deficiencies result from mutations of a structural gene for a sialidase localized to chromosome 10q23 and/or chromosome 6. Chromosome 6 may be responsible for deficiency of a protective protein required for activity of enzymes coded for by a gene on chromosome 20.

Fucosidosis

Clinical Features

Phenotypes differ greatly in severity and features. Type I fucosidosis is a severe, progressive neurologic disorder; type II resembles the Hurler phenotype with survival into the second, third, or fourth decade; type III has adult onset and may be the same as type II. Types I and II occur in the same family. Severely affected infants (type I) develop psychomotor retardation and hypotonia during infancy, then hypertonia and spasticity, tremor, and mental deterioration. They have thick skin and excessive sweating and may lose gallbladder function. Facial coarsening, radiographic bone changes, and organ enlargement are mild. Cardiac enlargement may occur. Some die before age 5 years; others (type II) have onset of symptoms in the second year of life with more markedly coarsened facial features and greater resemblance to Hurler's syndrome. These patients also deteriorate mentally and die at approximately age 5 years. Patients with infantile or juvenile onset have a milder course, with coarsened facial features, skeletal changes, dwarfing, and skin changes resembling the angiokeratoma of Fabry disease. Survival into the third decade is expected. Angiokeratoma is characteristic of patients with longer survival. In addition to Fabry disease and fucosidosis, angiokeratoma corporis diffusum also occurs in sialidosis and in β-mannosidosis. Type I and type II fucosidosis may not be independent diseases but rather represent a continuous clinical spectrum. Taken together, the percentage of cases with various clinical features are progressive mental (95%) and motor (87%) deterioration, coarse facies (79%), growth retardation (78%), recurrent infections (78%), dysostosis multiplex (58%), angiokeratoma corporis diffusum (52%), visceromegaly (44%), and seizures (38%).

Diagnosis

All phenotypes have marked deficiency of the lysosomal enzyme α-L-fucosidase. Diagnosis is established by finding abnormal oligosaccharides in urine and showing decreased α-L-fucosidase in serum, leukocytes, and cultured skin fibroblasts. Radiographs show mild dysostosis multiplexes that are most marked in the pelvis, hips, and spine.

Biochemical and Molecular Features

In fucosidosis, the lysosomal enzyme α-L-fucosidase is deficient in serum, leukocytes, and cultured skin fibroblasts. The α-L-fucosidase structural gene, *FUCA1*, has been mapped to human chromosome 1p34–p36. The gene has been cloned and sequenced. Several mutations in the α-L-fucosidase gene have been described in fucosidosis.

Alpha-Mannosidosis

Clinical Features

The clinical picture of α-mannosidosis is varied. Patients with a severe form have hepatomegaly, splenomegaly, severe infections, and early death. Severely affected patients look similar to patients with mucolipidosis I. Some have slower progression with greater dysmorphism, corneal opacities, and longer survival. Others have presented with marked mental defect, striking gingival hyperplasia, and survival into the third decade or longer. Facial dysmorphism, skeletal involvement, and organ enlargement are not important features in these patients. This more common mild form shows either no clinical abnormalities or nonspecific abnormalities in the first year of life (psychomotor delay, speech delay, or frequent infections), and only later do these patients develop sensorineural hearing loss, ataxia, mild then moderate to severe mental defects, coarse facial features, and dysostosis multiplex. Affected individuals have short stature and may survive into adulthood without hepatomegaly. The cognitive and language impairment do not correlate with the amount of residual α-mannosidase activity measured with an artificial substrate.

Diagnosis

Diagnosis requires a high index of suspicion, findings of abnormal urinary oligosaccharides, and demonstration of decreased α-mannosidase in leukocytes and cultured skin fibroblasts. The most notable radiographic finding is dense thickening of the calvaria. Dysostosis multiplex tends to be mild and in some cases decreases in prominence with the age of the patient.

Treatment

Bone marrow transplantation has been attempted for α-mannosidosis but was not successful.

Biochemical and Molecular Features

Patients with α-mannosidase have deficiency of lysosomal acid α-mannosidase. Several mannosidases are known, and their genetic origins, relationships, and natural substrate specificities are not well understood. A full-length cDNA sequence for a human lysosomal α-mannosidase gene has been cloned that appears to represent the human lysosomal α-mannosidase precursor.

Beta-Mannosidosis

Clinical Features

β-Mannosidosis presents with mental retardation, angiokeratoma, and tortuousness of conjunctival vessels. Hearing loss is sometimes associated. Intrafamilial heterogeneity is noted.

Diagnosis

The oligosacchariduria is characteristic and the enzyme defect can be shown in plasma, leukocytes, and fibroblasts. Heterozygotes can be detected and prenatal diagnosis is possible. Lectin histochemistry on paraffin-embedded tissue sections can distinguish between α-mannosidosis, β-mannosidosis, fucosidosis, and sialidosis.

Biochemical and Molecular Features

Oligosaccharides accumulate in cells and in urine. The deficient enzyme is lysosomal acid β-mannosidase. The gene responsible for human β-mannosidase has been neither mapped nor cloned.

Aspartylglycosaminuria

Clinical Features

Affected children may appear normal up to 5 years of age, when they develop progressive somatic and mental changes that include the following facial features: a depressed nasal bridge, anteverted nostrils, broad nose, broad face, and rosy cheeks. Skeletal changes include thickening of the skull, cranial asymmetry, short neck, joint hypermobility, thinned cortex of the long bones, short stature, and thoracic or lumbar scoliosis. Diarrhea, frequent respiratory infections, and rash may be associated. Development first slows then regresses, leading to severe mental defects in adults. Episodic hyperactivity, psychotic behavior, speech defects, and seizures may occur. Some patients have subcapsular, crystal-like lens opacities. Macroglossia, cardiac murmur, and hernia may occur. Inheritance is autosomal recessive.

Diagnosis

Diagnosis is confirmed by showing aspartylglycosamine in urine and deficiency of aspartylglucosaminidase (*N*-aspartyl-β-glucosaminidase). Aspartylglycosaminuria is detected in amniotic fluid, making prenatal diagnosis possible. The main radiographic findings are thickening of the calvaria, osteochondrosis of the vertebrae leading to wedge-shaped vertebral bodies with narrowing of the intervertebral spaces, and generalized osteoporosis. Cranial asymmetry may be noted. The cortex of the long bones is thin. Kyphosis or scoliosis may be associated.

Biochemical and Molecular Findings

Aspartylglycosamine is the chief storage material in tissues. The disease results from deficiency of the lysosomal enzyme aspartylglucosaminidase (*N*-aspartyl-β-glucosaminidase), an amidase that cleaves aspartylglycosamine. The aspartylglucosaminidase gene has been localized to the long arm of human chromosome 4, possibly in the q23–q27 region. The gene has been cloned and sequenced, and mutations responsible for aspartylglycosaminuria have been identified.

WOLMAN DISEASE

Wolman disease (WD) and cholesteryl ester storage disease (CESD) are caused by a deficiency of human lysosomal cholesteryl ester lipase (HLAL)/lysosomal acid lipase/cholesteryl ester hydrolase (CEH) that causes an abnormal accumulation of cholesteryl esters and triglycerides in tissues.

Clinical Features

WD is an autosomal recessive disease with onset in infancy. The early symptoms are failure to thrive, diarrhea, vomiting, malabsorption, and organomegaly. Death usually occurs before age 6 months, although hyperalimentation prolongs life. Lipid accumulation in liver, spleen, intestines, and lymph nodes is a direct cause of death. Plasma total cholesterol and low density lipoprotein (LDL) concentrations are elevated and high density lipoprotein concentrations are decreased. Hepatic biopsy show enormous increases in lipid droplets containing cholesterol esters, and assay for lysosomal CEH enzyme in skin fibroblasts showed reduced levels.

CESD has a milder clinical presentation and course than WD. Organomegaly, found incidentally, may be the initial feature in an otherwise healthy infant. Older children have progressive organomegaly, short stature, and hypercholesterolemia. Young adults may present with premature atherosclerosis. The serum cholesterol and triglyceride concentrations are elevated and the HDL concentration is reduced. Showing reduced lysosomal cholesterol ester hydrolase in circulating mononuclear cells establishes the diagnosis.

Biochemical and Molecular Features

Cholesterol is an essential constituent of cell membrane as well as the important structural component of steroids and bile. Cholesterol is available to cells from either endogenous or exogenous sources. Endogenous synthesis occurs in the microsomes, whereas the major exogenous source is from LDL. Lysosomal cholesterol ester hydrolase plays a critical role in that pathway. The lysosomal acid cholesterol ester hydrolase (HLAL) gene in WD and CESD has been cloned, expressed, and sequenced; it has been localized to chromosome 10q23.2–3. Two mutational changes have been identified in WD. One results in a premature stop codon and a truncated HLAL enzyme; the other causes a disrupted structure and dysfunctional enzyme activity. In CESD, the mutation produces a truncated mRNA.

Multisystem Lipid Storage Myopathy

The biochemical abnormality in metabolizing triglycerides in this condition is the opposite of WD. In WD, the cellular uptake of exogenous triglyceride by the liver is blocked, whereas endogenously synthesized triglycerides are normally catabolized. In multisystem lipid storage myopathy, only endogenously synthesized triglyceride is impaired

CERAMIDASE DEFICIENCY: FARBER LIPOGRANULOMATOSIS

Ceramidase deficiency (Farber lipogranulomatosis) is transmitted as an autosomal recessive trait. Deficient activity of the lysosomal enzyme acid ceramidase leads to the accumulation of ceramide, an intermediate in the synthesis and degradation of many sphingolipids and glycolipids.

Clinical Features

The main clinical features are painful and deformed joints, subcutaneous nodules, and hoarseness that may progress to aphonia caused by laryngeal involvement of periarticular tissues in the larynx. Hypotonia, muscular atrophy, and ataxia result from ceramide and glycolipid storage in anterior horn cells, autonomic ganglia, brain stem, cerebellum, and retinal ganglion cells. The disorder has been tentatively subdivided into seven forms (Table 6.3). In the most common form, the onset of feeding and respiratory difficulties is at 2 weeks to 4 months. Death occurs during the first year of life.

Table 6.3
Farber disease phenotype.

	Type 1, Classic	*Type 2, Intermediate*	*Type 3, Mild*	*Type 4, Neonatal, Visceral*	*Type 5, Neurologic, Progressive*	*Type 6, Combined with Sandhoff*	*Type 7, Prosaposin Deficiency*
Number of cases	27	6	5	3	4	1	1
Age of onset	2 wks–4 mos	Neonatal–9 mos	2.5–20 mos	Neonatal	1 yr–2.5 yrs	6 wks	Neonatal
Mean age of death	1.2 yrs	4.7 yrs	16–30 yrs	7 wks–6 mos	35 mos		4 mos
Mean age last follow-up	2.4 yrs	38 mos–6 yrs	9–29 yrs		20 mos–5.5 yrs	13 mos	
Nodules	100%	100%	100%	33%	100%	+	0
Joint involvement	100%	100%	100%	33%	100%	+	0
Hoarseness	100%	100%	100%	33%	66%	+	
Large liver	47%	33%	0%	100%	33%	+	+
Large spleen	12%	17%	0%	100%	33%	0	+
Lung infiltrates	76%	0%	0%	2/2	0%	0	
Macular cherry-red spot	12%	0%	0%	0%	66%	+	
Corneal opacities	6%	17%	0%	33%	0%	0	
Cataracts	6%	0%	0%	0%	0%	0	
Lower motor neuron involvement	71%	17%	1/1	—*	66%	—	
CNS normal	26%	67%	60%				
CNS impaired	42%	17%	40%				+
CNS progressive dysfunction	11%	17%			100%	+	
CNS: insufficient information	21%			100%			

CNS = central nervous system.
*Information not available.

Diagnosis

The clinical triad of arthropathy, subcutaneous nodules, and hoarseness in a young child is pathognomonic of Farber disease. Diagnosis is achieved by measuring acid ceramidase activity in leukocytes, cultured skin fibroblasts, or amniocytes or by showing the impaired degradation of ceramides in cultured skin fibroblasts.

Biochemical and Molecular Features

The accumulation of ceramide in Farber disease is caused by deficiency of acid ceramidase. Ceramide accumulation causes the granulomatous reaction, whereas the accumulation of ceramide and complex glycolipids accounts for neuronal storage. The addition of ceramides to fibroblasts of affected patients causes the cells to develop large lysosomal inclusions that contain the curvilinear structures characteristic of the disease.

The granuloma formation and histiocytic response in the nodules, joints, lungs, and lymph nodes are a response to ceramide accumulation. The accumulation of ceramide in neuronal cytoplasm is presumed to be a direct consequence of the degradative defect, with the accumulation of gangliosides and glycolipids a secondary phenomenon because ceramide is part of the degradative pathway of these substances.

Treatment

Farber disease patients should be candidates for bone marrow transplantation, because most children appear unaffected at birth. Experience indicates, however, that the nervous system involvement cannot be altered by bone marrow transplantation. This may not apply when nervous system function is unimpaired and nodule formation is the major cause of disability. Other forms of therapy are supportive. The laryngeal and pulmonary involvement requires close supervision. Physical therapy, analgesics, and corticosteroids may provide some relief for the joint involvement, and cosmetic surgery may be offered for particularly disfiguring lesions.

NIEMANN-PICK DISEASES GROUP

Two distinct metabolic derangements are encompassed by the term *Niemann-Pick disease*: In the first group (types A and B Niemann-Pick disease), excessive quantities of sphingomyelin accumulate in many organs and tissues. In the second group (type C Niemann-Pick disease), the accumulation of sphingomyelin is modest and the main defect is storage of unesterified cholesterol.

Type A and Type B Niemann-Pick Disease

Clinical Findings

Infants with type A Niemann-Pick disease have organomegaly and profound, rapidly progressing neurologic damage. Organomegaly usually appears within the first months of life and always by age 6 months. The skin is discolored and takes on a brownish yellow hue. A cherry-red spot of the macula in seen in half of these infants. Discoloration of the lens capsule and retinal opacification sometimes occur. Feeding difficulties are frequent and may be accompanied by vomiting or fever and occasionally diarrhea. Psychomotor deterioration progresses inexorably. Developmental motor milestones are rarely reached. The patients become hypotonic and flaccid. Seizures are rare. Survival beyond the second year is unusual.

Type B Niemann-Pick disease does not affect the nervous system. Hepatomegaly is marked and splenomegaly less severe. Liver dysfunction is always impaired, but signs of hypersplenism are not prominent. Lung involvement is common and characterized by recurring pulmonary infections and radiographic evidence of diffuse infiltration. The retina shows a characteristic macular halo syndrome consisting of perimacular and circumferential accumulation of reddish brown granular material.

Diagnosis

Large, lipid-laden Niemann-Pick cells are present in the liver, spleen, lymph nodes, adrenal cortex, and bone marrow in both types A and B Niemann-Pick disease.

Biochemistry and Molecular Features

Sphingomyelin is the principal accumulating lipid. Sphingomyelin is a major component of the plasma membrane of all cells and a prominent constituent of erythrocyte stroma. It is also one of the principal phospholipids of the myelin sheath. The quantity of sphingomyelin in various organs may rise as much as 50-fold over normal.

Other lipids stored are bis(monoacylglycero)phosphate, cholesterol, glucocerebroside, lactosylceramide, and ganglioside GM_3.

Patients with both type A and type B Niemann-Pick disease have a profound deficiency of acid sphingomyelinase activity in all of their organs and tissues. It is generally not possible to discriminate between types A and B Niemann-Pick disease by measuring sphingomyelinase activity in white blood cells or extracts of cultured skin fibroblasts. Type B patients have slightly more residual sphingomyelinase activity than type A patients. The slightly greater residual sphingomyelinase activity in the type B patients is sufficient to catalyze the hydrolysis of the sphingomyelin that is undergoing turnover in the nervous system.

The gene for sphingomyelinase has been localized to region p15.1–4 of human chromosome 11. It has been cloned, and the nucleotide sequence has been determined. Approximately a dozen mutations have been identified in patients with type A disease. The mutations seen in type B disease are different.

Treatment

Treatment for patients with type A Niemann-Pick disease is limited to supportive measures. Liver transplantation has been attempted and the recipient died. Because of the propensity to hyperlipidemia and the possibility of early-onset coronary artery disease, type B patients with elevated circulating lipids should be treated with gemfibrozil. Liver transplantation in a patient with type B disease provided some improvement in clinical status but is unlikely to be of permanent benefit. Enzyme replacement and gene therapy strategies are both being considered but are not yet available. Both are more likely to be beneficial in patients with type B disease.

Type C Niemann-Pick Disease

Clinical Findings

Type C Niemann-Pick disease is an autosomal recessive disorder characterized by gradual, progressive neurologic deterioration. Organomegaly is usually present. Neonatal jaundice is common and may be associated with cholestasis and giant cell hepatitis. The hepatic disease is self-limited, but the neurologic disease is progressive.

Phenotypic variation is considerable, even within the same sibship. The age of onset ranges from birth to 55 years. Most patients become symptomatic in childhood. The most prevalent neurologic signs are vertical supranuclear gaze paresis, ataxia, and cognitive impairment. Other features are seizures, extrapyramidal dysfunction (dystonia, tremor, or choreoathetosis), and pyramidal tract dysfunction (hyperreflexia and spasticity). Progressive dysarthria and dysphagia eventually develop. Choking and aspiration are common late in the course and lead to malnutrition and repeated pulmonary infections. One-third of patients have seizures. Death usually occurs in the teens or early 20s from aspiration and intercurrent pulmonary infection.

Diagnosis

The triad of vertical gaze paresis, organomegaly, and foam cells in the bone marrow virtually establishes the clinical diagnosis of type C Niemann-Pick disease. Magnetic resonance imaging (MRI) shows demyelination. Spleen and liver cells are infiltrated with foam cells that stain for cholesterol, phospholipid, and glycolipids. Foam cells, called *sea-blue histiocytes,* are almost always present in the bone marrow. A confirmatory test is the determination of the rate of cholesterol esterification in cultured skin fibroblasts or lymphocytes. Affected children show a delay in the formation of cholesterol ester.

Biochemistry and Molecular Biology

Type C Niemann-Pick disease is characterized by excessive intracellular quantities of unesterified cholesterol that is derived from extracellular sources. Although the primary biochemical defect is unknown, abnormal intracellular cholesterol processing is the consistent metabolic alteration in cultured skin fibroblasts. The partial reduction of sphingomyelinase activity sometimes found in cultured skin fibroblasts derived from patients with type C Niemann-Pick disease is due to inhibition of this enzyme by cholesterol. One of the unanswered aspects of type C Niemann-Pick disease is the extensive accumulation of glucocerebroside in the brain that occurs along with the increase in cholesterol and modest elevation of sphingomyelin. The mutated gene responsible for most cases is localized to the pericentric region of human chromosome 18q11.

Treatment

No specific therapy is available for patients with this disorder. Seizures are controlled with anticonvulsants appropriate for the type of episode.

GLUCOSYLCERAMIDE LIPIDOSIS: GAUCHER DISEASE

Three clinical phenotypes are currently recognized in patients with Gaucher disease. Type 1 Gaucher disease is the most common type. The term is reserved for patients without central nervous system (CNS) involvement.

Clinical Features

Type 1 Gaucher disease (the chronic non-neuronopathic form) begins in infancy, but many children are asymptomatic except for enlarged spleens until the second decade. Despite variability in age at onset and severity of symptoms, the most consistent signs are those associated with hypersplenism (i.e., splenomegaly, anemia, thrombocytopenia, and leukopenia). The abdomen is protuberant and intermittent severe abdominal pain may occur secondary to splenic infarctions. Other features include liver enlargement and impaired function, acute episodes of bone pain, and deformities of the lower femur. Aseptic necrosis of the femoral head and compression fractures of the thoracic and lumbar vertebrae are common and may lead to severe pain and restriction of mobility.

Type 2 Gaucher disease (the acute neuronopathic form) was previously called the *infantile form*. Organomegaly is evident within the first 6 months, often by 3 months. The CNS is extensively involved, and progressive neurologic damage is the principal cause of death. Cranial nerve nuclei and the pyramidal tracts are damaged. The appearance of trismus, strabismus, and retroflexion of the head is common. Hyperactive reflexes, extensor plantar responses, and progressive spasticity are constant findings. Horizontal supranuclear gaze palsy is commonly present. Feeding problems and difficulties in handling secretions appear as the disease progresses. Seizures may occur. The infant becomes hypotonic and apathetic. The mean age of death is 9–12 months, but some live for 2 years. The cause of death is usually aspiration pneumonia or apnea secondary to laryngospasm or disruption of brain stem respiratory control centers.

Type 3 Gaucher disease (the subacute neuronopathic form) was previously called the *juvenile form*. The liver, spleen, and bone marrow are involved. Two clinical subtypes are observed. The first group is characterized by a progressive neurologic syndrome in adolescence or early adulthood that includes cognitive decline, myoclonic and generalized tonic-clonic seizures, and horizontal supranuclear gaze palsy. Systemic disease is not severe. The second group presents with horizontal supranuclear gaze palsy as the sole neurologic sign during childhood. The subsequent clinical course is marked by aggressive systemic disease, with death in childhood or adolescence from hepatic or pulmonary complications.

Pathologic Features

The spleen in patients with Gaucher disease contains enlarged histiocytes engorged with lipid. These histiocytes are known as *Gaucher cells*. They are also present in bone marrow. The cortices of the bones become demineralized, and there is extensive endosteal scalloping. Remodeling of the long bones is frequent and leads to flaring of the distal femoral metaphysis (Erlenmeyer flask deformity). Fractures involving the neck of the femur are common, and compression fractures of the vertebrae can produce progressive myelopathy.

Changes in blood chemistries include increased activity of serum acid phosphatase and angiotensin-converting enzyme. The blood glucocerebroside concentration is increased 10-fold.

In the brain, closely packed Gaucher cells are observed in perivascular (Virchow-Robin) spaces, even in type 1 without neurologic signs. In type 2 Gaucher disease, the brain is infiltrated with scavenger cells of hematogenous origin that are involved in neuronophagia.

Biochemical and Molecular Features

A defect in glucocerebroside catabolism is the cause of Gaucher disease. The enzyme that catalyzes the hydrolytic cleavage of glucose from glucocerebroside is glucocerebrosidase. Glucocerebrosidase activity in type 2 disease is less than 1% of normal, whereas activity in type 1 disease is 5–29% of normal. The glucocerebrosidase gene has been localized to the long arm of chromosome 1q21. The full-length genomic clone for human glucocerebrosidase has been isolated and sequenced. Numerous mutations were anticipated in the glucocerebrosidase gene because of many phenotypic variations. In fact, two mutations account for approximately 80% of the mutant alleles. One occurs in exon 10 and is associated with neuronopathic Gaucher disease, either type 2 or type 3. The other is at exon 9 and is associated with type 1 Gaucher disease.

The catalytic activity of glucocerebrosidase is increased by supplemental factors such as phosphatidyl serine and gangliosides. Another factor is an activator, or cohydrolase. The preponderant activator of glucocerebrosidase is saposin C. Absence of saposins causes disease. The gene for saposins localizes to chromosome 10.

Diagnosis

Gaucher cells are frequently detected by sternal or iliac crest biopsy. The definitive diagnosis is made by determining glucocerebrosidase activity in leukocytes or cultured skin fibroblasts.

Treatment

Total or partial splenectomy provides only temporary relief of anemia, thrombocytopenia, and leukopenia. Orthopedic management of skeletal difficulties in patients with type 1 Gaucher disease is difficult. Joint prostheses and internal fixation of fractures are often required. Valproic acid (Valproate) provides the most benefit in the management of myoclonic seizures.

Intravenous glucocerebrosidase injections have proved successful in reversing all symptoms of type 1 disease without adverse effects. The enzyme is approved by the U.S. Food and Drug Administration for the treatment of patients. A recombinantly produced glucocerebrosidase is expected to eventually replace the use of human placental glucocerebrosidase. Enzyme replacement for types 2 and 3 Gaucher disease is still experimental.

KRABBE DISEASE (GLOBOID CELL LEUKODYSTROPHY)

Krabbe disease, or globoid cell leukodystrophy (GLD), is an autosomal recessive disorder affecting central and peripheral nervous system white matter caused by deficiency galactocerebrosidase (GALC) activity.

Clinical Features

Three stages occur in the progression of the infantile form of the disease. Stage I is characterized by general irritability, stiffness of limbs, arrest of mental and motor development, and episodes of temperature elevation without infection. During stage II, the patients are opisthotonic and have myoclonic-like jerks of the arms and legs, hypertonic fits, continued bouts of fever, and regression of any achieved abilities. In stage III, patients are decerebrate with no voluntary movements. They are hypotonic and cachectic and die of respiratory infections or cerebral hyperpyrexia. The average age of onset is 4 months and the average age at death is 13 months.

An increasing number of late infantile, juvenile, and adult cases are recognized. These have a variable phenotype. Older patients only have unexplained mental or motor deterioration.

Diagnosis

Enzyme concentration is measured in leukocytes or cultured skin fibroblasts. Prenatal diagnosis is available.

Biochemical and Molecular Diagnosis

GALC has specificity toward galactosylceramide, psychosine (galactosylsphingosine), monogalactosyldiglyceride, and lactosylceramide under specific assay conditions. Only the metabolism of the first two is important to the pathology of GLD. Globoid cells are composed of high concentrations of galactosylceramide. The gene for GALC has been mapped to human chromosome 14q31. Several different mutations have been identified in infantile and late infantile cases.

Treatment

Bone marrow transplantation has not been successful in the infantile and late infantile form. Long-lasting improvement has been shown in a few patients with juvenile-onset disease.

METACHROMATIC LEUKODYSTROPHY AND MULTIPLE SULFATASE DEFICIENCY: SULFATIDE LIPIDOSIS

The sulfatide lipidoses are a group of inherited diseases affecting brain myelin metabolism (Table 6.4). Metachromatic leukodystrophy (MLD) is an autosomal recessive disorder with six clinical variants. Most patients are equally divided between late infantile- and juvenile-onset MLD. Approximately one-fifth of patients have an onset in adolescence or later.

Clinical Features

Clinical signs of late infantile MLD usually appear between the ages of 15 months and 2 years. Affected children fall frequently and then lose the ability to walk secondary to peripheral neuropathy. Between 2 and 3 years of age, the ability to sit without support is lost and truncal titubation is observed. Speech becomes slow and less distinct, optic atro-

Table 6.4
Classification of the sulfatide lipidoses.

Type	*Age at Onset (yrs)*
Late infantile	1–2
Early juvenile	4–6
Late juvenile	6–12
Adult	>16
Multiple sulfatase deficiency	<1
Cerebroside sulfate sulfatase activator deficiency	<1–20s

phy develops, and tendon reflexes are diminished and lost. The arms remain hypotonic, but muscle tone increases in the legs. Sensitivity to touch may develop because of spinal root and peripheral nerve involvement. Eventually the child becomes quadriplegic and spastic, with decerebrate, decorticate, or dystonic posturing. The late stage is characterized by loss of speech, seizures, hypertonic fits, bulbar palsy, and blindness. Death occurs approximately 17 years after onset of symptoms.

The onset of juvenile metachromatic leukodystrophy is between ages 4 and 12 years. The initial features are a decline in school performance and gait disturbance. This is followed by confusion, slurred speech, and postural abnormalities. Spasticity and blindness develop. Tremor and seizures may be associated, but hearing is unimpaired. Peripheral neuropathy is common but not invariable. When onset is between ages 4 and 6 years, gait imbalance precedes the intellectual deterioration, whereas in the later-onset variant (6 to 10 years), cognitive, behavioral, and social difficulties precede the gait disturbance. Most patients with juvenile-onset MLD do not live into adulthood.

Adult metachromatic leukodystrophy is being recognized by the widespread use of MRI and enzymatic assays in psychiatrically disturbed adolescents and adults. Adult MLD begins insidiously in late adolescence or early adult life as cognitive or behavioral decline. Some patients present with depression or alcoholism. Pes cavus can be present from childhood. The gait becomes wide-based and ataxic, muscle tone increases, and tendon reflexes are hyperactive.

Multiple sulfatase deficiency affects the achievement of early developmental milestones. Walking is delayed, and in the second year, the child loses the ability to sit, stand, or speak. Staring spells, spasticity, and blindness occur in the third year. The facial features are coarsened, with a prominent forehead, midfacial hypoplasia, broad nose, upturned nares, and short neck. The skin is dry and flaky and the liver enlarged. Skeletal abnormalities include rib flaring, rounding and beaking of the lumbar vertebrae, and deformities of the acetabulum.

Sulfatide activator protein deficiency is a rare disorder. The onset is in infancy or early childhood. The main features are developmental delay followed by developmental regression. Most progress to severe mental retardation, seizures, spasticity, and quadriparesis.

Diagnosis

The cerebrospinal fluid protein concentration increases as the disease progresses in the late infantile and early juvenile forms and may exceed 100 mg/dl. Spinal fluid protein concentrations may not be elevated in the later-onset cases. Slowing of nerve conduction velocity occurs in the late-onset form of juvenile MLD and in adult MLD even in the absence of clinical features of polyneuropathy.

An MRI T2-weighted image shows confluent areas of high signal intensity in the periventricular white matter. Early on, the arcuate fibers are preserved and the subcortical white matter in the frontal regions are preferentially involved, especially in adolescent- and adult-onset cases. T2-weighted images also reveal a bright signal in the internal capsule and corticospinal tract and a low-intensity signal for the basal ganglia and thalamus.

A definitive diagnosis requires the determination of arylsulfatase activity in leukocytes or cultured skin fibroblasts. The amount of residual enzyme activity directly correlates with the age of onset of the disease.

Biochemical and Molecular Features

The major accumulating lipid in MLD is cerebroside sulfate (sulfatide). It is a sulfated sphingoglycolipid consisting of equimolar amounts of sphingosine, fatty acid, galactose, and sulfate. Degradation of sulfatide is catalyzed by the lysosomal enzyme arylsulfatase A. The tissues of patients with the MLD are deficient in arylsulfatase A activity. Intracellular accumulation of sulfatide is greatest in cells from patients with late infantile MLD and least in cells from patients with adult MLD. The gene for arylsulfatase A is located on human chromosome 22 distal to q13. The most common mutation in patients with late infantile MLD is a G-to-A transition that eliminates the splice donor site at the start of intron 2. In adults with MLD, the most frequent mutation is a C-to-T transition that results in substitution of a leucine for proline in amino acid 426 in exon 8. Compound heterozygosity for these two genes correlates with the juvenile (intermediate) form of MLD.

Patients with multiple sulfatase deficiency also fail to degrade sulfatide. However, sulfatases in addition to arylsulfatase A are inactive. Deficiencies in their activity result in the accumulation of mucopolysaccharides and steroid sulfates.

Deficiency of the saposin B activator protein can also cause MLD. In spite of ample arylsulfatase A activity, cultured skin fibroblasts from patients with this form of MLD cannot degrade sulfatide in situ because of deficiency of the activator protein. The gene for prosaposin has been mapped to chromosome 10.

Treatment

Supportive care includes maintenance of adequate nutrition, passive physical therapy, and drugs to reduce spasticity. Bone marrow transplantation may be of benefit if the transplant is done before signs of nervous system involvement develop. It is more likely to benefit patients with juvenile or adult forms of MLD than a child with the more rapidly progressive late infantile form of the disease.

Correction of the arylsulfatase A deficiency has been accomplished in culture using retroviral and adenovirus-mediated transfer into primary fibroblasts from MLD patients. The availability of the mouse arylsulfatase A gene and its cDNA should facilitate the establishment of an animal model of MLD for in vivo trials of gene therapy in the future.

FABRY DISEASE: ALPHA-GALACTOSIDASE A DEFICIENCY

Fabry disease is an X-linked recessive disorder resulting from deficient activity of the lysosomal hydrolase α-galactosidase A.

Clinical Features

Disease onset in affected males usually occurs during childhood or adolescence. Early features are periodic crises of severe pain in the extremities (acroparesthesias) and the appearance of angiokeratoma, hypohidrosis, and characteristic corneal and lenticular opacities. With advancing age, progressive vascular glycosphingolipid deposition causes ischemia and infarction, leading to cardiac, cerebral, and renal vascular disease, with death typically occurring in the fourth or fifth decade of life. Affected individuals who are blood group B or AB have a more severe course because the blood group B substance also accumulates due to the deficient α-galactosidase A activity. Atypical variants of Fabry disease have sufficient residual enzyme activity to prevent or markedly delay the major features of the disease. Heterozygous females are usually clinically asymptomatic or only mildly symptomatic. Disease expression in most heterozygous females is limited to a few isolated angiokeratoma and keratopathy; however, a few heterozygotes are as severely affected as males.

Biochemical and Molecular Features

The α-galactosidase A gene localizes to the region Xq22. The gene is fully penetrant, but different mutations result in variable clinical expressivity in affected males. Deficient activity of the enzyme results in the accumulation of glycosphingolipids and glycoconjugates with terminal α-galactosyl moieties in most visceral tissues and body fluids. Fully affected males have no detectable α-galactosidase A activity.

Human α-galactosidase A is encoded by a single gene. Partial gene duplications and partial gene deletions account for 3% of cases. Approximately 75% of the mutations causing Fabry disease are missense or nonsense mutations. Other abnormalities include RNA-processing defects and small insertions and deletions and complex mutations. Most mutations have been confined to a single Fabry pedigree.

Diagnosis

The diagnosis is confirmed enzymatically by showing deficient α-galactosidase A activity in plasma, isolated leukocytes, tears, or cultured fibroblasts or lymphoblasts. Prenatal detection can be accomplished by showing deficient α-galactosidase A activity in chorionic villi obtained in the first trimester or in cultured amniocytes obtained by amniocentesis in the second trimester of pregnancy. Heterozygous females may have intermediate levels of enzymatic activity and accumulated substrate.

Treatment

The single most debilitating and morbid aspect of Fabry disease is the excruciating pain. Prophylactic administration of low maintenance dosages of phenytoin, carbamazepine, or both provides relief in hemizygotes and heterozygotes. Because renal insufficiency is the most frequent late complication in patients with this disease, chronic hemodialysis or renal transplantation have become life-saving procedures.

Replacement therapy using partially purified human enzyme has proved biochemically effective in pilot trials; however, sufficient enzyme has not been available to evaluate the clinical effectiveness in long-term replacement therapy. The high level expression of active human α-galactosidase A in mammalian cells has been achieved. Production of large amounts of the recombinant enzyme will permit future trials of replacement therapy.

SCHINDLER DISEASE: DEFICIENT ALPHA-*N*-ACETYLGALACTOSAMINIDASE ACTIVITY

Schindler disease is a autosomal recessive disorder resulting from deficient activity of α-*N*-acetylgalactosaminidase, the lysosomal glycohydrolase previously known as α-galactosidase B. It is one of a group of neuroaxonal dystrophies (Seitelberger disease, Hallervorden-Spatz syndrome, and neuroaxonal leukodystrophy) characterized by a common axonal lesion.

Clinical Features

Type I disease has three stages: (1) apparently normal development in the first 9–12 months of life; (2) a period of developmental delay followed by rapid regression starting in the second year of life; and (3) increasing neurologic impairment, resulting in cortical blindness, seizures, spasticity, decorticate posturing, and profound psychomotor retardation by age 4 years.

Skeletal radiography shows systemic, diffuse, and severe osteopenia and bilateral subluxation of the hips. MRI of the brain shows marked atrophy of the cerebellum, brain stem, and cervical spinal cord. Nerve conduction velocities are low normal.

Type II disease is primarily a cutaneous disorder with angiokeratoma corporis diffusum and glycopeptiduria. A disseminated petechiae-like eruption spreads slowly over the body, face, and limbs. The facies are slightly coarse with an enlarged nasal tip, depressed nasal bridge, and thick lips. Dilated blood vessels are present on the conjunctiva and in the fundi. Neurologic examination is normal except for a borderline intellect.

Biochemical and Molecular Features

Deficient activity of α-*N*-acetylgalactosaminidase is the specific enzymatic defect in types I and II disease. Heterozygotes for both types have approximately half-normal levels of activity. The α-*N*-acetylgalactosaminidase gene is located on chromosome 22q13. Mutations in the gene cause the expression of glycopeptides that are unstable.

Diagnosis

Type I disease is considered in children with developmental delay and regression in the first or second year, and type II disease is considered in adults with mild intellectual impairment and angiokeratoma. The ultrastructural demonstration of characteristic alterations in dystrophic axons in the myenteric plexus of biopsied rectal tissue or skin or the demonstration of lysosomal vacuoles in blood elements, sweat glands, and vascular endothelial cells should suggest the diagnosis of type I or II disease, respectively. Definitive diagnosis of both forms is made by showing deficient α-*N*-acetylgalactosaminidase activity in plasma, isolated leukocytes, or cultured lymphoblasts or fibroblasts.

Treatment

Curative treatment is not available. Supportive care should be implemented to optimize patient comfort.

BETA-GALACTOSIDASE DEFICIENCY: GM_1 GANGLIOSIDOSIS, MORQUIO B DISEASE, AND GALACTOSIALIDOSIS

Genetic β-galactosidase deficiency causes two distinct clinical phenotypes that were previously classified as different diseases: GM_1 gangliosidosis and Morquio B disease. GM_1 gangliosidosis is primarily a neurologic disorder, whereas Morquio B disease is primarily a skeletal disease. Galactosialidosis shares clinical features with GM_1 gangliosidosis.

GM_1 Gangliosidosis

Clinical Features

It is customary to divide the phenotype into infantile, juvenile, and adult forms according to the time of onset and the rate of progression. Onset of the infantile form is by 6 months, although facial and bony abnormalities are often recognized at birth. Infants appear dull and hypotonic with retarded psychomotor development. Developmental regression follows and is associated with spasticity and seizures. Eventually patients become deaf and blind and are totally unresponsive to external stimuli. Macular cherry-red spots are common. The entire clinical course rarely exceeds 2–3 years, and death occurs as a result of concurrent infections. White matter and peripheral nerve involvement is relatively minor. Many clinical features are similar to those in mucopolysaccharidoses, including facial deformity, macroglossia, radiologic bone abnormalities, and visceromegaly.

The late infantile or juvenile form of the disease begins after 1 year of age, with milder neurologic signs and slower progression. Systemic involvement is less prominent or absent. Survival beyond 10 years is the rule.

The adult or chronic form is variable. Clinical onset can be any time from childhood to 30 years or older. Slowly progressive dysarthria, gait difficulties, dystonic movements, and other extrapyramidal signs are prominent. Intellectual impairment is mild to moderate. Macular cherry-red spots, facial abnormalities, and visceromegaly are not associated.

Biochemical and Molecular Features

GM_1 gangliosidosis is characterized by the massive accumulation of GM_1 ganglioside in the brain. Small amounts of GM_1 ganglioside are also stored in viscera, but the main storage materials are heterogeneous galactose-rich fragments of varying molecular weights derived from glycoproteins, keratan sulfate, and other carbohydrate-containing materials. The underlying cause of GM_1 gangliosidosis is a genetic deficiency of the lysosomal acid β-galactosidase. The cDNA clone has been isolated and characterized and the gene assigned to chromosome 3p21.33. Eight specific mutations are known to cause GM_1 gangliosidosis. Table 6.5 lists the disease-causing mutations in the acid β-galactosidase gene known at this time.

Diagnosis

The enzyme deficiency is readily demonstrated in fibroblasts.

Morquio B Disease

Clinical Features

Morquio B disease was originally classified as a form of mucopolysaccharidosis because of its clinical and pathologic similarity to other forms of Morquio disease. Progressive skeletal dysplasia starts during the first years of life and is most prominent in vertebral and pelvic bones. Many patients have short stature similar to those with other forms of Morquio disease. Severe spinal deformities are common. Odontoid hypoplasia is always present and is potentially fatal because of cervical cord compression. Mild corneal opacity, mild organomegaly, and cardiac lesions are common.

Biochemical and Molecular Features

Excessive amounts of galactose-containing materials and keratan sulfate are excreted in the urine. The first two steps of keratan sulfate degradation are desulfation by *N*-acetylgalactosamine 6-sulfatase ("galactose-6-sulfatase") and then cleavage of the β-galactosidic bond by β-galactosidase. A genetic block at the first step causes Morquio disease type A, whereas blockage of the second step causes type B disease. Deficient activities of β-galactosidase can be shown in tissues. Because the fundamental enzymatic defect is the same as in GM_1 gangliosidosis, it is likely that the mutations underlying these disorders differentially affect the specificity of the enzyme toward natural substrates. The capacity of the β-galactosidase from Morquio B patients to hydrolyze GM_1 ganglioside is activated by the natural activator protein saposin 1, but it cannot be activated to hydrolyze the β-galactose residue from keratan sulfate.

The cDNA coding for acid β-galactosidase has been cloned and sequenced and the genomic organization of the β-galactosidase gene characterized. The gene is located on chromosome 3, and one mutation has been found to cause Morquio B disease.

Table 6.5
Identified mutations in acid β-galactosidase that cause GM_1 gangliosidosis or Morquio B disease.

Mutation	*mRNA*	*Phenotype When Homoallelic*
GM_1 gangliosidosis	+	Likely infantile
20-bp insertion from intron 2, caused by a base insertion in the 5' donor region duplication of exons 11 and 12 in mRNA	+ (large)	Infantile
Arg^{49}→Cys	±[a]	Infantile?
Ile^{51}→Thr	+	Adult
Thr^{82}→Met	+	Very mild adult?
Gly^{123}→Arg	+	Infantile
Arg^{201}→Cys	+	Juvenile
Arg^{208}→Cys	+ (decreased)	Infantile
Tyr^{316}→Cys	+	Infantile
Arg^{457}→Ter	–	Infantile
Arg^{457}→Gln	+	Infantile
Arg^{482}→His	+	Infantile
Arg^{482}→Cys	?	Likely infantile
Gly^{494}→Cys	+	Infantile
Trp^{509}→Cys	+	Infantile?[b]
Lys^{577}→Arg	+	Infantile
Arg^{590}→His	+	Juvenile or adult
Glu^{632}→Gly	+	Juvenile or adult
Morquio B		
20-bp insertion from intron 2, caused by a mutation at the 3' acceptor site	+	Juvenile Morquio B
Tyr^{83}→His	+	Juvenile Morquio B
Arg^{208}→His	?	GM_1/Morquio B intermediate
Pro^{263}→Ser		GM_1/Morquio B intermediate
Trp^{273}→Leu	+	Adult Morquio B[c]
Asn^{318}→His	?	GM_1/Morquio B intermediate

[a]Because this mutation was found in a heteroallelic patient and the abnormality in the other allele has not been identified, it is possible that the observed low mRNA level may be due to an mRNA-negative mutation in the other allele and that this mutation itself may generate a nearly normal amount of mRNA.
[b]This phenotype was found in a heteroallelic patient with Morquio B disease.
[c]One gene dose was sufficient for the Morquio B phenotype.

Galactosialidosis (Protective Protein [Cathepsin A] Deficiency)

Galactosialidosis is a genetic disorder entirely distinct from GM_1 gangliosidosis and Morquio B disease. The acid β-galactosidase gene is not affected in galactosialidosis. Deficiencies of both β-galactosidase and sialidase (α-neuraminidase) coexist. The mode of inheritance is autosomal recessive.

Clinical Features

The clinical phenotype of galactosialidosis is heterogeneous, ranging from an early-onset, severe, and rapidly progressive infantile form to a late-onset, slowly progressive adult form. The infantile form resembles infantile GM_1 gangliosidosis, with severe central nervous system involvement, macular cherry-red spots, visceromegaly, renal insufficiency, coarse facies, and skeletal abnormalities. The late infantile form is essentially a later-onset, milder phenotype of the infantile disease. The juvenile/adult form has a much higher incidence in Japan, and its main clinical features are slowly progressive central nervous system symptoms, including motor disturbance and mental retardation, skeletal abnormalities, dysmorphism, macular cherry-red spots, and angiokeratoma. Patients survive into adult life.

Biochemical and Molecular Features

The biochemistry of tissue constituents in patients with galactosialidosis is poorly defined. The storage materials in cultured fibroblasts and those excreted into urine are predominantly sialylated glycopeptides, similar to those found in sialidosis patients. The half-life of β-galactosidase is abnormally short but can be prolonged by addition of protease inhibitors. A 32-kD protein protects β-galactosidase and neuraminidase from proteolytic digestion within the lysosome. A genetic abnormality in this protective protein is the underlying cause of galactosialidosis. The human gene coding for the protective protein is on chromosome 20. Several specific mutations responsible for human galactosialidosis are known, and genotype-phenotype correlations have been established.

THE GM_2 GANGLIOSIDOSES

The inborn errors of GM_2 ganglioside metabolism cause GM_2 ganglioside to accumulate within the lysosomes of nerve cells. GM_2 ganglioside is normally degraded by the lysosomal enzyme hexosaminidase A acting in concert with a GM_2-activator protein. Late infantile, juvenile, and adult-onset forms of GM_2 gangliosidosis occur. The later the onset, the slower the progression and the more restricted the neurologic deficit. Differences in clinical expression may occur even within the same family.

Tay-Sachs Disease

Clinical Features

Tay-Sachs disease is the infantile form of the GM_2 gangliosidoses. Some children may startle easily in the newborn period and appear listless and hypotonic. Most appear normal at first and show normal early development only to begin regressing after 4–6 months of age. At this stage, a cherry-red macula is present. The whitish halo that surrounds the fovea is caused by lipid deposition in the bipolar ganglion cells of the retina. It accentuates the normal red color of the choroidal blood vessels that lie beneath the fovea. After 1 year of age, the child becomes progressively more lethargic and immobile, not speaking and not reaching for objects. Spasticity develops, and in the second year, small-amplitude myoclonic jerks are seen and are later followed by generalized tonic-clonic seizures. Sound, light, or touch stimuli precipitate decerebrate posturing. The subsequent course is one of neurologic deterioration to a vegetative state by age 2. Progressive cachexia, dehydration, and aspiration pneumonia lead to death, usually by age 4 or 5 years.

B_1 Variant

Clinical Features

The B_1 variant is a variable phenotype. The initial features may be gait or speech disturbances between ages 3 and 7 years, or feeding, sleeping, and gait disturbances from early infancy. All phenotypes are associated with progressive mental deterioration, and loss of speech and walking ability within a few years. Other features in some patients are cherry-red maculae, spasticity, hyperactivity, seizures, and tremor.

A chronic form of the B_1 variant with survival into the third and fourth decades has been described. The first symptom is behavioral changes noted between ages 5 and 11 years. Disturbances in speech and language follow. Spasticity develops but walking is maintained until the third decade. Another chronic form is characterized by proximal leg weakness, fasciculations, limitation of upward gaze, and extrapyramidal symptoms.

Late-Onset GM_2 Gangliosidosis

Clinical Features

Most patients with this disorder are of Ashkenazi Jewish ancestry. The predominant features are a motor neuron disease or a progressive ataxia. The term *adult-onset GM_2 gangliosidosis* is a misnomer. Early development is normal, but the child remains clumsy and unathletic, does not do well in physical education, and may not be able to ride a bicycle. Many patients develop a dysarthric nasal speech that does not improve with speech therapy. Academic performance in grade school is usually satisfactory, although some individuals are labeled as learning disabled. At some point during adolescence, proximal muscle weakness develops, and the youngster becomes aware of difficulty climbing stairs. Fasciculations become evident in the thighs, upper back, shoulders, and upper arms, and muscle cramps occur, especially at night. Less than half of patients develop psychiatric symptoms.

Treatment

The psychiatric symptoms are improved by lithium, carbamazepine, valproic acid, clonazepam, lorazepam, or a combination of these drugs, whereas they are generally worse after receiving haloperidol, chlorpromazine, or other phenothiazines.

Sandhoff Disease

The term *Sandhoff disease* is used to describe GM_2 gangliosidosis that results from a combined deficiency of hexosaminidase A and B.

Clinical Features

Juvenile Sandhoff disease begins after 1 year of age, with clumsiness and unsteady gait. Seizures, tremors, and dystonic posturing may occur. A cherry-red spot is not present in the macula. The late-onset, or adult, form follows much the same clinical course as late-onset GM_2 gangliosidosis with hexosaminidase A deficiency.

AB Variant

The AB variant refers to patients with GM_2 gangliosidosis who have normal activity of hexosaminidase A and B but lack the activator protein that induces the enzymatic degradation of GM_2 ganglioside by hexosaminidase A.

Biochemical and Molecular Genetics

Hexosaminidases A and B

Two forms of lysosomal hexosaminidase exist: hexosaminidase A (Hex A) and hexosaminidase B (Hex B). Hex A is composed of one α-subunit and one β-subunit, whereas Hex B is composed of two slightly different β-subunits. The gene for the α-subunit, known as *HEXA*, maps to chromosome 15q23–24. The gene for the β-subunit is *HEXB*, which maps to chromosome 5q11.2–13.3. Although they are encoded on separate chromosomes, the two genes have striking structural similarities.

GM_2 Activator

This small transport protein is delivered to the lysosome in the same manner as Hex A and Hex B. It acts to overcome the steric hindrance by adjacent lipid molecules that interferes with access of Hex A to membrane-bound GM_2. GM_{2A}, the gene encoding this protein, maps to chromosome 5q32–33, whereas a processed pseudogene has been localized to chromosome 3.

Mutations Affecting the α-Subunit

GM_2 gangliosidosis due to Hex A deficiency results from mutations in the α-subunit gene, *HEXA*. At least 75 alterations in its nucleotide sequence are now known, 65 of which are disease-causing mutations, mostly of the infantile type. The mutations found among Jews and non-Jews are different.

Mutations Affecting the β-Subunit

Mutations in the *HEXB* gene can result in deficiency of both Hex A and Hex B activity. One exception is a point mutation in *HEXB*, $A_{619}\rightarrow G$, that caused a motor neuron disease in an adult patient. (*HEXB* activity was absent and *HEXA* activity was 30–50% of normal.) Approximately 50% of patients with Sandhoff disease have a deletion in one or both *HEXB* alleles. Due to the absence of the promoter, no transcription or translation occurs, and the homozygote has the severe infantile form of Sandhoff disease.

Mutations Affecting the GM_2-Activator Protein

Two mutations in the GM_{2A} gene have been identified. Both involved a single substitution and were found in homozygous form in the cells of infantile AB variant patients.

Diagnosis

Serum and leukocyte assays detect most patients with a GM_2 gangliosidosis. Diagnosis of the rare patient who has the AB variant may be suspected on the basis of a skin biopsy showing lamellated bodies in axons of the dermal nerves. Tay-Sachs carrier testing by Hex A and B determination is being done in more than 50 laboratories worldwide. Since its introduction in 1970, the incidence of Tay-Sachs disease in the Jewish population has decreased by more than 90%.

The pregnancies of couples in which both parents have partial deficiency of Hex A can be monitored by chorionic villus biopsy or by amniocentesis. Hex A determinations are done on the fresh chorionic villus tissue and on cultured cells derived from this tissue or from the amniotic fluid.

Treatment

The goals of treatment are to maintain function and quality of life for the child with GM_2 gangliosidosis. Enzyme therapy has been attempted, but no trial has succeeded in delivering active Hex A to neurons and clearing GM_2 ganglioside from neurons.

For a more detailed discussion, see Matalon R, Kaul R, and Michals K. The Mucopolysaccharidoses and Mucolipidoses (Chapter 15; pp. 333–354); Johnson WG. Disorders of Glycoprotein Degradation: Sialidosis, Fucosidosis, Alpha-Mannosidosis, Beta-Mannosidosis, and Aspartylglycosaminuria (Chapter 16; pp. 355–369); Yatsu FM, Alam R. Wolman Disease (Chapter 17; pp. 371–378); Moser HW, Ceramide Deficiency: Farber Lipogranulomatosis (Chapter 18; pp. 379–386); Brady RO, Carstea ED, Pentchev PG. The Niemann-Pick Diseases Group (Chapter 19; pp. 387–403); Brady RO, Murray GJ, Barton NW. Glucosylceramide Lipidosis: Gaucher Disease (Chapter 20; pp. 405–420); Wenger DA. Krabbe Disease (Globoid Cell Leukodystrophy) (Chapter 21; pp. 421–431); Kolodny EH. Metachromatic Leukodystrophy and Multiple Sulfatase Deficiency: Sulfatide Lipidosis (Chapter 22; pp. 433–442); Desnick RJ, Eng CM. Fabry Disease: Alpha-Galactosidase A Deficiency (Chapter 23; pp. 443–452); Desnick RJ, Schindler D. Schindler Disease: Deficient Alpha-N-Acetylgalactosaminidase Activity (Chapter 24; pp. 453–462); Suzuki K. Beta-Galactosidase Deficiency: GM1 Gangliosidosis, Morquio B Disease, and Galactosialidosis (Chapter 25; pp. 463–471); Kolodny EH. The GM2 Gangliosidoses (Chapter 26; pp. 473–490), in RN Rosenberg, SB Prusiner, S DiMauro, RL Barchi (eds), **The Molecular and Genetic Basis of Neurological Disease** ***(2nd ed). Boston: Butterworth–Heinemann, 1997.***

7

Degenerative Disorders

CANAVAN DISEASE

Canavan disease is a spongy degeneration of the brain transmitted as an autosomal recessive trait that is prevalent among individuals of Ashkenazi Jewish extraction. Deficiency of the enzyme aspartoacylase causes excessive amounts of *N*-acetylaspartic acid to accumulate in body tissues and fluids.

Clinical Features

Three clinical variants are recognized: (1) a congenital form with onset at birth or shortly thereafter; (2) an infantile form, the most common, with onset after 6 months of age; and (3) a very rare juvenile form with onset after 5 years of age. It is difficult to ascertain whether the three forms are separate entities or a spectrum of clinical severity.

In the infantile form, delayed development and hypotonia may be noted at 3 months. Macrocephaly is common, although head circumference may not be greatly increased during infancy and may remain in the upper limit of normal. With time, spasticity develops and affected children may be diagnosed with cerebral palsy. Motor milestones are not attained during infancy, and seizures usually develop in the second year. Other associated features are optic atrophy, irritability, sleep disturbance, and intermittent fever. As the disease progresses, gastroesophageal reflux develops, causing feeding difficulty and poor weight gain. Swallowing deteriorates, and some nasogastric feeding or permanent feeding gastrostomy is required. Death usually occurs in the first decade.

Diagnosis

Magnetic resonance imaging (MRI) of the brain reveals diffuse white matter degeneration mainly affecting the cerebral hemispheres. This MRI finding may not be present until the second year. The diagnosis can be confirmed by brain biopsy, but a biochemical assay is now available. The histopathology shows spongy degeneration of the white matter, a finding that may also occur in homocystinuria, glycine encephalopathy, glutaric acidemia, and mitochondrial encephalopathies. Electron microscopy of the brain shows astrocytic swelling and elongated mitochondria, which are considered to be specific.

The biochemical diagnosis is made by showing excessive concentrations of *N*-acetylaspartic acid in the urine. The normal concentration is 23 ± 16.1 μmol/mmol creatinine, whereas in Canavan patients, the concentration is 1,440 ± 873.3 μmol/mmol creatinine. The concentration of *N*-acetylaspartic acid is also high in plasma, cerebrospinal fluid (CSF), and brain. Such high concentrations are specific for Canavan disease. Aspartoacylase activity can be measured in cultured skin fibroblasts. The activity in cultured fibroblasts of obligate carriers is about half or less of the activity found in healthy individuals, which makes carrier detection possible.

Biochemical and Molecular Features

The synthesis of *N*-acetylaspartic acid is catalyzed by L-aspartate-*N*-acetyltransferase (aspartoacylase), an enzyme found only in the central nervous system. Aspartoacylase hydrolyzes *N*-acetylaspartic acid to acetate and aspartate. The discovery of aspartoacylase deficiency in Canavan disease suggests that the hydrolysis of *N*-acetylaspartic acid is critical to the normal maintenance of the brain white matter. The cDNA and the gene for aspartoacylase have been cloned and the gene localized to the 17p13-ter region. Two point mutations account for 97% of cases among Ashkenazi Jews. A more diverse pattern of mutations is found in non-Jewish patients. Genotype-phenotype correlations are not apparent in non-Jewish cases. In three different patients homozygous for the same mutation, death occurred at the ages of 6 months, 15 years, and 32 years.

Prenatal diagnosis of Canavan disease using cultured amniocytes or chorionic villi samples for aspartoacylase is unsatisfactory because the concentration of the enzyme is low in these cells. Estimation of *N*-acetylaspartic acid in the amniotic fluid has been used successfully as a diagnostic marker in several pregnancies. Identification of mutations causing Canavan disease has made it possible to use DNA mutation analysis in the at-risk families.

GENETIC BASIS OF ATAXIA

Ataxia refers to the inability to fine-tune posture and movement in an orderly manner. Ataxia may be seen with any disorder that interrupts afferent or efferent cerebellar pathways but is unusual with pure cere-

Table 7.1
Hereditary ataxias.

- Disorders with known metabolic or other cause
  - Metabolic disorders
    - Progressive unremitting ataxia
      - Abetalipoproteinemia
      - Hexosaminidase deficiency
      - Cholestanolosis (cerebrotendinous xanthomatosis)
      - Leukodystrophies: metachromatic, late-onset globoid cell, adrenoleukomyeloneuropathy
      - Mitochondrial encephalomyopathies
      - Refsum disease
    - Intermittent ataxia
      - Pyruvate dehydrogenase deficiency
      - Hartnup disease
      - Intermittent branched-chain ketoaciduria
      - Deficiencies of urea cycle enzymes
  - Disorders characterized by defective DNA repair
    - Ataxia telangiectasia
    - Xeroderma pigmentosum
    - Cockayne syndrome
- Disorders of unknown cause
  - Early-onset cerebellar ataxia (onset before age 20 years)
    - Friedreich's ataxia
      - Early-onset cerebellar ataxia with associated features*
      - Marinesco-Sjögren syndrome
      - Ramsay Hunt syndrome
      - X-linked recessive spinocerebellar ataxia
  - Late-onset cerebellar ataxia (onset after age 20 years)
    - Machado-Joseph disease
    - Olivopontocerebellar atrophy
    - Pure cerebellar ataxia

*Hypogonadism, deafness, mental retardation, optic atrophy, cataracts, and pigmentary retinal degeneration.
Source: Modified from AE Harding. The Hereditary Ataxias and Related Disorders. Edinburgh: Churchill Livingstone, 1984.

bellar disease. Hereditary ataxias may involve only the cerebellum or may also involve the basal ganglia, the spinal pathways, and the peripheral nerves. Classifications based on phenotype or pathologic findings are inadequate. Affected families with genetic homogeneity have marked phenotype heterogeneity, and diverse molecular abnormalities cause similar phenotypes and neuropathologic features. A genotype classification for the inherited ataxias in which the chromosome location or genomic mutation defines the disorder is shown in Tables 7.1 and 7.2. Ataxias caused by lysosomal storage diseases are discussed in Chapter 6.

Table 7.2
Genotype classification of the spinocerebellar ataxias.

Name	*Locus*	*Phenotype*
SCA type 1 (autosomal dominant type 1)	6p22–p23 with CAG repeats	Ataxia with ophthalmoparesis; pyramidal and extrapyramidal findings
SCA type 2 (autosomal dominant type 2)	12q23–24.1 with CAG repeats	Ataxia with slow saccades and minimal pyramidal and extrapyramidal findings
SCA type 3 (autosomal dominant type 3) Machado-Joseph disease	14q24.3-qter; CAG repeats	Ataxia with ophthalmoparesis and variable pyramidal and extrapyramidal findings
SCA type 4 (autosomal dominant type 4)	16q22.1	Ataxia with normal eye movements, sensory axonal neuropathy, and pyramidal signs
SCA type 5 (autosomal dominant type 5)	Centromeric region of chromosome 11	Ataxia and dysarthria
Dentatorubropallidolouysian atrophy (autosomal dominant)	12p12-ter with CAG repeats	Ataxia, choreoathetosis, dystonia, seizures, myoclonus, and dementia
SCA type 7; spinocerebellar degeneration with retinal degeneration (autosomal dominant)	3p12–p21.1; Rhodopsin gene, CAG repeats	Ataxia with retinal degeneration
Friedreich's ataxia (autosomal recessive)	9q13–q21.1; GAA intron repeats	Ataxia, areflexia, extensor plantar responses, position sense deficits, cardiomyopathy, diabetes mellitus, scoliosis, foot deformities
	8q13.1–13.3	Same as the phenotype that maps to 9q but associated with vitamin E deficiency
		α-Tocopherol transport protein deficiency
Kearns-Sayre syndrome (sporadic)	mtDNA deletion and duplication mutations	Ptosis, ophthalmoplegia, pigmentary retinal degeneration, cardiomyopathy, diabetes mellitus, deafness, heart block, increased cerebrospinal fluid protein levels, ataxia

Name	*Locus*	*Phenotype*
Myoclonus epilepsy and ragged-red fiber syndrome (maternal inheritance)	Mutation in mtDNA of $tRNA^{lys}$ at 8344; also a mutation at 8356	Myoclonic epilepsy, ragged-red fiber myopathy, ataxia
Mitochondrial encephalopathy lactic acidosis and stroke syndrome (maternal inheritance)	$tRNA^{leu}$ mutation at 3243; also at 3271 and 3252	Headache, stroke, lactic acidosis, ataxia
Leigh's disease (subacute necrotizing encephalopathy; maternal inheritance or autosomal recessive)	mtDNA complex V deficit (adenosine triphosphatase gene at 8993) or mitochondrial protein synthesis defect (both maternally inherited) or complex IV defect (autosomal recessive)	Obtundation; hypotonia; cranial nerve defects; respiratory failure; hyperintense signals on T2-weighted magnetic resonance imaging in basal ganglia, cerebellum, or brain stem; ataxia
Episodic ataxia type 1 (autosomal dominant)	12p; potassium channel gene, *KCNA1*	Episodic ataxia for minutes; ataxia provoked by startle or exercise; facial and hand myokymia; cerebellar signs not progressive; ataxia responds to phenytoin
SCA type 6 or episodic ataxia type 2 (autosomal dominant)	19p; α, voltage-dependent Ca^{++} channel protein; CAG repeats with progressive cerebellar atrophy; point mutations with episodic ataxia or familial hemiplegic migraine	Episodic ataxia for days; ataxia provoked by stress, fatigue; downgaze nystagmus; cerebellar atrophy results; ataxia responds to acetazolamide

SCA = spinocerebellar ataxia.

Source: Modified from RN Rosenberg, ST Iannaccone. Genetic Neurological Diseases. In RN Rosenberg, DE Pleasure (eds), Comprehensive Neurology. New York: Wiley, 1998.

Abetalipoproteinemia

Abetalipoproteinemia (ABL) is a progressive, unremitting ataxia characterized by the absence of serum β-lipoprotein and a reduction in plasma chylomicrons, very low-density lipoproteins (VLDLs), and low-density lipoproteins (LDLs), rending the tissues deficient in vitamin E, which is transported in the liver by VLDL.

Clinical Features

A celiac syndrome comprised of abdominal distention, diarrhea, and foul-smelling stools develops during infancy. This is followed by a neurologic syndrome of progressive truncal and extremity ataxia, dysarthria, and nystagmus. Proprioception is lost, as are tendon reflexes. Peroneal muscle wasting is associated with distal sensory loss. The onset of the neurologic syndrome occurs by age 10 years in one-third of cases.

Pathologic Features

The posterior columns and spinocerebellar tracts are demyelinated, and neuronal loss occurs in the anterior horn cells, the cerebellar molecular layer, and cerebral cortex. Chylomicrons are absent in intestinal biopsy.

Laboratory Features

β-Lipoprotein is absent on serum protein electrophoresis, acanthocytes are seen on peripheral blood smears, and the chylomicrons, VLDLs, and LDLs are absent. Blood cholesterol concentrations range from 20 to 50 mg/dl and triglyceride concentrations range from 2 to 13 mg/dl. The blood concentration of fat-soluble vitamins A, E, and K is low, and the urine concentration of mevalonic acid is increased.

Axonal neuropathy is demonstrated by nerve conduction velocities. The somatosensory evoked potential test is abnormal in all but the least affected patients. Visual evoked potentials may also be abnormal. The electroretinogram is abnormal early in the disease.

Biochemical Features

The most likely defect is the failure of β-apoprotein synthesis. β-Apoproteins are necessary for chylomicron formation, which are necessary for the transport of lipids. The transfer of cholesterol esters and triglycerides between high-density lipoproteins (HDLs) and VLDLs is reduced by 50% and 66%, respectively.

The neurologic manifestations may be caused by the peroxidation of unsaturated myelin phospholipids. In ABL, the activity of the degradative enzyme, platelet-activating factor acetyl hydroxylase, is only found in HDL, and its half-life is prolonged. This in turn causes a deficiency in VLDL, which is needed to transport vitamin E in the plasma. Deficiency of vitamin E is presumed to cause peripheral neuropathy.

Genetics

ABL is an autosomal recessive disease. The defect does not appear to be in the apolipoprotein β gene. No major insertions or deletions have been identified. The primary defect may be a post-translational defect in the processing or secretion of the apolipoprotein β gene.

Therapy

Replacement of fat-soluble vitamins, especially A and E, often prevents the development of some symptoms or the progression of the disease. Vitamin replacement is most effective when initiated at an early age and has limited value in adults.

Cerebrotendinous Xanthomatosis

Cerebrotendinous xanthomatosis is a rare autosomal recessive disease characterized by elevated plasma cholestanol and accumulation of cholestanol in xanthomas of the tendons, lungs, and brain in spite of a normal or low plasma cholesterol level.

Clinical Features

Cerebrotendinous xanthomatosis has an insidious onset in childhood and follows an unpredictable course. It is arbitrarily divided into three stages:

1. Affected children have borderline intelligence and usually show mental deterioration. Some maintain normal intelligence into adult life.
2. During the second and third decades, progressive spasticity and ataxia develop secondary to progressive leukodystrophy associated with development of cataracts and tendon xanthomas.
3. The final stage is characterized by enlargement of the xanthomas and severe neurologic deterioration involving the gray and white matter of the cerebrum, cerebellum, and spinal cord.

Diagnosis

The diagnosis is difficult to establish in the first stage. The disease should be considered in any young adult with tendon xanthomas, cataracts, low or borderline intelligence, and ataxia. The diagnosis is confirmed by measuring the concentration of cholestanol in plasma and particularly in xanthomas, skin, or adipose tissue. High concentrations of seven α-hydroxylated bile acids are found in the urine. MRI shows demyelination in the cerebral white matter.

Biochemical and Genetic Features

Most patients show normal plasma concentrations of cholesterol, triglyceride, and phospholipid, but plasma cholestanol concentrations are increased 10–40 times the upper limit of normal. Free esterified cholestanol in the brain is increased from its normal trace amount to 20–25% of the total free sterols. Cerebral and cerebellar cholesterol content is also increased, primarily because of increased cholesterol esters. Peripheral nerves show that 20% of the total sterols is cholestanol, 59% of which is esterified cholestanol. Ninety percent of the total sterols in tendon xanthoma is cholesterol and 10% is cholestanol. The enzymatic defect is a block in bile acid synthesis. Mutations in the sterol 27-hydroxylase gene (*CYP27*), located on chromosome 2, underlie the disease.

Therapy

Oral chenodeoxycholic acid (750 mg/day) improves dementia in most patients and may resolve pyramidal and cerebellar dysfunction in some. The improvement can be documented with neuroimaging studies. Therapeutic intervention reverses the process by changing the course of sterol deposition in the nervous system. Cataract extraction may partially relieve the visual symptoms, and surgical removal of tendon xanthomas may help relieve pain and discomfort.

Refsum Disease

Heredopathia atactica polyneuritiformis, or Refsum disease, is an autosomal recessive disorder of lipid metabolism characterized by the accumulation of phytanic acid, a 20-carbon branched fatty acid. Infantile Refsum disease is a peroxisomal disorder and is discussed in Chapter 5.

Clinical Features

Refsum disease is characterized by the slowly progressive development of neurogenic hearing loss, atypical retinitis pigmentosa, ichthyosis-like skin changes, ataxia, and a peripheral neuropathy. Onset is in childhood. Examination of the CSF shows albuminocytologic dissociation.

Biochemical Features

The primary defect is a deficiency of phytanic acid oxidase. Blood concentrations of phytanic acid range between 10 and 50 mg/dl (normal is 0.2 mg/dl or less). Fatty material is deposited in all organs including the brain, which is rich in phytanic acid. Indirect evidence localizes phytanic acid oxidase to peroxisomes (see Chapter 5).

Treatment

Phytanic acid is mainly of exogenous origin and derived from dietary phytol ingested in the form of nuts, spinach, and coffee. A diet low in phytol and phytanic acid decreases the plasma concentration. Periodic plasma exchanges decrease body stores of phytanic acid. The decrease in phytanic acid is accompanied by increased conduction velocities, return of reflexes, and improvement in sensation and objective coordination.

Related Disorders

Elevated blood phytanic acid concentrations also occur in several genetic peroxisomal disorders (see Chapter 5) and were described in a man who developed progressive cerebellar ataxia at the age of 21 years. Vibration sense, position sense, and stereognosis were impaired, and tendon reflexes were absent. The CSF protein concentration was elevated, and MRI showed cerebellar atrophy. His sister had a similar clinical syndrome, except that serum phytanic acid concentrations were normal. Asymptomatic heterozygotes may have elevated blood concentrations of phytanic acid.

Hartnup Disease

Hartnup disease is an autosomal recessive disorder of neutral amino acid transport that causes an intermittent cerebellar ataxia.

Clinical Features

Intermittent cerebral dysfunction, characterized by intermittent personality change, psychosis, migraine-like headaches, photophobia, and intermittent cerebellar ataxia, develops by age 10 years. Attacks are precipitated by fasting. Dystonia, responsive to trihexyphenidyl, was described in a 6-month-old girl. Most patients have normal mental development and are asymptomatic. Those with a low summed plasma amino acid value for the group of amino acids sharing the Hartnup transport system are at risk for progressive cognitive decline and symptoms of disease. In addition to neurologic dysfunction, affected individuals have photosensitive, red, scaly pellagra-like rash, a change in hair texture, and a constant aminoaciduria.

Biochemical Features

The aminoaciduria is secondary to decreased renal absorption, resulting in increased excretion of indican, indole-3-acetic acid, indole-3-acryllylglycine, and indole-3-acetyl-C-glutamine. The concentration of neutral amino acids in the stool is increased, as are CSF concentrations of 5-hydroxy indole acetic acid, a metabolite of serotonin. Hartnup disease shows genetic heterogeneity. Tissue-specific phenotypes may be confined to the kidney and intestine or to the intestine alone.

Therapy

Adequate caloric intake is essential. Nicotinic acid depletion may play a role in Hartnup disease but cannot be the primary determinant because pellagra does not cause a specific hyperaminoaciduria. It is not established that nicotinic acid reverses all phenotypic manifestations of Hartnup disease. Oral tryptophan ethyl ester raised serum and CSF tryptophan concentrations to normal in one child. The patient's chronic diarrhea resolved and body weight increased by 26%.

Intermittent Branched-Chain Aminoacidurias

Maple syrup urine disease is transmitted as an autosomal recessive trait. The basic defect is in the enzyme branched-chain amino acid decarboxylase (see Chapter 17).

Clinical Features

Complete absence of the enzyme results in the classic form with neonatal onset. The clinical phenotype includes opisthotonos, intermittent hypertonicity, and vomiting. The serum and urine concentrations of branched-chain ketoacids (leucine, isoleucine, valine) are increased. An isoleucine derivative is responsible for the characteristic odor.

Variant forms have residual amounts of branched-chain ketoacid decarboxylase activity. One is characterized by intermittent ataxia, behavioral changes, and seizures. Mild to moderate mental retardation may be associated. The onset is usually before 1 year of age. The amount of enzyme activity does not predict the clinical course.

Biochemical and Molecular Features

Five distinct molecular phenotypes are distinguished based on messenger RNA and protein subunit contents. The complete primary structure of the E1 β subunit has been deduced. Three overlapping cDNA clones encoding the E1 subunit have been identified.

Treatment

Treatment consists of restricting the dietary intake of branched-chain amino acids. Peritoneal dialysis is highly effective. Some patients respond to thiamine supplementation.

Urea Cycle

Urea cycle enzyme defects are relatively common and are often associated with intermittent ataxia (see Chapter 17). Deficiency of each of the five enzymes of the urea cycle are known causes of disease. All are transmitted as autosomal recessive traits, except for ornithine transcarbamylase deficiency, which is X-linked. Newborns with complete deficiency of one urea cycle enzyme are normal at birth but develop symptoms of hyperammonemia during the first 10 days of life. These symptoms include feeding difficulties, impaired level of consciousness, vomiting, and seizures. The urea cycle includes five separate enzyme steps that convert two amino nitrogen moieties and 1 mole of carbon dioxide to one molecule of urea. Carbamyl phosphate synthetase and ornithine transcarbamylase are in the mitochondrial membrane, and the other three enzymes are in the cytoplasm.

Carbamyl-Phosphate Synthetase Deficiency

Carbamyl-phosphate synthetase deficiency is a rare disorder that presents in the newborn with hyperammonemia, obtundation, and dehydration.

Ornithine Transcarbamylase Deficiency

Ornithine transcarbamylase deficiency (OTC) is the most common urea cycle defect. The OTC gene maps to the short arm of the X chromosome. Intermittent ataxia occurs in males. Clinical severity is variable in females depending on random inactivation of the X chromosome. A variant of OTC deficiency is the syndrome of hyperornithinemia, hyperammonemia, and homocitrullinuria, which is characterized by protein intolerance, mental retardation, seizures, and episodic attacks of ataxia and stupor in adolescents and young adults. It is inherited as an autosomal recessive disorder, and the basic defect is in the transport of ornithine into mitochondria.

Adult-onset disease occurs in males with partial OTC deficiency. The main features are episodes of nausea, vomiting, and bizarre behavior. OTC activity is one-fourth of normal. Treatment consists of restricting dietary protein, supplementing the diet with essential amino acids and citrulline, and activating alternative pathways of waste-nitrogen synthesis and excretion with sodium benzoate and sodium phenylacetate. Patients with the disease show a deletion of a substantial portion of the OTC gene.

Argininosuccinic Acid Synthetase Deficiency (Citrullinemia)

The clinical manifestations of argininosuccinic acid synthetase deficiency include neonatal, late infantile, childhood, and early adult-onset forms. The neonatal form is characterized by lethargy, tachypnea, vomiting, irritability, and failure to thrive in the first days after birth, then proceeds to seizures, coma, and death. Citrulline concentrations in serum, urine, and CSF are significantly elevated. Hyperammonemia is expected. Other laboratory findings are metabolic acidosis, hypocalcemia, hypoglycemia, elevated serum glutamic-oxaloacetic transaminase, and hyperammonemia.

Argininosuccinase Deficiency

Argininosuccinase deficiency is associated with argininosuccinic aciduria. Neonatal, subacute, and late-onset forms result from allelic modifications of the enzyme. The neonatal type includes failure to thrive, lethargy, seizures, coma, hepatomegaly, and dry, brittle hair (*trichorrhexis nodosa)*. The hair disorder may be related more directly to the low-protein diet. Moderate mental retardation is characteristic in older children. One-third have ataxia and seizures. Hyperammonemia and elevated argininosuccinic acid concentrations in serum, urine, and CSF are characteristic. Argininosuccinase is deficient in liver, fibroblasts, and amniotic fluid cells. Oral arginine supplementation aids in the formation of argininosuccinic acid. The enzyme locus is assigned to chromosome 7.

Arginase Deficiency (Argininemia)

Newborns with arginase deficiency develop seizures, vomiting, and failure to thrive proceeding to mental retardation, spastic paraplegia, ataxia, and hepatomegaly. Arginine values and arginase activity are intermediate in heterozygotes.

Ataxia Telangiectasia

Ataxia telangiectasia is a disorder of DNA repair and replication. Although usually sporadic in occurrence and isolated in families, the pattern is consistent with autosomal recessive inheritance.

Clinical Features

A slowly progressive cerebellar ataxia develops during infancy and affected children never walk. The ataxia involves both trunk and limbs and is associated with dysarthria, extensor plantar responses, myoclonic jerks, and a sensory neuropathy with areflexia. Oculomotor apraxia is a very frequent feature. Telangiectatic lesions involving the conjunctivae, malar eminences, earlobes, and upper neck develop during childhood. Most children have an associated immunodeficiency that first causes recurrent bronchopulmonary infections and later is associated with lymphatic and reticuloendothelial system cancer. Also described are thymic hypoplasia with cellular and humeral (IgA and IgG_2) immunodeficiencies, premature aging, and endocrine disorders such as insulin-dependent diabetes mellitus.

Biochemical and Molecular Features

Glutamic acid is reduced in the brain. γ-Aminobutyric acid (GABA) content is greatly reduced in the dentate nucleus, and GABA receptor binding is reduced by 70% in the cerebellar cortex. Phosphorylethanolamine is also greatly reduced in the cerebellar cortex and inferior olivary nucleus. Linkage analysis localizes the ataxia telangiectasia gene to chromosome 11q22–23.

Diagnosis

The combination of ataxia and oculomotor apraxia beginning during infancy, especially when associated with recurrent bronchopulmonary infections, should suggest the diagnosis. The telangiectasias develop later and are not present at the time of diagnosis. Serum protein electrophoresis shows deficiency of IgA and IgE. Serum α-fetoprotein levels are elevated.

Treatment

Early and aggressive treatment of sinopulmonary infections is mandatory, but repeated radiation should be avoided because it leads to early development of malignancy.

Xeroderma Pigmentosum

Xeroderma pigmentosum (XP) is a rare autosomal recessive disorder caused by an inability to repair DNA that has been damaged by ultraviolet (UV) radiation.

Clinical Features

XP is characterized by sunlight hypersensitivity, skin cancers, and neurologic deterioration. The skin manifestations include prolonged erythema, edema, and blistering on minimal skin exposure; freckling, dry, scaly skin; and telangiectasia. Basal cell and squamous cell carcinomas and malignant melanomas are common. Noncutaneous features are dwarfism, hypogonadism, progressive mental deterioration, microcephaly, ataxia, spasticity, choreoathetosis, nerve deafness, axonal neuropathy, and seizures.

Biochemical and Molecular Features

Two distinct biochemical forms of XP exist. One is characterized by defective nucleotide excision and comprises nine genetic complementation groups that probably represent a different defective DNA-repair gene. The other is defective in postreplication repair and is referred to as the *XP variant form*. Neurologic involvement is always associated with the DNA nucleotide-excision defective form.

Cockayne Syndrome

Cockayne syndrome is a disorder of defective DNA repair.

Clinical Features

Neonatal onset of Cockayne syndrome predicts early death. Age of onset in most cases is in infancy or childhood. The characteristic features are a bird-headed facies, dwarfism, mental retardation, optic atrophy, neural deafness, skin hypersensitivity to sunlight, cataracts, and retinal pigmentary degeneration. Neurologic examination shows cerebellar, pyramidal, and extrapyramidal deficits. Normal pressure hydrocephalus and peripheral neuropathy may be associated. Prenatal diagnosis is accomplished by showing that amniotic cells exposed to UV radiation have abnormal RNA synthesis.

Friedreich Disease

Friedreich disease (FRDA) has been the prototype of hereditary ataxias. It is transmitted as an autosomal recessive trait.

Clinical Features

The onset of FRDA is before 25 years of age. The main features are a progressive staggering gait, frequent falling, and titubation. The legs are more involved than the arms. Less common presenting features are dysarthria, progressive scoliosis, foot deformity, nystagmus, or cardiopathy. The neurologic examination shows nystagmus, loss of fast saccadic eye movements, truncal titubation, dysarthria, dysmetria, and ataxia of limbs and trunk. The plantar responses are extensor, tendon reflexes are absent, and weakness is greater in distal than proximal muscles. Vibratory and proprioceptive sensations are often depressed in the legs. The median age of death is 35 years. Women have a better prognosis; the 20-year survival rate is 100% in women and 63% in men. Cardiac involvement, characterized by cardiomegaly, symmetric hypertrophy, and conduction defects, approaches 90%. Moderate mental retardation or psychiatric syndromes are sometimes associated, but diabetes occurs in 20% of patients.

Biochemical and Molecular Features

Classic FRDA maps to 9q13–q21.1. Triplet GAA expanded repeats in intron 1 of the FRDA gene result in loss of expression of the frataxin protein. Frataxin is greatly reduced in spinal cord and selected brain regions. An inverse relationship exists between the number of repeats and the age of onset. The vitamin E–deficient form of FRDA maps to 8q13.1–q13.3 and is caused by loss of function of the α-tocopherol transport protein.

Several studies have suggested a defect in pyruvate metabolism. Blood pyruvate concentrations are elevated in response to an oral glucose load. The abnormal pyruvate response may be explained by enzymatic defects in mitochondrial malic enzyme, pyruvate dehydrogenase complex, α-ketoglutarate dehydrogenase complex, and lipoamide dehydrogenase.

Treatment

A high-fat diet has been suggested to provide substrate and bypass the error in sugar metabolism. Thiamine, steroids, physostigmine, choline, and lecithin may also benefit selected patients. Vitamin E therapy has not been determined to be therapeutic in vitamin E–deficient patients.

Marinesco-Sjögren Syndrome

Clinical Features

Marinesco-Sjögren syndrome is rare and begins in early childhood. Progressive cerebellar ataxia is associated with cataracts, mental retardation, multiple skeletal abnormalities, hypogonadotrophic hypogonadism, and cataracts.

Biochemical Features

The pathophysiology of Marinesco-Sjögren syndrome is not understood. It may be a lysosomal storage disorder caused by an unknown enzymatic defect.

Machado-Joseph Disease

Machado-Joseph disease (MJD) is transmitted as an autosomal dominant trait. It is believed to have originated among the Portuguese and spread worldwide during the age of exploration.

Clinical Features

Three clinical types of MJD represent variation in the expressivity and penetrance of the same mutant gene. Type I (amyotrophic lateral sclerosis-parkinsonism-dystonia) has its onset before age 20 years. The neurologic syndrome includes limb weakness and spasticity affecting the legs more than the arms and is often associated with dystonia of the face, neck, trunk, and limbs. Patellar and ankle clonus are common, as are extensor plantar responses. The gait is slow and stiff, with a slightly broadened base and lurching from side to side. The gait is more spastic than ataxic. Truncal titubation is absent. Pharyngeal weakness and spasticity cause difficulty with speech and swallowing. Horizontal and vertical nystagmus are prominent. Fast saccadic eye movements are lost and upward gaze is impaired. Fasciculations of the face and tongue, without atrophy, are common and early features.

Type II (ataxic type) begins in the second to fourth decades and is characterized by true cerebellar deficits, including dysarthria and gait and limb ataxia, along with corticospinal and extrapyramidal deficits such as spasticity, rigidity, and dystonia. Type II is the most common form of the disease. Ophthalmoparesis, upward gaze deficits, and facial and lingual fasciculations are also present, as in type I disease. Type II shares features with olivopontocerebellar degeneration, from which it must be differentiated.

Type III (ataxic-amyotrophic lateral sclerosis type) presents in the fifth to seventh decades of life with a pancerebellar disorder, including dysarthria, gait, and extremity ataxia. Distal sensory loss to pain, touch, vibration, and position senses, as well as distal atrophy are prominent. The tendon reflexes are depressed or absent, and no corticospinal or extrapyramidal findings occur. Intelligence is always normal.

Biochemical and Molecular Features

The gene locus for MJD has been assigned to 14q24.3–q32 by genetic linkage. CAG unstable repeat expansions occur in the MJD gene. The expanded CAG repeats encode for polyglutamine. The mechanism has not been established.

Treatment

Specific treatment is not available. Palliative therapy with antiparkinsonian medications, antispasmodics, and trimethoprim-sulfamethoxazole is somewhat effective.

Olivopontocerebellar Atrophy (Spinocerebellar Atrophy Types 1 and 2)

Late-onset, dominantly inherited ataxias are difficult to classify because of pathologic and clinical heterogeneity. Olivopontocerebellar atrophy (OPCA) is a collection of disorders that produce progressive cerebellar dysfunction and show a reduction of neurons in the inferior olivary nuclei of the medulla, and in the basis pontis, cerebellar cortex, and the deep cerebellar nuclei.

Clinical Features

Limb and truncal ataxia with dysmetria and dysarthria progressively develop in the second or third decades. Spasticity associated with clonus, hyperreflexia, and extensor plantar responses develop later. Nystagmus, optic nerve atrophy, and loss of fast saccadic eye movements may occur. A late occurrence of atrophy and fasciculations involving the facial, lingual, and mastication muscles is secondary to loss of lower motor neurons. Sensory involvement in a distal distribution may occur. Mild intellectual deterioration may occur late in the course. Ophthalmoplegia, extrapyramidal signs, and optic atrophy with vision loss may occur.

Biochemical and Molecular Features

The spinocerebellar ataxia type 1 (SCA1) gene maps to 6p22–p23 and shows a highly polymorphic CAG repeat in this region. Larger repeats correlate with earlier age of onset of SCA1. SCA2 maps to 12q23–q24.1 and is also associated with CAG repeats.

Diagnosis

The development early in life of progressive symmetric involvement of cerebellar function, followed by progressive symmetric development of spasticity, is characteristic of OPCA. Abnormality of eye movement, minimal intellectual impairment, and muscle atrophy with distal sensory loss complete the picture. MRI shows cerebellar and pontine atrophy. CSF studies are normal.

Treatment

Specific therapy for the underlying disease is not available.

HUNTINGTON'S DISEASE

Huntington's disease (HD) is transmitted as an autosomal dominant trait.

Clinical Features

The mean age of onset of motor symptoms in HD is approximately 40 years, but onset can be in childhood. The initial features are chorea, personality change, and dementia. Behavioral and personality disorders in at-risk individuals may occur because of alterations in family structure as well as because of the disease itself. Onset before age 20 is associated with a rapid, severe course, whereas onset after 60 years is associated with slow progression. Death occurs usually 15–20 years after onset of motor symptoms.

Some observant patients notice problems with motor control before the onset of chorea. These include unexplained falls, slight unsteadiness in walking, a tendency to drop objects, or a change in handwriting. Cognitive impairment is frequently evident at the onset of chorea. Most experience a change in personality; increased tendency to anxiety, anger, or frustration is common, along with withdrawal from social interaction and interests. Some exhibit a hypersomatization disorder, alcohol abuse, antisocial behavior, aimless wandering, or occasionally a hypomanic state.

Clinical Variants

Late-onset disease refers to patients who develop chorea after age 60. They usually are affected less severely by HD. *Juvenile HD* often presents with progressive rigidity without chorea. The gene is usually inherited from an affected father. *Early psychosis* is the development of disabling thought and behavioral disorders years before the diagnosis of HD.

Biochemical and Molecular Features

Population and archival studies have suggested that the overwhelming majority of HD cases worldwide are descended from one or more mutations originating in northwestern Europe in the fourteenth or fifteenth century. The gene for HD is located on the short arm of chromosome 4. It contains a $(CAG)_n$ trinucleotide repeat that is expanded and unstable. The gene encodes a protein called *huntingtin,* which contains an elongated polyglutamine tract near the amino terminus. The function of the normal huntingtin protein is unknown. Except for juvenile-onset patients, who have the largest number of repeats, the size of the expanded CAG in an individual patient does not predict age of onset or clinical severity.

Treatment

Specific treatment is not available, but genetic testing is available to confirm the clinical diagnosis and can aid individuals at risk for HD in planning their future. Disordered emotional control is perhaps the most common and difficult management issue. Clonazepam, fluoxetine, valproic acid, neuroleptics, β-adrenergic antagonists, or carbamazepine can be of limited benefit in controlling this behavior.

INHERITED DISORDERS OF THE BASAL GANGLIA

Huntington's disease is the prototype of an inherited disorder in which gene expression primarily targets the basal ganglia. This section reviews other disorders of the basal ganglia for which an inherited basis has been established or is suspected.

Neuroacanthocytosis

Clinical Features

In neuroacanthocytosis (NA), the onset of symptoms is usually in the fourth or fifth decade but may begin in childhood or as late as the seventh decade. Men are affected twice as frequently as women and more severely. In some families, a few individuals have acanthocytosis but very mild or absent neurologic abnormalities. The appearance of acanthocytes usually precedes the neurologic features. Movement disorders develop in nearly all familial cases of NA. Such disorders usually are hyperkinetic and consist of chorea, tics, dystonia, and orofacial dyskinesias. Akinetic-rigid features, dysarthria, and dysphagia may develop as NA progresses. Gradually advancing cognitive impairment is characteristic, and affective illness, obsessive-compulsive disorder, and personality change are common. Generalized seizures occur in approximately 40% of patients. Reduced or absent muscle tendon reflexes indicate an associated axonal neuropathy. Average life span is approximately 14 years from onset of illness.

Biochemical and Molecular Features

Most affected families show an autosomal dominant or recessive pattern of inheritance. Sporadic cases occur and may be underreported. An X-linked mode of transmission for NA has also been suggested by the near absence of male-to-male transmission, the 2:1 male-to-female occurrence, and the observation that males are more severely affected than females. In further support of this notion are the occasional associations of NA with the McLeod phenotype, which has been linked to a locus on the short arm of the X chromosome.

Diagnosis

Acanthocytes are mature erythrocytes characterized by multiple, irregularly arranged, spiny or blunt projections. Acanthocytes are best detected on a fresh blood smear using conventional light or phase-contrast microscopy. MRI of the brain shows variable degrees of caudate and cerebral atrophy.

Parkinson's Disease

Parkinson's disease (PD) has not been viewed traditionally as a genetic disorder. Considerable attention has been accorded recently to the notion that PD derives from a common pathology caused by diverse etiologies.

Clinical Features

The clinical syndrome of idiopathic PD is characterized by bradykinesia associated with asymmetric onset of rigidity and resting tremor and the development of postural instability. The onset of clinical features of PD may begin as early as the third decade. Although the pathologic features are the same in early- and late-onset PD, patients with onset before age 50 years appear to have a more favorable prognosis.

Biochemical and Genetic Features

The main chemical abnormality is dopamine depletion in the striatum. Familial clustering of cases occurs. The prevalence of PD is increased among siblings of affected probands, particularly in early-onset PD. Large kindreds of autosomal dominant PD, with and without dementia or depression, have also been described.

Considerable investigative attention has been accorded to apolipoprotein (Apo) genotypes, particularly the apolipoprotein E allele (ApoE), which has been established as a susceptibility gene for late-onset familial and sporadic Alzheimer's disease. Although the cause or causes of PD have not been established, accumulating knowledge suggests that genetic predispositions, perhaps also involving aging genes, may interact with environmental events over a period of years to set in motion a cascade of pathophysiologic mechanisms, perhaps mediated by oxidative mechanisms, which leads to nigral degeneration and the emergence and progression of PD.

Treatment

Treatment of PD includes the use of dopamine agonists and dopamine replacement therapy.

Gilles de la Tourette Syndrome

Clinical Features

Gilles de la Tourette syndrome (TS) is a hereditary disorder characterized by motor and verbal tics, with age of onset younger than 21 years and lasting more than 1 year. Tics are brief stereotyped movements or sounds. They are not constantly present, except when extremely severe, and occur in a background of normal motor activity. Other phenotypic expressions of the TS phenotype are attention deficit disorder and obsessive-compulsive disorder.

Molecular and Biochemical Features

TS is inherited as an autosomal dominant trait with incomplete and sex-specific penetrance. Affected males are more likely to show tics and attention deficit disorder; affected females are more likely to have obsessive-compulsive disorder. Bilineal transmission (from both maternal and paternal sides) is common and may determine severity of illness. The prevailing notion regarding the neurochemical mechanism for tics in TS is supersensitivity of central dopamine receptors. This hypothesis is suggested by low CSF concentrations of the dopamine metabolite homovanillic acid, the improvement after treatment with dopamine receptor antagonists, and the clinical worsening after use of dopaminergic drugs, such as amphetamines.

Diagnosis

TS is a clinical diagnosis. A family history of tics, attention deficit disorder, or obsessive-compulsive disorder is particularly useful in establishing the diagnosis.

Treatment

Dopamine receptor antagonist drugs, such as haloperidol and pimozide, are the most effective tic-suppressing medications. Drugs that inhibit serotonin reuptake, including fluoxetine and clomipramine, are often effective agents for the treatment of obsessive-compulsive disorder.

Dystonia

Dystonia is classified as symptomatic, secondary to another disease, and idiopathic or genetic. This section focuses on genetic dystonia. Dystonia is sustained muscle contraction, frequently causing twisting and repetitive movements or abnormal postures. Dystonic movements may occur at rest or when engaged in voluntary motor activity (action dystonia). Dystonia at rest usually indicates a more severe form than action dystonia. Idiopathic or primary torsion dystonia may be inherited as autosomal dominant, autosomal recessive, and X-linked recessive traits (Table 7.3). Several distinct forms are readily distinguished by age at onset, diurnal fluctuation of symptoms, and responsiveness to specific medications. Almost all are transmitted as autosomal dominant traits.

Clinical Features

Childhood Onset without Marked Diurnal Fluctuation. Childhood-onset dystonia without marked diurnal fluctuation was originally called *dystonia musculorum deformans*. The age of onset clusters at

Table 7.3
Forms of hereditary primary dystonia.

Autosomal dominant forms
Childhood onset without marked diurnal fluctuation
(classic hereditary dystonia)
Dopa-responsive dystonia
Childhood onset with marked diurnal fluctuations
(Segawa type)
Dystonia-parkinsonism
Adult onset
Paroxysmal dystonic choreoathetosis
Myoclonic dystonia
Autosomal recessive form
Spanish gypsies
X-linked recessive forms
Filipino type (Lubag)
With deafness

approximately 9 years. Initial leg involvement rapidly progresses to generalized and disabling dystonia. Age of onset and clinical features can vary within a single family. The disorder is transmitted by autosomal dominant inheritance with a 30% penetrance.

Childhood Onset with Marked Diurnal Fluctuation. Typical patients with childhood-onset dystonia with marked diurnal fluctuation are normal in the early morning but develop increasing dystonia as the day progresses. Other distinguishing features are responsiveness to levodopa therapy and a pronounced female preponderance. As in other forms of childhood-onset primary dystonia, symptoms begin in the legs and the disease appears to be inherited in an autosomal dominant fashion with reduced penetrance.

Dystonia-Parkinsonism. Childhood-onset dystonia in association with parkinsonism may present with rigidity, bradykinesia, postural imbalance, hypomimia, and tremor. The disorder is inherited as an autosomal dominant trait with variable penetrance. Initial symptoms are in the legs. The condition is usually responsive to levodopa, and progression during adulthood is minimal. Cases of childhood-onset dystonia-parkinsonism, with or without diurnal fluctuations, may be grouped together as *dopa-responsive dystonia.*

Adult-Onset Dystonia. The adult-onset form of primary dystonia usually starts in the arms. Progression is slow and often not severe. Some cases of adult-onset dystonia respond to levodopa. Autosomal dominant inheritance with high penetrance and marked variability of expression is the rule.

Paroxysmal Dystonic Choreoathetosis. Two forms of paroxysmal dystonia are recognized depending on whether the paroxysms are exertion-induced: paroxysmal kinesiogenic dystonia (PKD) and paroxysmal nonkinesiogenic dystonia (PNKD). PKD is a seizure disorder and responds to anticonvulsant therapy. PNKD is an ion channel defect characterized by episodic attacks of dystonia, choreoathetosis, or both. Episodes last from minutes to hours and occur a few times each day. Attacks are precipitated by fatigue, cold, emotional states, and alcohol or caffeine ingestion. Affected individuals are asymptomatic between episodes. The age of onset ranges from infancy to early adulthood.

Molecular Neurobiology

Genetic linkage studies have localized the genes for both Jewish and non-Jewish autosomal dominant childhood-onset dystonia to chromosome 9q32–q34 (the *DYT01* gene). Families with adult cervical/cranial-onset dystonia do not show linkage to the same gene region. Autosomal dominant dopa-responsive dystonia maps to chromosome 14q. X-linked dystonia localizes to the pericentromeric region of the X chromosome (*DYT-3* gene) by linkage analysis.

Treatment

The treatment of these dystonic conditions is largely empiric. The best results are obtained with high-dose anticholinergic therapy. The autosomal dominant forms with marked diurnal variation or associated parkinsonism usually respond to levodopa therapy. Some adult-onset cases may respond to levodopa as well. Paroxysmal dystonic choreoathetosis is best treated with benzodiazepines or L-tryptophan, whereas PKC usually responds to anticonvulsant therapy.

ALZHEIMER'S DISEASE

Alzheimer's disease (AD) is the largest single cause of late-life dementing illness in the United States, accounting for more than 50% of cases.

The clinical and pathologic features probably result from several pathophysiologic processes. Both genetic and environmental factors play a role in the expression of the disease.

Clinical Features

AD is characterized by the gradual development of profound dementia. The onset of symptoms usually begins in the seventh and eighth decades of life (late-onset or senile-onset AD). Less than 10% begin before age 65, and some as early as the fourth and fifth decades (presenile AD). Profound dementia develops in 2–10 years, and life expectancy is significantly reduced. Early signs include deficits in attention, concentration, orientation, memory, and abstract reasoning. Language difficulties begin with impaired naming, progress to fluent aphasia, and eventuate in mutism. Praxis difficulties are detected early as constructional dyspraxia: the inability to draw simple geometric figures. They progress to dressing dyspraxia and ultimately to inability to perform ordinary activities of daily living, to self-feed, and to walk. Psychiatric symptoms are frequent, occurring most often in the early or middle stages of the disease, and include depressive symptoms, suspiciousness, delusions, and visual hallucinations.

Early in the course, neurologic examination is normal except for cognitive dysfunction. Later, symmetric mild hyperreflexia and primitive reflexes, such as palmomental, snout, and grasp, may be demonstrated. Behavioral disturbances, such as wandering and aggression, are more common in the middle and late stages of the disease. Urinary and fecal incontinence are late features, as are myoclonus, bradykinesia, and rigidity. Terminally, patients appear mute and decorticate and tend to develop flexion contractures. Death is usually due to sepsis after pulmonary or urinary tract infection.

Diagnosis

Criteria for the diagnosis of *probable* AD include the following:

- Dementia established by clinical examination and documented by the Mini-Mental State Exam (MMSE), Blessed Dementia Scale, or some similar examination, and confirmed by neuropsychological tests
- Deficits in two or more areas of cognition
- Progressive worsening of memory and other cognitive functions
- No disturbance of consciousness
- Onset between ages 40 and 90 years

- Absence of systemic disorders or other brain diseases that by themselves could account for the progressive deficits in memory and cognition

The diagnosis of *possible* AD includes the development of a dementia syndrome in the absence of other disorders sufficient to cause dementia and in the presence of variations in onset, presentation, or clinical course. Possible AD may be diagnosed in the presence of a second disorder sufficient to produce dementia that is not thought to be the cause of the dementia. The diagnosis of *definite* AD requires autopsy confirmation.

The Lewy body variant of AD, also called *senile dementia of the Lewy body type*, accounts for 7–30% of dementia cases. The course of illness may be more rapid than in AD, with intermittent delirious states, visual and auditory hallucinations, and delusions. Extrapyramidal symptoms may develop early in the course. Lewy bodies are found throughout the cerebral cortex in addition to numerous senile plaques (SPs). Neurofibrillary tangles (NFTs) are not prominent.

Risk Factors

The major risk factor for late-onset AD is age. The prevalence doubles every 5 years between the ages of 65 and 85. Major risk factors are having an affected first-degree relative or trisomy 21 or inheriting the ε4 allele of apoliprotein E (ApoE-ε4), which seems to promote earlier expression of the disease. Inheritance of the ε4 allele may also modify nongenetic risk factors, such as head injury. Inheritance of the ApoE-ε2 allele appears to reduce the risk of AD by delaying onset.

Pathologic Features

NFTs and SPs are central to the neuropathologic definition of AD, but neither their etiology nor their role in disease progression is completely understood. NFTs are intraneuronal accumulations of paired helical filaments. SPs consist of varying proportions of dystrophic neurites and extracellular amyloid. Dystrophic neurites are probably derived from both axons and dendrites, and most contain paired helical filaments similar to those that constitute NFTs in neuronal cell bodies. The amyloid found in SPs as well as in cerebral blood vessels in AD is a unique 39– to 43–amino acid peptide termed *Aβ*, which is able to self-aggregate into 8-nm fibrils. The Aβ peptide derives from a much larger precursor, termed *amyloid precursor protein* (APP), which resembles a cell surface receptor in structure. The brain in late-stage AD is characterized not only by abundant SPs and NFTs in specific regions but also by death of specific neuronal populations. More severe cholinergic deficits occur in patients with the ApoE-ε4 genotype, and patients with different ApoE genotypes may have different responses to cholinergic drugs.

Genetic Features

Most cases of AD are sporadic. In the early-onset form, approximately 10% of families show inheritance consistent with autosomal dominant transmission. Genetic mapping of the early-onset AD genes show that candidate genes mapping to chromosomes 21q, 14q, and 1q account for virtually all inherited early-onset forms of the disease. Eighty percent of early-onset familial AD maps to chromosome 14q24.3, and a causal gene, presenilin 1, has been identified. Mutations in the APP gene on chromosome 21 lie in or around the Aβ region of APP, suggesting the possibility that these mutations could affect the processing and aggregation of Aβ. AD in families of Volga-German ancestry is rare. The locus is at 1q31–42 and the causal gene is presenilin 2.

Whereas several genes have been identified as candidates in autosomal dominant transmission of early-onset AD, no such inherited mutations have yet been described for the much more common late-onset form of the disease.

Treatment

Attempts at augmenting cholinergic neurotransmission have made use of acetylcholinesterase (AChE) inhibitors, cholinergic agonists, ACh precursors, and ACh-releasing agents. The reversible AChE inhibitor tacrine was approved by the U.S. Food and Drug Administration in 1993 for the treatment of AD. Most studies of this drug report modest positive results in cognitive measures without major improvements in activities of daily living.

Selegiline, a monoamine oxidase-B inhibitor, improves performance on attention, memory, and learning tasks. Studies to improve cognitive function by combining selegiline and tacrine show contradictory results.

Nootropics are drugs thought to enhance cognition by ameliorating cellular metabolic processes. Piracetam, the prototype nootropic, may, in high doses, slow cognitive deterioration in AD. Acetyl-L-carnitine (ALC) is a naturally occurring substance involved in mitochondrial energy processing. Double-blind placebo-controlled studies suggest that ALC slows cognitive deterioration in AD. Donepezil, an AChE inhibitor, has been shown to improve patient attention and mental focus.

For a more detailed discussion see Matalon R, Kaul R, Michals K. Canavan Disease (Chapter 27; pp. 493–502); Conner KE, Rosenberg RN. The Genetic Basis of Ataxia (Chapter 28; pp. 503–544); Koroshetz WJ, Martin JB. Huntington's Disease (Chapter 29; pp. 545–564); Shoulson I, Kurlan R. Inherited Disorders of the Basal Ganglia (Chapter 30; pp. 565–579); Morrison-Bogorad M, Weiner MF, Rosenberg RN, Bigio E, White CL III. Alzheimer's Disease (Chapter 31; pp. 581–600); Selkoe DJ, Cellular and Molecular Biology of the Beta-Amyloid Precursor Protein and Alzheimer's Disease (Chapter 32; pp. 601–611); Goedert M, Trojanowski JQ, Lee VM-Y. The Neurofibrillary Pathology of Alzheimer's Disease (Chapter 33; pp. 613–627), in RN Rosenberg, SB Prusiner, S DiMauro, RL Barchi (eds), **The Molecular and Genetic Basis of Neurological Disease** *(2nd ed). Boston: Butterworth–Heinemann, 1997.*

8

Multiple Sclerosis

Multiple sclerosis (MS) is the prototypic demyelinating disease in humans. It is an inflammatory disorder believed to result from an autoimmune response directed against myelin proteins and other unidentified antigens. An underlying genetic susceptibility in concert with an undefined environmental exposure is believed to play a role in the pathogenesis.

CLINICAL FEATURES

The onset may be sudden or develop slowly over months or years. Common features are weakness of one or more limbs, visual blurring caused by optic neuritis or diplopia, sensory disturbances, vertigo or dizziness, bladder or bowel disturbances, and cognitive disorders. Several clinical forms of MS are identified. Relapsing-remitting MS is characterized by recurrent attacks of neurologic dysfunction that evolve over days or weeks and are followed by complete, partial, or no recovery. Secondary progressive MS begins as a relapsing-remitting disease but evolves into a gradually progressive course. The progressive phase may begin shortly after disease onset or may be delayed for years or decades. Primary progressive MS is characterized by gradual progression of disability from onset; periods of apparent disease stability may occur, but there are no distinct relapses. This form accounts for less than 15% of all MS and is more common in men. Onset is after age 40 years.

Fifteen years after diagnosis, approximately 20% of all MS patients have no functional limitation, 70% are limited or unable to perform major activities of daily living, and 75% are not employed.

PATHOLOGIC FEATURES

The main feature of MS is the *plaque*; a well-demarcated lesion characterized by complete myelin loss, an absence of oligodendrocytes, and relative sparing of axons. However, the location and size of plaques do not correlate with clinical severity. Plaques are multiple, generally asymmetric, and usually concentrated in the deep white matter. New plaques have perivascular and parenchymal infiltration of T cells and macrophages, and myelin breakdown that appears mediated by the infiltrating cells. B cells and plasma cells are rare. Evolving lesions are traversed by axons with marked irregular beading. Astrocytic proliferation occurs, and lipid-laden macrophages containing myelin debris are prominent. Progressive fibrillary gliosis follows, and mononuclear cells gradually disappear. Oligodendrocyte proliferation is sometimes present initially, but the cells are destroyed as gliosis progresses. Chronic lesions show complete or nearly complete demyelination, dense gliosis, and loss of oligodendroglia.

The earliest event in plaque development is increased permeability of the blood-brain barrier associated with inflammation. Myelin is the primary target of the pathologic immune reaction. Oligodendrocytes are preserved in early lesions of relapsing MS but not in chronic lesions or in early aggressive cases. Later, oligodendrocytes and astrocytes at the periphery of the plaque proliferate. These oligodendrocytes continue to function as myelinating cells. When inflammation decreases, the edema disappears and conduction is restored. Remyelination is not essential to remission. Astrogliosis in MS is considerable compared to other conditions. It occurs not only in and around the plaque but also in normal-appearing white matter. Astrocytic proliferation is probably triggered by cytokines elaborated as part of the inflammatory response.

Upregulation of major histocompatibility complex (MHC) molecules has been proposed as a marker of plaque activity. Class I MHC antigens are identified in plaque tissue on endothelial cells, infiltrating lymphocytes, and astroglia, whereas class II determinants are expressed on endothelial cells, macrophages, and microglia. High expression of MHC class II molecules in MS brains suggests that the local microenvironment may be enriched in MHC-activating factors such as interferon-gamma (IFN-γ), and that antigen is possibly presented to T cells. Many silent plaques are devoid of T-cell infiltrates, however, and class II MHC antigens may be expressed at high levels on reactive microglia.

NATURE OF INFILTRATING T CELLS

T cells in the parenchyma and in the perivascular cuffs consist of CD8 (suppressor/cytotoxic) cells and CD4 (helper/inducer) cells. Most CD4/CD8 T cells in MS brains bear the common form of the antigen cell receptor—that is, the α/β heterodimer. The T cell receptor (TCR) is expressed on the surface of mature T lymphocytes that subserves T cell recognition by fragments of antigen associated with MHC molecules. Complementary determining regions (CDR), specifically CDR3 regions, play a critical role in peptide recognition. Modeling of the trimolecular interaction between the TCR, the MHC-antigen presenting molecules, and bound antigenic peptide suggests that the CDRs, CDR1 and CDR2, of the TCR interact primarily with the alpha helical regions of the MHC and provide the structural framework and topology for the interaction of a particular CDR3 region, (N)Jα and (N)Dβ(N)Jβ, with the peptide bound in the MHC cleft.

IMMUNOLOGY

Cellular and Humoral Studies in Multiple Sclerosis

The candidate antigenic targets of the autoimmune response are the quantitatively major myelin proteins myelin basic protein (MBP) and proteolipid protein (PLP), the minor myelin protein myelin oligodendrocyte glycoprotein, and myelin lipids or nonmyelin proteins of the central nervous system. MBP is the most likely candidate because it is known to be highly encephalitogenic (immunogenic) in animal models of autoimmune demyelination. The TCR molecules that appear to be derived from MBP-reactive T cells have been identified in lesions of MS. MBP-reactive T cells can be recovered from the circulation of MS patients but not from the circulation of controls when selected under conditions that permit only expansion of cells that carry mutations in a marker gene; this suggests that these cells have undergone chronic stimulation in vivo. T cells reactive against both MBP and PLP appear to be concentrated in CSF compared with their frequency in peripheral blood, suggesting that they home selectively to the CNS in MS patients. In addition to autoreactive T cells, autoantibodies may play a role in the pathogenesis of MS. Most MS patients have an increased concentration of intrathecally synthesized immunoglobulin in the central nervous system. The specificity of these antibodies is unknown.

Role of Cytokines

During the process of lesion formation, cytokines, growth factors, and other small molecules such as nitric oxide induce and regulate critical cell functions, including cell recruitment and migration, cell proliferation, and cell death. Several cytokines regulate the activation, differentiation, and proliferation of T lymphocytes. Under their influence, cells differentiate into two major pathways. T helper (h) 1 cells produce interleukin (IL)-2, IL-3, tumor necrosis factor-beta (TNF-β), and IFN-γ. Th2 cells produce IL-3, IL-4, IL-5, and IL-10. A third subset of T cells, Th0, with a pattern of cytokine production overlapping both Th1 and Th2, may represent a precursor population. In contrast to Th1 cells, Th2 cells depend on IL-4 rather than IL-2 for their autocrine growth and can proliferate to anti-CD3 antibodies in the absence of accessory cells. Several proinflammatory cytokines are detected in brain, peripheral blood, and CSF of MS patients; these may constitute a functional network that regulates the cellular interactions operating in MS.

Establishment of Inflammatory Foci

In experimental allergic encephalitis (EAE), the establishment of inflammatory lesions and clinical disease is a multistep event. The first step requires that activated T cells cross the blood-brain barrier. Activated lymphocytes that bear a memory phenotype, suggesting previous activation by antigen, become attached to appropriate receptors on endothelial cells at parajunctional areas, adjacent to the endothelial tight junctions and then pass directly into the interstitial matrix. Next, specific CD4+ T cells are reactivated in situ by fragments of myelin antigens presented in the framework of MHC class II molecules on the surface of antigen-presenting cells (macrophages, microglia, and perhaps astrocytes). This leads to a second wave of inflammatory recruitment and clinical EAE. Proinflammatory cytokines such as TNF-α and IFN-γ are probably key mediators of the full inflammatory response. Encephalitogenic, myelin-specific T cells may not be capable of mediating symptomatic EAE in the absence of this secondary leukocyte recruitment. T cells and antibodies may act synergistically to promote demyelination.

VIROLOGY

Experimental demyelinating disease can result from chronic viral infection of oligodendrocytes in animals, and the possibility of an environmental exposure in MS is suggested by epidemiologic studies. Measles virus and a human retrovirus related to human T-cell leukemia (HTLV)-1 have been suspected but never proved as causes. Several nonviral microorganisms or their toxins, including prions, have been implicated in demyelination but never confirmed. Mechanisms that may explain a pathogen-MS interaction are polyclonal activation of T and B cells, infection and destruction of regulatory cells, exposure of sequestered or modified antigens, and molecular mimicry. *Molecular mimicry* refers to the initiation of an autoimmune response because of sequence or structural homologies between a self-protein and a protein in a viral or bacterial pathogen.

Superantigens are associated with numerous human diseases, such as food poisoning, toxic-shock syndrome, and scalded skin syndrome. The involvement of exogenous superantigens as etiologic agents in several autoimmune diseases is the subject of active investigation. Many autoimmune diseases are exacerbated, and perhaps even preceded, by infections.

EPIDEMIOLOGY

MS is twice as common in females than in males. Onset is typically in early to middle adulthood. Ten percent of cases begin before age 18 years. Onset as early as age 2 years or as late as the eighth decade of life has been reported. Mean age of onset in men is slightly later than in women. In general, MS is a disease of temperate climates. In both the northern and southern hemispheres, the prevalence of MS decreases with decreasing latitude. These data support a possible environmental effect, an effect also supported by migration data. Children born to parents who have migrated from a high-risk area to a low-risk area have a lower lifetime risk than their parents. The converse is also true. Some migration studies suggest that the critical time of the suspected exposure occurs before age 15 years. The final evidence for an environmental effect on MS is derived from a small number of apparent point epidemics that have been reported. The most convincing occurred among the native population of the Faroe Islands, off the coast of Scotland, after the British military occupation during World War II.

GENETICS

Evidence of a genetic effect on susceptibility to MS is found in studies of different ethnic groups and in family, adoption, and twin studies. Differences in the prevalence of MS among different ethnic groups that reside in the same environment support an underlying genetic predisposition. The highest reported prevalence of MS, estimated at 250 cases per 100,000 population, occurs in the Orkney Islands, north of Scotland. MS is also highly prevalent throughout northern Europe, in particular Ireland and Scandinavia. In the United States, the prevalence is higher among whites than in other racial groups. MS is uncommon in Japan (2 per 100,000) and among black Africans. The low risk in these groups has been thought to represent genetic resistance. Japanese-Americans residing in Hawaii are at higher risk for MS than are their counterparts in Japan. The prevalence of MS in black Americans is approximately one-third that in white Americans.

Familial aggregation occurs in MS, resulting in an increased risk among first-, second-, and third-degree relatives of patients. The most convincing data that susceptibility to MS is inherited are derived from studies of twins. The risk of MS to a monozygotic twin of an MS patient is approximately 20–25%, whereas the risk to a fraternal twin is similar to the risk to a nontwin sibling. Analysis of pooled data from MS families suggests that a simple model of inheritance is unlikely. It is likely that susceptibility is determined by multiple interacting loci (polygenic inheritance), each with a relatively small contribution to overall risk.

Candidate Genes

Most attempts to identify the MS susceptibility genes focused on those polymorphic genes whose products participate in the immune response, such as the genes constituting the MHC on chromosome 6, TCR genes on chromosomes 7 and 14, and immunoglobulin genes. Suggestive correlations between certain alleles at these loci and the presence of MS have been described, but the results are conflicting.

For a more detailed discussion see Seboun E, Oksenberg JR, Hauser SL. Molecular and Genetic Aspects of Multiple Sclerosis (Chapter 34; pp. 631–660), in RN Rosenberg, SB Prusiner, S DiMauro, RL Barchi (eds),* The Molecular and Genetic Basis of Neurological Disease *(2nd ed). Boston: Butterworth–Heinemann, 1997.

9

Neuro-Oncology

ONCOGENES

Oncogenes are mutant versions of normal growth regulatory genes. The normal cellular sequences involved in regulation of growth and differentiation from which oncogenes are derived are called *proto-oncogenes*. Normal cell proliferation is under the intrinsic control of proto-oncogenes (positive regulators) and tumor suppressor genes (negative regulators). Oncogenes encode proteins that are classified into seven types based on their physiologic function: growth factors, receptors and nonreceptor protein-tyrosine kinases, receptors lacking protein kinase activity, membrane-associated G proteins, cytoplasmic protein-serine kinases, cytoplasmic regulators, and nuclear transcription factors.

Proto-Oncogene Activation

Three different genetic alterations activate proto-oncogenes implicated in human neoplasms: (1) functional mutations within the coding sequences, (2) transcriptional activation due to chromosomal translocation or adjacent insertion of proviral sequences, and (3) increased expression as a result of an increase in the number of copies or amplification of oncogenes.

Central Nervous System Tumors

Gliomas and medulloblastomas are the two most common types of central nervous system (CNS) tumors in adults and children. Low-grade gliomas include astrocytomas, oligodendrogliomas, and ependymomas. Malignant gliomas are anaplastic astrocytoma and glioblastoma multiforme (GBM). Medulloblastomas are also called primitive neuroectodermal tumors. All three mechanisms of oncogene activation occur in gliomas. The most common mechanism of activation in gliomas and medulloblastomas is gene amplification of the proto-oncogenes epidermal growth factor receptor gene (*EGFR*) and C-*MYC* genes.

Amplification, rearrangement, and overexpression of the *EGFR* gene is seen in approximately 40% of GBMs. *EGFR* amplification appears to be important in tumor progression because amplification is almost exclusively seen in high-grade gliomas. However, attempts to correlate *EGFR* amplification with survival rate have been largely negative. Approximately 10% of high-grade tumors exhibit amplification of the *CDK4* gene, which is involved in the regulation of cell cycle. Amplification of *MDM2*, *GLI*, and *PDGFR-α* genes is seen in isolated cases. Expression of a variety of growth factors is documented in subgroups of tumors, and autocrine stimulation pathways may play a role in aggressive growth. The C-*MYC* gene is amplified in a few primary medulloblastomas, but the incidence is higher in medulloblastoma-derived cell lines.

NEUROBLASTOMA

Etiology

Neuroblastoma is almost exclusively a disease of childhood. It is thought to arise in neuroblasts, primitive neural crest–derived cells that differentiate along a neuronal pathway. Most neuroblastoma tumor cell lines correspond to cells differentiating along a chromaffin lineage, the major neural crest–derived cell type in the mature adrenal medulla. In contrast, differentiation in vivo is invariably along a ganglionic pathway.

Clinical Features

Most neuroblastomas arise in the adrenal medulla and other sites of known sympathetic nervous system tissue. Eighty-five percent are in the abdomen and 15% in the thoracic cavity. Low-stage, anatomically limited disease is most common in young children. Metastatic disease is present at presentation in 60–70% of patients. Neuroblastoma disseminates most commonly to the cortex of long and flat bones, regional lymph nodes, liver, bone marrow, and subcutaneous tissue. The clinical findings at presentation depend on the location of the tumor. Children with disseminated neuroblastoma are often cachexic, pale, and in substantial pain from marrow and bone metastases. Thoracic neuroblastomas are often identified as a posterior mediastinal mass found incidentally on chest radiographs. Occasional tumors occur as a paraspinal mass that invades the intervertebral foramina ("dumbbell tumor"), causing signs of spinal cord compression. Primary thoracic tumors can also cause superior vena cava syndrome, persistent watery diarrhea, or Horner's syndrome. The syndrome of opsoclonus-myoclonus is an immune-mediated response to thoracic or abdominal neuroblastoma.

Genetic Features

Nearly 80% of neuroblastomas have a chromosomal abnormality. The most common abnormality is a deletion or rearrangement of the short arm of chromosome 1. In some tumors, the deleted 1p material is preferentially replaced by material from chromosome 17q, resulting from an unbalanced 1;17 translocation. The chromosomal rearrangements in neuroblastomas of greatest importance are homogeneously staining regions (HSRs) and double minute (DM) chromosomes, indicating gene amplification. The N-*myc* gene, which has considerable homology to the cellular proto-oncogene c-*myc*, is amplified within HSRs and DM chromosomes found in neuroblastoma-derived cell lines and tumor specimens and has considerable clinical significance.

Molecular Biology

The tumor appears to arise in close association with a disturbance of the differentiation of primitive neural crest cells. Neurotrophic factors acting through specific cell surface receptors play a critical role in the survival and differentiation of normal sympathetic neuroblasts. However, their role in the pathogenesis of neuroblastoma is uncertain. Analysis of the expression of neurotrophic factors and their receptors in neuroblastoma tumors provides prognostic information. Expression of Trk A, the high-affinity receptor for nerve growth factor, is strongly predictive of a favorable outcome. Many aggressive neuroblastomas, especially those with N-*myc* amplification, express both Trk B and its ligand BDNF. The almost mutually exclusive expression of Trk A and Trk B and the different outcomes associated with these two markers suggest a role for these receptors in tumorigenesis.

Insulin-like growth factor II (IGF II) is a major mitogenic signal for the growth of neuroblastoma tumor cells. IGF II expression is detected in infiltrating and adjacent normal tissues, including normal adrenal cortical tissue. Many proto-oncogenes, especially N-*myc*, are expressed in neuroblastoma tumor cell lines and tissue specimens. Amplification of N-*myc* is regarded as a marker of poor prognosis.

Treatment

Low-grade tumors are treated by surgical excision alone. Radiation therapy is added for somewhat higher-grade tumors, and chemotherapy is reserved for the highest-grade tumors that are not resectable.

PERIPHERAL NEUROEPITHELIOMA

Peripheral neuroepithelioma is also called *adult neuroblastoma, peripheral neuroblastoma,* and *primitive neuroectodermal tumor of the chest wall.*

Clinical Features and Treatment

Peripheral neuroepithelioma occurs at all ages, with a peak in the second decade. The initial features of thoracic peripheral neuroepithelioma are pleural-based masses with or without pleural effusion and rib erosion. Spinal cord compression from a paraspinal mass is a less common presentation. Peripheral neuroepithelioma tends to recur locally, although it can be metastatic to the lungs and bones either at presentation or at recurrence. The typical survival of patients with metastatic disease is approximately 8 months even when a multimodality approach to therapy consisting of surgery, radiation, and chemotherapy is used. Aggressive treatment for patients with metastatic disease or with tumors recognized as likely to recur include ablative chemotherapy with bone marrow rescue.

Genetic Features

Approximately 85% of tumors show a characteristic chromosomal translocation, rcp(11;22)(q24;q12). As a consequence of this translocation, the region of a gene coding the NH_2-terminal portion of a newly described, ubiquitously expressed protein of unknown function, termed *EWS,* is fused to a distal region of the FLI-1 gene, which encodes a member of the Ets transcription factor family. The chimeric EWS–FLI-1 molecule is important in the oncogenesis of neuroepithelioma. Detection of chimeric EWS–FLI-1 transcripts is the basis of a sensitive and specific diagnostic assay.

NEUROFIBROMATOSIS TYPE 1

Neurofibromatosis type 1 (NF1) is also called *Von Recklinghausen disease* and mainly affects the skin and peripheral nerves. It is transmitted by autosomal dominant inheritance.

Genetic Clues to Pathogenesis

The high and uniform frequency of NF1 worldwide is compatible with both a low phenotypic burden and a high mutation rate. The high mutation rate (approximately 1 per 10,000 meioses per generation) suggests that the locus is large, that it has an intrinsically high susceptibility to mutation, or both. More than 90% of the nondeletion mutations are derived from the father. For large deletions, maternal and paternal origins are almost equal in frequency. Expression of the mutation is the same whether one parent is affected or the mutation is new. The variable expressivity of a mutant NF1 gene appears to be determined by nongenetic factors. Penetrance is complete once the mutation occurs. A predecessor syndrome exists in which NF1 features are limited in terms of type or distribution.

Clinical Features

Pigmentation abnormalities are the most consistent and earliest features of NF1. Café-au-lait spots (CLS) occur in 99% of patients and freckling in at least 75% of adult patients. Although six or more CLS indicate the diagnosis of NF1, the number is usually larger after 1 year of age. CLS are unlikely to be seen on the face, and the largest ones are more likely on the buttocks. Otherwise, the distribution of CLS over the body is random. Freckling is seen in skin folds or where there is frequent friction.

Almost all patients with NF1 have cutaneous neurofibromas, particularly on the upper trunk and arms. Adult females have a high likelihood of neurofibromas on the nipples or areolae, and the shins are spared in both sexes. The absence of subcutaneous fat may decrease likelihood that cutaneous neurofibromas develop. Diffuse plexiform neurofibromas are congenital lesions, whereas cutaneous and subcutaneous neurofibromas as well as nodular plexiform neurofibromas generally develop during or after the second decade. Many neurofibromas increase in size, but growth is not inevitable. An acceleration of neurofibroma growth occurs during puberty and pregnancy and after trauma.

CNS tumors of NF1 are almost all astrocytomas, and most are restricted to the optic pathway. The entire optic pathway is at risk; the frequency of such tumors is approximately 15%. The treatment of optic pathway gliomas is not established. Cerebral and spinal cord gliomas or astrocytomas occur with increased frequency in NF1, but malignant tumors are the most important complications of NF1 because they contribute substantially to mortality.

Molecular Features

Chromosome 17q11.2.7 is the site of the NF1 gene. The gene product is neurofibromin, which is a member of a family of proteins called *guanosine triphosphatase (GTPase)–activating proteins (GAPs)*. GAP proteins down-regulate small GTPase proteins. One of these, the p21-ras proto-oncogene, a target for neurofibromin down-regulation has a tumor suppressor function. Ras is a central proto-oncogene that, when mutated to become an oncogene, is expressed in as many as 30% of human malignancies. Ras proteins are in their active form when bound to GTP and inactive when bound to GDP. Neurofibromin and other GAP proteins accelerate this conversion of ras from its active GTP-bound confirmation to its inactive GDP-bound form.

The NF1 gene is thought to be a tumor suppressor gene. Tumor suppressor genes are genes whose expression is sufficiently reduced in tumors that they are no longer able to suppress cell growth. Individuals born with NF1 harbor one mutated copy of the NF1 gene in all cells in their body. A second somatic mutation must occur in the remaining "normal" copy of the NF1 gene to render both copies nonfunctional.

Diagnostic Testing

The purpose of a molecular test is to identify the presence of a mutation, and the test is primarily indicated when the issue is family planning. The test is not needed to confirm the clinical diagnosis of NF1. The protein truncation assay, with a 70% mutation detection rate, is best—and perhaps solely—useful for childbearing decisions.

Treatment

The treatment of NF1 is a matter of minimizing symptoms, generally in a nonspecific manner (e.g., using anticonvulsants for seizures, ventriculoperitoneal shunting for hydrocephalus, surgical removal of tumor, radiotherapy for optic pathway gliomas).

NEUROFIBROMATOSIS TYPE 2

The key feature of NF2 is the presence of CNS tumors, almost always including bilateral acoustic neuromas (actually vestibular schwannomas). NF2 is an autosomal dominant disorder occurring at an estimated frequency of 1 per 50,000. The genetic defect is on chromosome 22q.

Clinical Features

The hallmark of NF2 is the development of bilateral vestibular schwannomas derived from Schwann cells surrounding the vestibular branch of the eighth cranial nerve. Vestibular schwannomas are inherited with a penetrance of at least 95%. The risk for an offspring of an affected parent is almost 50%. The main clinical features of vestibular schwannomas is deafness. Other typical tumors associated with NF2 include meningiomas, gliomas, ependymomas, trigeminal nerve schwannomas, and spinal nerve root schwannomas. Vestibular schwannomas and meningiomas in NF2 occur at an earlier age (typically in the second and third decades) than their sporadic counterparts (fourth and fifth decades). Astrocytomas of the brain, particularly of the optic pathway, are distinctly unusual.

Skin tumors are predominantly schwannomas, although at least occasionally neurofibromas may also be present. Diffuse plexiform neurofibromas are unusual. Skin hyperpigmentation is very variable, ranging from none to faint patches to typical CLS. When present, the hyperpigmented patches may be much larger than is typical of NF1. Freckling is not a feature of NF2. Ocular findings are typically posterior subcapsular cataracts.

In addition to a careful neurologic examination, studies especially useful for either diagnosis or ongoing assessment of clinical status include cranial magnetic resonance imaging scans and brain stem auditory evoked response testing or other measurements of eighth cranial nerve function.

Genetic Clues to Pathogenesis

NF2 is an autosomal dominant trait with its locus in the 11.2 band of the long arm of chromosome 22. One-half of all cases are probably new mutations, in contrast to no more than one-third for NF1. Although its penetrance is nearly 100%, the expression of the NF2 mutation is extremely variable. Genetic heterogeneity is well established, with schwannomatosis shown to be an allelic form. Both very mild and severe forms of ordinary NF2 are also candidates to be allelic alternatives.

Pathologic Clues to Pathogenesis

Neurofibromas from patients with NF1 and NF2 have the same histologic appearance. Fibromas in patients with NF2, however, show loss of heterozygosity for chromosome 22 DNA markers, and fibromas in patients with NF1 show no loss of heterozygosity for chromosome 17 DNA markers. The relatively consistent finding of schwannomas at the entrance or exit from bony foramina may indicate that Schwann cells at the junction in this position are different, or that mechanical forces at the foramina contribute a stimulus to proliferation of local Schwann cells, which, when coupled with a somatic mutation, leads to neoplastic proliferation.

Molecular Features

The NF2 gene is on chromosome 22q11.2 and codes for a 2.2-kb messenger RNA and a 595-amino-acid protein called *MERLIN*. The sequence of MERLIN shows a striking sequence similarity to a family of proteins that link cell membrane glycoproteins with the actin filaments and may be involved in remodeling of cell shape. Mutations in the MERLIN gene have been demonstrated for both NF2-related and sporadic meningiomas, NF2-related and sporadic schwannomas, breast cancer, and colon cancer.

Diagnostic Testing

NF2 molecular testing can detect approximately 90% of all the mutations. The main point of the test is to document the absence of the mutant gene. Children born to an individual with NF2 should be screened to determine the need for close follow-up.

Treatment

The treatment of NF2 is largely the treatment of tumors to minimize their adverse effects. The primary approach is surgical. Chemotherapy for meningiomas and ependymomas is sometimes indicated, but it has no role in the treatment of schwannomas.

VON HIPPEL-LINDAU DISEASE

von Hippel-Lindau (VHL) disease is a devastating hereditary tumor syndrome involving multiple organ systems. It is an inherited autosomal dominant trait with almost complete penetrance. Both genders are affected equally.

Clinical Features

VHL disease is characterized by an inherited susceptibility to cerebellar and spinal cord hemangioblastomas, angiomas of the retina, multifocal and bilateral renal cell carcinoma, pheochromocytoma, islet cell tumors of the pancreas, and multiple cysts of the kidney, pancreas, ovaries, and other organs. These lesions may appear in any combination or sequence in an individual with the VHL phenotype. The most frequent cause of death in VHL disease is renal cell carcinoma. The initial features are variable and the age of onset is from the first to the seventh decades.

Molecular Features

The VHL gene is on the tip of chromosome 3p. The sequence of the cloned human VHL cDNA predicts a protein with no significant sequence or potential structural homology to any known protein. Mutations have been identified in 40–75% of VHL families examined. Approximately 15% of these are large deletions or rearrangements within the gene.

Some families are predisposed primarily to renal cell carcinomas in combination with retinal angiomas and hemangioblastomas of the CNS, whereas others show predominantly pheochromocytomas in combination with the same CNS tumors. Three VHL subtypes are recognized: type 1, VHL disease without pheochromocytoma; type 2A, VHL disease with pheochromocytoma; and type 2B, VHL disease with pheochromocytoma and renal cell carcinoma. Nearly all families with VHL type 2 possess missense mutations within the gene, whereas families with VHL type 1 have small insertions, deletions, or premature stop codons, all of which predict truncated proteins.

VHL mutations have been detected not only in renal cell carcinomas and other tumor types from patients with VHL, but also in 30–60% of sporadic renal cell carcinomas. The VHL gene is mutated even in families with only renal cell carcinoma. The VHL gene is structurally or functionally inactivated in most sporadic renal cell carcinomas and is therefore the most frequently mutated gene in this tumor type.

For a more detailed discussion see Rasheed BKA, Bigner SH. Oncogenes in Neuro-Oncology (Chapter 35; pp. 663–674); Lasorella A, Israel MA. Tumors of Neuronal Cell Origin (Chapter 36; pp. 675–681); Kley N, Seizinger BR. Hereditary Tumor Syndromes of the Nervous System: The Neurofibromatosis Type 2 and von Hippel-Lindau Tumor Suppressor Genes (from Gene Cloning to Function) (Chapter 37; pp. 683–692); Riccardi VM, Gutmann DH. The Clinical and Molecular Genetics of Neurofibromatosis Types 1 and 2 (Chapter 38; pp. 693–712), in RN Rosenberg, SB Prusiner, S DiMauro, RL Barchi (eds), **The Molecular and Genetic Basis of Neurological Disease** ***(2nd ed). Boston: Butterworth–Heinemann, 1997.***

10

Ion Channel Disorders

Muscle contraction occurs when signals arriving at the neuromuscular junction are successfully coupled to the release of Ca^{2+} from the sarcoplasmic reticulum. This coupling requires the spread of an action potential across the muscle fiber surface membrane and into the T-tubular system and the activation of signaling molecules at the t-system triad. Should this process fail, muscle paralysis results in spite of normal neuromuscular junctions and contractile protein function. Each step in the pathway from activity at the neuromuscular junction to eventual muscle contraction involves membrane ion channels.

Three cation channels that play central roles in skeletal muscle excitation are the voltage-dependent sodium channel, the L-type voltage-gated calcium channel, and the calcium channel. The coding region for the skeletal muscle sodium channel (SCN4) is located on chromosome 17q23, and the gene for the skeletal muscle chloride channel (ClC-1) is on chromosome 7q35. The sodium channel controls the conductance changes responsible for the membrane action potential, whereas the calcium channel links membrane excitation to intracellular calcium release. Diseases that affect muscle membrane excitability can be divided into two groups: those in which the sarcolemma is hyperexcitable, responding to normal depolarizations with long trains of action potentials (myotonic discharges), and those in which the membrane is intermittently hypoexcitable, leading to muscle weakness or paralysis. Either phenotype can result from abnormalities in a single key membrane protein, and conversely, similar signs and symptoms may be caused by defects in a number of different channel proteins.

MYOTONIA CONGENITA

Myotonia is impaired muscle relaxation after voluntary contraction caused by an electrical instability of the muscle plasma membrane. A single stimulus leads to a train of action potentials instead of a single action potential. These "myotonic runs" cause the defect in muscle relaxation.

Clinical Features

Myotonia congenita is characterized only by myotonia. It is not precipitated by cold or by high potassium concentration, and dystrophy is not associated. An autosomal dominant form, Thomsen's disease, and an autosomal recessive form, Becker myotonia, are recognized. In both forms, myotonia is worse after rest following voluntary contraction and improves after continued exercise. In addition to the difference in inheritance, the two disorders differ clinically by the age of onset, by the spreading of myotonia to different muscle groups, and by a typical transitory muscle weakness in the recessive form. Myotonia congenita must be distinguished from autosomal dominant myotonic dystrophy, in which weakness and systemic disturbances are present, paramyotonia congenita, in which myotonia is precipitated by exposure to cold, and hyperkalemic periodic paralysis.

Biochemical and Molecular Features

Both the recessive and the dominant forms of myotonia congenita are the result of mutations in the skeletal muscle chloride channel ClC-1. Chloride conductance is unusually high in skeletal muscle and accounts for approximately 70–80% of the resting conductance of its plasma membrane. Because the equilibrium potential for chloride is close to the resting potential, it stabilizes the membrane potential. Chloride conductance contributes significantly to the repolarization of muscle action potentials and is essential for the electrical stability of the muscle fiber. Inhibition of muscle chloride channels is responsible for the myotonic run.

More than 20 different disease-causing mutations are identified in the human ClC-1 gene, and many more may exist. Certain mutations in the same gene lead to recessive disease and others to dominant disease. A total loss-of-function mutation will probably reduce muscle chloride conductance to approximately 50% in a heterozygote. This level of conductance is still sufficient to ensure muscle membrane stability. The fact that total loss of function of the gene product of one allele results in recessive disease implies that the dominant mutations found in Thomsen's disease must interfere with the functional expression from the normal allele.

THE PERIODIC PARALYSES

The periodic paralyses are transmitted by autosomal dominant inheritance and characterized by intermittent episodes of weakness or paralysis, often with apparently normal muscle function between attacks. The episodes of weakness are often accompanied by shifts in serum potassium concentration. During an attack, the concentration may consistently fall (hypokalemic periodic paralysis), rise (hyperkalemic periodic paralysis), or remain unchanged (normokalemic periodic paralysis). Some families also express occasional myotonic features, whereas in other cases myotonia is the principal complaint and the paralytic episodes are rare (paramyotonia congenita).

Clinical Features

Hypokalemic periodic paralysis is the most common form. Paralytic episodes usually begin during early childhood and often have their onset during the night. Attacks of weakness can be so severe as to cause transitory quadriplegia. Respiration is not usually impaired. Episodes last from hours to days and are precipitated by rest after exercise, cold exposure, excitement, and carbohydrate loading. Administration of glucose and insulin will often trigger paralysis and can be used as a provocative test. The administration of oral potassium can shorten the duration of attacks and reduce the frequency of future attacks.

In hyperkalemic periodic paralysis, episodes of weakness or paralysis begin in the first decade and may decline in frequency with age. Attacks are more frequent but are briefer in duration and milder in severity than in the hypokalemic form. Residual weakness may linger after attacks, and some individuals develop irreversible myopathic weakness. Attacks may be precipitated by rest after exercise, immobility, potassium ingestion, irregular diet, cold exposure, or emotional stress. Myotonia, an associated feature in some families, may occur only after cold exposure or at normal ambient temperature.

Individuals affected with paramyotonia congenita have myotonic symptoms on cold exposure and little or no symptoms in a warm environment. Onset is in childhood and improvement may occur with age. Cooling greatly increases the severity of the myotonic stiffness and can lead to weakness and even paralysis. Both myotonia and paralysis are reversible with rewarming, after a lag of minutes to hours. A common complaint is myotonic stiffness of the facial muscles during cold weather. Unlike other myotonic disorders, the myotonia in paramyotonia congenita is worse after continued exercise.

Biochemical and Molecular Features

Mutations in the calcium channel gene are responsible for hypokalemic periodic paralysis, whereas mutations in the sodium channel gene (SCN4A) have been identified in hyperkalemic periodic paralysis and paramyotonia congenita. An atypical form of painful myotonia congenita has been linked to SCN4A (see Sodium Channel Myotonia).

Sodium Channel Myotonia

The sodium channel myotonias (SCMs) resemble myotonia congenita in their clinical and electrophysiologic features but are associated with sodium rather than chloride channel gene mutations.

Clinical Features

The symptoms of SCMs resemble dominantly inherited myotonia congenita. In some families, the myotonia fluctuates in intensity from day to day, and in others, myotonia is associated with muscle pain. Paralytic episodes or weakness do not occur. The myotonia improves with exercise.

Molecular Features

SCN4A point mutations have now been identified in several SCMs.

MALIGNANT HYPERTHERMIA

Malignant hyperthermia (MH) is inherited as an autosomal dominant mutation. It is a disease of abnormal Ca^{2+} regulation.

Clinical Features

An MH crisis is a response to the administration of potent inhalational anesthetics and depolarizing skeletal muscle relaxants. It is characterized by a rising end tidal CO_2, skeletal muscle rigidity, tachycardia, unstable and rising blood pressure, hyperventilation, cyanosis, a falling Pao_2 (arterial oxygen tension), an increasing $Paco_2$ (arterial carbon dioxide tension), lactic acidosis, and, eventually, fever. Cellular damage causes electrolyte imbalance with an early rise in serum potassium and calcium concentrations, then a fall, and finally, a marked rise in the serum and urine concentrations of creatine kinase and myoglobin. Without immediate treatment, death occurs within minutes of ventricular fibrillation, within hours of pulmonary edema or coagulopathy, or within days of neurologic damage (postanoxic cerebral edema) or obstructive renal failure from the release of myoglobin into the circulation.

Individuals who have MH reactions may have had previous uneventful general anesthesias. Why a crisis is not precipitated by a first exposure is uncertain, but it may be that an additional environmental trigger, other than anesthetic agents, is needed to initiate a reaction.

Emergency Treatment

When MH occurs, the triggering anesthetic should be stopped immediately, the gas machine changed, or if this is not possible, the soda lime, corrugated anesthetic tubing, and ventilating bag must be changed. The antidote, dantrolene, should be administered at a dosage of 1 mg/kg/minute until muscle tone softens; fever, heart rate, and respiratory rate decline significantly toward normal; and blood gas concentrations normalize. Regular insulin may be infused if serum potassium and blood glucose concentrations are elevated. Furosemide and mannitol are infused to prevent the onset of acute renal failure and to prevent muscle and brain edema. These practices have lowered the death rate from MH episodes from more than 80% to less than 7%.

Diagnostic Tests

Several tests have been developed to determine susceptibility to MH. The most sensitive is the in vitro testing of muscle fascile contracture to caffeine or halothane. These tests are based on the premise that the muscle from MHS individuals might be more sensitive to agents inducing contractures. Problems with such tests are that they are invasive and expensive to perform. The false-positive error rate is significant and the false-negative error rate is small. They are rarely used in clinical practice; instead, patients thought to be at risk are pretreated with dantrolene.

Biochemical and Molecular Features

Blood chemistry studies showed that lactic acidosis, presumably originating in glycogenolysis and glycolysis, and the release of K^+, Mg^{2+}, and Ca^{2+} from muscle occur within seconds of the time that halothane reaches the muscle. The interaction of actin and myosin is regulated by Ca^{2+} and that Ca^{2+} regulation is mediated through the Ca^{2+} binding protein troponin. Muscle Ca^{2+} concentrations are regulated by the activities of Ca^{2+} pumps and channels located in the sarcoplasmic reticulum and transverse tubular systems. Ca^{2+} also controls glycolysis in muscle through its activation of phosphorylase kinase. A defect in Ca^{2+} regulation, leading to the chronic elevation of Ca^{2+} within the sarcoplasm, could induce muscle contracture, extensive glycolysis, and enhanced mitochondrial oxidation of glycolytic end products. These various reactions, leading to high turnover of ATP, could be responsible for the elevated temperatures associated with MH episodes.

MH could be caused by any abnormality in the regulation of intracellular Ca^{2+} concentrations. Therefore, mutations in genes encoding the Ca^{2+} pump, the Ca^{2+} release channel, or other proteins of excitation-contraction coupling might be at fault. Abnormalities in the Ca^{2+} pump have been ruled out, but abnormalities in the Ca^{2+} release channel have been substantiated. Ca^{2+} release channels have been cloned from skeletal (ryanodine receptor 1 [RYR1]), cardiac (RYR2), and nonmuscle (RYR3) sources. A defect in the Ca^{2+} release channel could account for all the features of MH. If the Ca^{2+} release channels had longer open times in the presence of anesthetic agents, intracellular Ca^{2+} might be chronically elevated, resulting in muscle contracture and activation of the first steps in glycogenolysis through activation of phosphorylase kinase. RYR1 has been linked to human MH on chromosome 19q13.1.

CENTRAL CORE DISEASE

Central core disease (CCD) has been linked to mutations in the RYR1 gene. It is inherited as an autosomal dominant trait with variable penetrance.

Clinical Features

CCD is a nonprogressive myopathy that presents as infantile hypotonia. Proximal muscle weakness is the main feature. Other variable features are pes cavus, kyphoscoliosis, foot deformities, congenital hip dislocation, and joint contractures. Most children with the genetic abnormality show the typical phenotype, but as many as 40% are asymptomatic.

The muscle histology is diagnostic. Oxidative enzyme activity is absent in central regions of skeletal muscle cells. Ultrastructure studies show disintegration of the contractile apparatus, ranging from blurring and streaming of the Z lines to total loss of myofibrillar structure. The sarcoplasmic reticulum and transverse tubular systems are greatly increased in content and are less well structured. NADH-tetrazolium reductase reactions show circular areas that are called *central cores.*

Mitochondria are depleted in the cores but may be enriched around the surfaces of the cores.

Molecular Features

An important feature of CCD is its close association with susceptibility to MH. Analysis of RYR1 cDNA sequences in several CCD families led to the discovery of four mutations that are linked to CCD, MH, or both. The CCD mutations might cause altered Ca^{2+} regulation that leads to disorganization of the contractile proteins in the central core, a proliferation of sarcoplasmic reticulum and transverse tubules, and a loss of functional mitochondria. This results in damage to the interior of the cell, with loss of mitochondrial function and structural abnormalities that lead to muscle weakness and atrophy.

EPISODIC ATAXIA AND MYOKYMIA

The episodic ataxias (EAs) are neurologic disorders characterized by attacks of ataxia, lasting minutes to hours, brought on by physical and emotional stress. Between attacks, only minimal neurologic abnormalities are present. Most EAs are transmitted by autosomal dominant inheritance.

Clinical Features

Two distinct clinical syndromes are recognized: EA-1 and EA-2. EA-1 is characterized by episodes of ataxia, lasting seconds to minutes; feelings of weightlessness; and sometimes tremor. Some patients also have myokymia and twitching of small muscles, both during and between attacks. Myokymia is not always seen on physical examination of facial and hand muscles but is usually detected by EMG as spontaneous, repetitive discharges in distal muscles. It arises from abnormal excitability of the peripheral nerve. Most individuals with EA-1 have mild symptoms that do not impair reasonably normal functioning. Some have contractures of their Achilles tendons that may require surgical treatment. Paroxysmal kinesiogenic choreoathetosis (PKC) is an associated feature in some patients. PKC, which lasts a few seconds, is characterized by dystonic posturing or choreoathetotic movements precipitated by sudden movement.

EA-2 differs from EA-1 in that episodes of ataxia generally last minutes to hours. Nystagmus is often present both during and between attacks, and the initially mild episodic cerebellar dysfunction may progress to chronic involvement similar to that seen in the spinocerebellar ataxias. Myokymia is never present. Patients with both forms of EA, but especially EA-2, often respond to acetazolamide with a decrease in the frequency and severity of attacks.

Molecular Features

Mutations in K^+ channel genes on chromosome 12p13 are associated with EA-1. The gene for EA-2 maps to chromosome 19p13. Although no ion channel genes have yet been localized to human chromosome 19p13, it seems likely that many such genes remain to be mapped.

TREATMENT

All of the autosomal dominant periodic neurologic diseases (EA-1, hyperkalemic and hypokalemic periodic paralyses, and paramyotonia congenita) may be prevented with prophylactic use of acetazolamide.

For a more detailed discussion see Jentsch TJ. Myotonia Congenita (Chapter 39; pp. 715–721); Barchi RL. Molecular Pathology of the Periodic Paralyses (Chapter 40; pp. 723–731); MacLennan DH, Phillips MS, Britt BA. The Molecular and Genetic Basis for Malignant Hyperthermia and Central Core Disease (Chapter 41; pp. 733–748); Litt M, Nutt JG. Episodic Ataxia and Myokymia (Chapter 42; pp. 749–753), in RN Rosenberg, SB Prusiner, S DiMauro, RL Barchi (eds),* The Molecular and Genetic Basis of Neurological Disease *(2nd ed). Boston: Butterworth–Heinemann, 1997.

11

The Genetic Epilepsies

Seizures are paroxysmal, transitory disturbances in cerebral function associated with an abnormal, synchronous discharge of cortical neurons. The term *epilepsy* refers to recurrent seizures of any cause. Some are genetic (idiopathic) and some are symptomatic of brain injury or acquired neurologic disorders.

CLASSIFICATION

The cellular pathophysiology of seizures in humans is unknown. Current classifications are based on observation of the behavioral manifestations of seizures and, when possible, on their correlation with concurrent electroencephalogram (EEG) activity. Two types of classification systems are used. The first is based on seizure type (Table 11.1) and the second is based on the concept of the *epilepsy syndrome*, a constellation of clinical, historical, and electrophysiologic features that describes a patient population (Table 11.2).

The International Classification of Epileptic Seizures uses behavioral and electrophysiologic data to classify seizures. The fundamental difference among seizures is described as *partial* versus *generalized* onset. Partial seizures are further subdivided into simple, complex, and secondarily generalized. A simple partial seizure can have motor, sensory, autonomic, or psychic components but lacks impairment of consciousness. Complex partial seizures impair consciousness. Secondary generalization implies spread from the initiating focus to the remainder of the nervous system. Generalized seizures are defined by an inability to identify a seizure focus by clinical features or EEG. The two most common seizure phenotypes, staring and tonic-clonic, can be either partial or generalized in onset.

The International Classification of Epileptic Syndromes is based on epilepsy type rather than seizure type. This classification also uses partial

Table 11.1
International Classification of Epileptic Seizures.

- Partial seizures (seizures beginning locally)
  - Simple partial seizures (consciousness not impaired)
    - With motor symptoms
    - With somatosensory or special sensory symptoms
    - With autonomic symptoms
    - With psychic symptoms
  - Complex partial seizures (with impairment of consciousness)
    - Simple partial onset followed by impairment of consciousness with impairment of consciousness at onset
  - Partial seizures evolving to secondary generalized seizures
- Generalized seizures (convulsive or nonconvulsive)
  - Absence
    - Typical absences
    - Atypical absences
  - Myoclonic seizures
  - Clonic seizures
  - Tonic seizures
  - Tonic-clonic seizures
  - Atonic seizures
- Unclassified epileptic seizures

Source: Modified from Commission on Classification and Terminology of the International League Against Epilepsy (ILAE). Proposal for revised clinical and electroencephalographic classification of epileptic seizures. Epilepsia 1981;22:489.

Table 11.2
International Classification of Epilepsies and Epileptic Syndromes.

- **Localization-related (focal, local, partial) epilepsies and syndromes**
  - Idiopathic with age-related onset
    - Benign childhood epilepsy with centrotemporal spikes
    - Childhood epilepsy with occipital paroxysms
  - Symptomatic
    - This category comprises syndromes of great individual variability, which will mainly be based on anatomic localization, clinical features, seizure types, and etiologic factors (if known)
- **Generalized epilepsies and syndromes**
  - Idiopathic with age-related onset, listed in order of age
    - Benign neonatal familial convulsions
    - Benign neonatal convulsions
    - Benign myoclonic epilepsy in infancy
    - Childhood absence epilepsy (pyknolepsy)
    - Juvenile absence epilepsy
    - Juvenile myoclonic epilepsy (impulsive petit mal)
    - Epilepsy with grand mal seizures (GTCS) on awakening

Other generalized idiopathic epilepsies, if they do not belong to one of the above syndromes, can still be classified as generalized idiopathic epilepsies
Idiopathic and/or symptomatic, in order of age or appearance
West syndrome (infantile spasms)
Lennox-Gastaut syndrome
Epilepsy with myoclonic-astatic seizures
Epilepsy with myoclonic absences
Symptomatic
Nonspecific etiology
Early myoclonic encephalopathy
Specific syndromes
Epileptic seizures may complicate many disease states
Epilepsies and syndromes undetermined as to whether they are focal or generalized
With both generalized and focal seizures
Neonatal seizures
Severe myoclonic epilepsy in infancy
Epilepsy with continuous spike-waves during slow-wave sleep
Acquired epileptic aphasia (Landau-Kleffner syndrome)
Without unequivocal generalized or focal features
This heading covers all cases where clinical and EEG findings do not permit classification as clearly generalized or localization-related, such as in many cases of sleep grand mal
Special syndromes
Situation-related seizures
Febrile convulsions
Seizures related to other identifiable situations such as stress, hormonal changes, drugs, alcohol, or sleep deprivation
Isolated, apparently unprovoked epileptic events
Epilepsies characterized by specific modes of seizure precipitation
Chronic progressive epilepsia partialis continua of childhood

Source: Modified from Commission on Classification and Terminology of the International League Against Epilepsy. Proposal for revised classification of epilepsies and epileptic syndromes. Epilepsia 1989;30:389.

(localization-related) versus generalized as a first step. A distinction is then made between idiopathic and symptomatic groups. Idiopathic usually means a genetic predisposition, whereas symptomatic indicates that a second disorder is known or suspected.

The Electroencephalogram

EEG abnormalities are used in classification schemes. EEG "traits" may be present in asymptomatic relatives of patients with epilepsy, and these have been used as markers of disease for pedigree analysis. Specific EEG patterns are highly correlated with, and may be used to define, specific types of epilepsy, such as the generalized 3-Hz spike–slow wave discharge occurring in childhood absence epilepsy (CAE), the photoconvulsive response (PCR) frequently present in the primary generalized epilepsies, or the characteristic centrotemporal focal discharge in benign epilepsy of childhood with rolandic spikes.

THE GENETICS OF GENERALIZED EPILEPSIES AND SYNDROMES

Benign Familial Neonatal Convulsions

Clinical Features

Benign familial neonatal convulsions (BFNC) is an epilepsy syndrome with onset usually in the first week after birth, but can begin as late as 4 months. The seizures may be focal or generalized clonic or tonic seizures. Seizure frequency is 1–40 per day, with a duration of 30 seconds to 3 minutes. Generalized EEG abnormalities are usual, but focal onset is also possible. Other laboratory studies are normal. The seizures usually stop within months of onset, but as many as 3–16% of children have neurologic sequela such as learning disabilities, epilepsy, and developmental delays indicating phenotypic heterogeneity.

Genetic Features

BFNC is usually transmitted as an autosomal dominant trait with high penetrance, but autosomal recessive inheritance may also occur. In several large BFNC pedigrees, a locus has been identified on the long arm of chromosome 20. This locus is designated *EBN1*. In two other families, in which individuals had seizures beyond 1 year, subsequent epilepsy, and asymptomatic obligate carriers, linkage to the *EBN1* locus was established in one but not the other, suggesting genetic as well as phenotypic heterogeneity. The family that did not map to the *EBN1* locus showed linkage to chromosome 8q. This locus is designated *EBN2*. In one large kindred that mapped to *EBN1*, seizures and learning disabilities persisted in 16% and 7%, respectively. The DNA markers for the α-4-subunit of the nicotinic acetylcholine receptor may colocalize to *EBN1*.

Benign Infantile Familial Convulsions

Clinical Features

Children with benign infantile familial convulsions have seizure onset between age 4 and 8 months. The seizures are characterized by behavioral arrest, slow horizontal deviation of head and eyes, cyanosis, and generalized hypertonia with unilateral or bilateral limb jerks or both. The interictal EEG is normal, but the ictal EEG shows onset in one posterior quadrant or the other followed by secondary generalization. Neuroimaging studies are normal and the prognosis is excellent. Seizures always stop, and psychomotor decline is not reported.

Genetic Features

Autosomal dominant transmission is suspected. Despite the similarities to the syndrome of BFNC, the *EBN1* and *EBN2* loci have been excluded.

Juvenile Myoclonic Epilepsy

Clinical Features

The onset of juvenile myoclonic epilepsy (JME) is between 8 and 20 years. The seizures are myoclonic jerks, usually in the morning on awakening, which may proceed to generalized tonic-clonic seizures (GTCS). The onset of GTCS may precede the myoclonic jerks. Absences occur at a variable rate; frequent absences may indicate a genetically distinct syndrome. The most common EEG abnormality is 4- to 6-Hz bilaterally symmetric, polyspike-wave complexes, or 2- to 3-Hz spike-wave complexes. JME is estimated to account for 4–11% of individuals with epilepsy.

Genetic Features

A high incidence of JME as well as of several other generalized seizure types occurs in families of individuals with JME. Twin studies have not been reported. The incidence of abnormal EEGs is approximately 11–12% in siblings and parents who do not have seizures.

The mode of inheritance of JME may be dominant, with 70–90% penetrance, or recessive. A two-locus model provides a better fit for the data on affected individuals than a simple mendelian dominant or recessive single locus. Linkage studies on many families with JME indicate a locus on chromosome 6p. The locus is called *EJM1*. Some families with JME do not show linkage to chromosome 6p. The syndrome of adolescent-onset grand mal seizures on awakening, however, has been linked to *EJM1*, whereas a similar syndrome of adolescent-onset grand mal seizures that occur at any time is not linked to *EJM1*.

Childhood and Juvenile Absence Epilepsy

Clinical Features

Childhood absence epilepsy (CAE) occurs predominantly in children between the ages of 4 and 8 years and is characterized by multiple absences, which may be accompanied by brief clonic movements, especially of mouth or hands. Approximately 40–50% of individuals may develop GTCS. The EEG shows characteristic 3-Hz spike-wave discharges; faster and slower frequencies are also seen. Children with CAE are usually intellectually and neurologically normal. CAE accounts for 13–17% of individuals with epilepsy and has a female preponderance (60–75%). Absence seizures respond well to ethosuximide or valproate, although only valproate is also effective against GTCS. Some children (25%) outgrow both seizure types by adolescence, some stop having absence but have GTCS, and others continue to have both types of seizures throughout life.

The onset of juvenile absence epilepsy (JAE) is 8–10 years of age and overlaps in clinical and EEG features with CAE. In contrast to CAE, the absences are less frequent and produce less impairment of consciousness. GTCS usually occur within several years of onset. The EEG may show the typical 3-Hz spike-wave of CAE or a 4- to 5-Hz generalized spike-wave more characteristic of JME. Cognitive outcome is excellent, but complete seizure control is difficult to achieve, and the likelihood of seizures in adult life is greater than with CAE.

Genetic Features

Spike-wave bursts without clinical seizures are common among family members. Only one-fourth of mothers of affected children who have abnormal EEGs experience seizures. Concordance rates for monozygotic twins with absence epilepsy is 75% for absence seizures and 84% for 3-Hz spike-wave. This indicates a high degree of penetrance. Autosomal dominant inheritance is probable. CAE and JAE do not show linkage to the *EJM1* locus on chromosome 6, and CAE does not show linkage to the site on chromosome 21 associated with progressive myoclonus epilepsy.

Severe Myoclonic Epilepsy in Infancy

Clinical Features

Severe myoclonic epilepsy in infancy is characterized by the combination of mixed myoclonic or clonic seizures, GTCS, and complex partial seizures (CPS). The onset is usually before age 2, and the early seizures are often associated with a febrile illness. These seizures may partially respond to valproate but are generally intractable. Psychomotor retardation is common. Whether this occurs as a result of the intractable seizures or if both are due to a common underlying cause is not established.

Genetic Features

A family history for seizures, febrile and nonfebrile, occurs in up to half of cases. One pair of monozygotic twins showed a similar onset and pattern of seizures. The mode of inheritance and chromosomal localization are not known.

Early Childhood Myoclonic Epilepsy

Clinical Features

Early childhood myoclonic epilepsy (ECME), or epilepsy with myoclonic astatic seizures, consists of atonic drop attacks with or without myoclonic jerks, absences, or GTCS. ECME may be a genetically based epilepsy with some overlap with JME and severe myoclonic epilepsy in infancy. The EEG shows 2- to 3-Hz spike-wave or polyspike-wave complexes, or 4- to 6-Hz polyspike-wave complexes. The children are intellectually and neurologically normal and have normal neuroimaging studies. The seizures usually respond to valproate.

Genetic Features

Twenty percent of families with ECME had some form of epilepsy, usually idiopathic primary generalized epilepsy.

Progressive Myoclonus Epilepsies

The progressive myoclonus epilepsies (PME) include Lafora disease, Unverricht-Lundborg (U-L) disease, ceroid lipofuscinosis, the sialidoses, and mitochondrial encephalopathies (see Chapter 4). These disorders are characterized by a general neurologic deterioration associated with both sporadic nonepileptic myoclonus and epileptic seizures, which can be myoclonic, clonic, tonic, or generalized tonic-clonic. These syndromes have in common the progressive nature of the neurologic deterioration (e.g., myoclonus, dementia, ataxia) as well as autosomal dominant and recessive modes of inheritance (except for mitochondrial encephalomyopathies, which are transmitted by maternal inheritance).

Progressive Myoclonus Epilepsy: Lafora Type

PME of the Lafora type is a rapidly progressive syndrome that often begins in the mid-teens with generalized tonic-clonic or myoclonic seizures. Later, a relatively rapid deterioration in intellectual function occurs, sometimes accompanied by psychotic symptoms. Muscle atrophy is also seen. These individuals have periodic acid-Schiff–positive inclusion bodies (containing acid mucopolysaccharides) throughout the gray matter of the central nervous system (CNS), in skeletal and heart muscle, and in liver. Within the brain, the cerebellum, olives, red nucleus, substantia nigra, thalamus, and cortex are most involved. The course tends to be rapid. Inheritance is believed to be autosomal recessive. PME of the Lafora type has been mapped to the long arm of chromosome 6. Efforts to associate this phenotype to the *EPM1* locus were not successful.

Progressive Myoclonus Epilepsy: Unverricht-Lundborg and Related Syndromes

The characteristic phenotype includes onset between age 6 and 15 years and progressive (but variable) cognitive decline associated with GTCS. U-L disease was first described in Finland but has since been reported among several ethnic groups. Baltic and Mediterranean PME is distinguished from U-L disease by slightly different clinical features, whereas all three differ from Lafora disease in lacking the pathologic features (Lafora bodies). The Baltic myoclonus epilepsy syndrome is important to recognize because phenytoin may accelerate the neurologic deterioration.

U-L disease and related disorders are transmitted as autosomal recessive traits. U-L disease maps to chromosome 21q using linkage analysis. The locus is designated *EPM1*. Baltic and Mediterranean PME have an identical chromosomal localization, as does PME in other ethnic groups. Haplotype markers indicate that more than one mutation may occur in this region. The mutation responsible for PME of the U-L type (*EPM1*) was identified in the gene encoding cystatin B.

Progressive Myoclonus Epilepsy: Northern Epilepsy Syndrome

The northern epilepsy syndrome was described in 11 Finnish families derived from two ancestral pedigrees. The most common age at onset is between 5 and 7 years, but may be as early as infancy. GTCS predominate with or without CPS. Seizure frequency peaks during adolescence and then declines in the third decade. Clonazepam is the most effective anticonvulsant. Mental deterioration is a constant feature by 30 years of age and is accompanied by progressive impairment of fine motor tasks, equilibrium, and gait. Neuroimaging shows initial brain stem and cerebellar atrophy followed by generalized cortical atrophy. Linkage analysis has mapped the disease locus, designated *EMR,* to the short arm of chromosome 8.

Progressive Myoclonus Epilepsy: Ceroid Lipofuscinoses

The neuronal ceroid lipofuscinoses are a group of disorders named for the storage material (lipofuscin) found within neurons, conjunctiva, liver, rectum, and lymphocytes. The age of onset ranges from the neonatal period to adult life, with considerable variation in seizure type and severity, cognitive deterioration, associated neurologic symptoms (e.g., blindness, ataxia), and life expectancy. The late infantile, juvenile, and adult forms have myoclonic seizures as a prominent part of the syndrome.

All types are believed to be transmitted as autosomal recessive traits, although the adult form may also be transmitted as an autosomal dominant trait. The juvenile onset form (Batten's disease), presenting at 4–10 years of age with severe atypical absence and GTCS, maps to a locus on chromosome 16p designated *CLN3*. The infantile form, which is phenotypically distinct from the other PME syndromes, has been linked to chromosome 1p and is designated *CLN1*. The late infantile form (*CLN2*) is distinct from *CLN1* and *CLN3* markers, whereas a subtype of the late infantile form has been mapped to 13q and designated *CLN5*. These disorders show how a similar pathologic marker may not be predictive of either phenotypic or genetic homogeneity.

Progressive Myoclonus Epilepsy: Sialidosis Type 1

Sialidosis type 1 syndrome is also referred to as *cherry-red spot myoclonus* due to the macular appearance associated with the stimulus-sensitive massive myoclonus. Onset is after age 7 years. Neuraminidase deficiency is associated with both sialidosis types 1 and 2. This disorder has been mapped to chromosome 10q23 [141].

THE GENETICS OF LOCALIZATION-RELATED EPILEPSIES

Benign Epilepsy of Childhood with Rolandic Spikes

Clinical Features

Benign epilepsy of childhood with rolandic spikes (BECRS) may be the most common childhood epilepsy, occurring in 25% of epileptic children. Development, neurologic examination, and neuroimaging studies are normal. The interictal EEG consistently shows normal background activity and a characteristic unihemispheric or bihemispheric, shifting monomorphic epileptiform discharge, usually with an amplitude maximum over the inferior rolandic cortex. This neuroanatomic localization is consistent with the clinical seizures that are characterized by hemifacial or lingual tingling or twitching, drooling, and a motor-based inability to speak. The seizures are predominantly nocturnal but may be diurnal. In some patients, the focal discharge secondarily generalizes to a hemiclonic or GTCS. The prognosis is excellent, as most seizures are easily controlled by a single medication, and the epilepsy completely resolves in at least 95% of cases by 20 years of age.

Genetic Features

A family history of epilepsy is cited in 9–68% of cases. Age-related penetrance is strongly suggested by the appearance of the seizures and the EEG trait at approximately 4 years and resolution of the seizures and the EEG abnormality by the end of adolescence. Siblings of affected children often have seizures other than BECRS. The EEG may serve as a marker for epileptogenicity in both symptomatic and unaffected family members, but the epileptiform abnormality may not be the same in all affected members. Autosomal dominant inheritance with age-dependent, variable penetrance is the likely mode of inheritance, but a polygenic basis is also reasonable.

The fragile X syndrome has some EEG similarities with discharges seen in BECRS. The *fraX* site has been screened for and excluded. The *EJM1* locus has also been excluded.

Benign Epilepsy with Occipital Paroxysms

Several partial epilepsies localize to the occipital lobes. At least one is familial and considered to be a discrete epilepsy syndrome. These syndromes can have overlapping clinical or EEG features but different outcomes and genetic features.

Clinical Features

Childhood epilepsy with occipital paroxysms (CEOP) is a localization-related, idiopathic syndrome. The initial feature is blindness or phosphenes that are followed by hemiclonic seizures and sometimes GTCS, often followed by headache. The EEG shows bilateral or unilateral occipital spike-wave discharges that attenuate with eye opening. Developmental status, neurologic examinations, and neuroimaging studies are normal.

Idiopathic photosensitive occipital lobe epilepsy is an age-related syndrome with onset between 5 and 17 years in which photic-induced seizures are characterized by visual phenomena, headache, abdominal pain, head turning, and, occasionally, secondary generalization. Seizures can be controlled with medication and by avoidance of provoking stimuli in most patients. Development is normal.

A third occipital lobe epilepsy syndrome that occurs in otherwise normal children also has occipital paroxysms with eye opening. However, the clinical seizures are different. All seizures are nocturnal and characterized by tonic deviation of the eyes and vomiting. Onset is before 8 years and seizures stop after 12 years. Headache is not part of the syndrome.

Genetic Features

There are at least three occipital epilepsy syndromes with a benign outcome. The genetic basis for each of these syndromes is not established.

Autosomal Dominant Nocturnal Frontal Lobe Epilepsy

Clinical Features

Autosomal dominant nocturnal frontal lobe epilepsy was originally described as a sleep disorder. Seizures usually occur during drowsiness or the first few or last few hours of sleep. Onset is usually before age 20 years. Seizures vary in severity and recurrence but tend to occur in clusters. Auras may be somatosensory, special sensory, psychic, and autonomic. Motor activity is tonic, clonic, and hyperkinetic. Neurologic examination and neuroimaging studies are normal. Interictal EEG is usually normal. Ictal EEG may show bihemispheric, frontally predominant spike-wave discharges, or it may be normal.

Genetic Features

The disorder is transmitted as an autosomal dominant trait with high penetrance. In one multigenerational family, linkage was found at locus chromosome 20q. The gene for the α-4 subunit of the nicotinic acetylcholine receptor also maps to this locus, making it the first human genetic epilepsy for which an associated gene has been identified.

Rolandic Epilepsy and Speech Dyspraxia

Clinical Features

Rolandic epilepsy and speech dyspraxia syndrome was described in one family with nine affected family members. Seizure onset is before age 10 years. The seizures are exclusively nocturnal in most affected individuals and are characterized by tonic and clonic contractions of the arms, facial jerks, and occasional secondary generalized convulsions. Other prominent features include auras (fright, oral/hand paresthesia), preservation of consciousness with difficulty talking, and stuttering. The interictal EEG of affected family members is characterized by sharp-wave–slow-wave complexes in a unilateral or bilateral centrotemporal distribution with a horizontal dipole. Deficits in speech production (dyspraxia), receptive language processing, and naming were documented.

Genetic Features

Pedigree analysis demonstrated an autosomal dominant mode of inheritance with 100% penetrance. In addition, the severity of the speech and seizure disorders increased with each successive generation (*anticipation*).

Partial Epilepsy with Auditory Features

Clinical Features

In partial epilepsy with auditory features, age at onset is 8–19 years, and cognition is normal. Seizures are infrequent. Partial onset occurs in most cases, and half of affected individuals have auditory phenomena.

Genetic Features

The trait appears to be inherited by autosomal dominant transmission, with a 70% penetrance. Linkage analysis indicates a region on chromosome 10q that includes genes for several types of adrenergic receptors and glutamate metabolism.

Familial Temporal Lobe Epilepsy

Clinical Features

A hereditary temporal lobe epilepsy has been described in a series of 13 unrelated families. Affected individuals have relatively infrequent and mild simple or complex partial seizures and secondarily GTCS. The partial seizures often have psychic, autonomic, or sensory symptoms. EEGs show occasional focal sharp- and slow-wave complexes in temporal leads. MRI is normal. Most patients are well controlled with antiepileptic medication.

Genetic Features

Inheritance patterns indicate autosomal dominant inheritance with age-dependent penetrance.

Acquired Partial (Focal) Epilepsy

Some acquired epilepsies may have a genetic basis. A possible genetic predisposition exists for the development of focal epilepsy after brain tumors and brain trauma and in infantile hemiplegia.

Acquired partial or focal epilepsy can be defined as epilepsy that occurs in an otherwise clinically normal individual after a specific provocation (e.g., head trauma, stroke, brain tumor) and is characterized by focal (or partial) seizures with or without secondary generalization. The partial seizures can be simple or complex. Focal spikes or slowing is seen on EEG in locations that correspond to the focal symptomatology. Individuals with partial epilepsy comprise approximately 70% of adults and 40% of children with epilepsy. In approximately 70% of individuals with partial epilepsy, a specific cause can be determined. Pathologic examination of the brain often shows lesions that are presumed to be the cause of the epilepsy. Individuals with partial epilepsy are often the most refractory to pharmacologic treatment. Some patients with intractable partial epilepsy are effectively treated with resective surgery, and it is by examination of the diseased temporal lobe that specific pathologic diagnoses can be made.

Genetic Features

Relatives of individuals with acquired partial epilepsy have an increased prevalence of seizures. Children with focal motor or psychomotor seizures have a history of seizures in approximately 20% of first-degree relatives. Several mechanisms could explain why acquired partial epilepsy could have a genetic component. Small changes in any component of neuronal excitability could be aggravated by a brain injury in such a way as to promote the development of epilepsy.

THE GENETICS OF EPILEPSIES THAT OCCUR AS PART OF SPECIAL SYNDROMES

Febrile Convulsions

Clinical Features

Febrile convulsions are seizures associated with fever, occurring between the ages of 1 month and 7 years, that are not symptomatic of recognized acute neurologic illness. Simple febrile seizures are brief, generalized, and not repetitive. Complex febrile seizures are prolonged (>30 minutes), focal, or recurrent within 24 hours. Simple febrile seizures in otherwise normal infants have only a 2% risk of later epilepsy. Children with complex febrile seizures are at higher risk for developing epilepsy.

Genetic Features

Febrile seizures occur in 2% of children. Males and females are equally affected. A familial predisposition exists, and autosomal dominant inheritance is suspected.

Pyridoxine-Dependent Seizures

Clinical Features

Pyridoxine-dependent seizure disorder is the only human epilepsy that is known to be caused by a specific biochemical disorder. The seizures are secondary to a greater than normal requirement for pyridoxine by dependent enzymes within the CNS. This state is to be distinguished from pyridoxine deficiency in which the cofactor is missing due to inadequate dietary intake or impaired gastrointestinal absorption. Diagnosis of both syndromes is made by noting a rapid improvement in an epileptiform EEG and attending seizures in response to intravenous administration of pyridoxine. Affected individuals must be maintained on a lifelong daily oral dose of pyridoxine. Seizures recur days to months after discontinuation of the vitamin.

Genetic Features

Small pedigrees have indicated that siblings of the proband either had documented pyridoxine-dependent seizures or a history consistent with the diagnosis. An autosomal recessive mode of inheritance is suspected.

Seizures Associated with Inherited Phacomatoses

See Chapters 9 and 14.

For a more detailed discussion see Dichter MA, Buchhalter JR. The Genetic Epilepsies (Chapter 43; pp. 757–783), in RN Rosenberg, SB Prusiner, S DiMauro, RL Barchi (eds), **The Molecular and Genetic Basis of Neurological Disease** ***(2nd ed). Boston: Butterworth–Heinemann, 1997.***

12

Neuropathies and Neuronopathies

INHERITED MOTOR NEURON DISEASES

Inherited motor neuron disorders are classified according to whether they involve the upper motor neuron, the lower motor neuron, or both.

Disorders of the Upper and Lower Motor Neurons

Dominant (Adult-Onset) Amyotrophic Lateral Sclerosis

Amyotrophic lateral sclerosis (ALS) is a rapidly progressive, uniformly lethal, paralytic disorder caused by the death of motor neurons in the brain, brain stem, and spinal cord.

CLINICAL FEATURES. Onset can occur at any age in adult life. Death from respiratory paralysis usually occurs within 3–5 years. In those cases in which lower motor neurons are involved first, the initial features are weakness, muscle atrophy (amyotrophy), fasciculations, and cramps; if corticospinal motor neurons are involved first, the initial features are spasticity (such as exaggerated tendon reflexes, stiffness, and scissoring of the gait), or stiffening and slowness of movement. Bilateral corticobulbar involvement causes release of emotional reflexes, termed *pseudobulbar affective changes,* in which behavioral responses to emotional stimuli are inappropriately intensified. Except in the most exceptional cases, sensory function, cognition, and memory are spared.

ALS typically begins focally and asymmetrically, then spreads, often in an anatomic pattern, indicating dissemination among contiguously located groups of motor neurons. It may begin in one hand and foot and then spread up the arm, subsequently involving either the contralateral arm and hand, or the ipsilateral leg and foot. With time, all limb and bulbar motor function is involved in a pattern consistent with upper and lower motor neuron disease.

Genetic Features. Sporadic ALS accounts for 90% of cases, and familial ALS (FALS) accounts for the other 10%. FALS is transmitted as an autosomal dominant trait. Both forms are clinically and pathologically the same and probably share a common pathogenetic mechanism. Twenty percent of FALS families have mutations in the gene for cytosolic, copper/zinc superoxide dismutase (*SOD1*) encoded on chromosome 21q. More than 30 *SOD1* mutations have been reported in FALS pedigrees. Mutations in the gene encoding the heavy subunit of neurofilament (NF-H) are sometimes present in individuals with apparently sporadic ALS. *SOD1* converts the superoxide anion $O_2^{\bullet}$ to hydrogen peroxide (H_2O_2). After this "dismutation" reaction, H_2O_2 is detoxified by conversion to water by either catalase or glutathione peroxidase. FALS associated with mutations in *SOD1* may be a disorder of free radical homeostasis, entailing oxidative cytotoxicity that induces a pathologic process of cell death within motor neurons. Sporadic ALS could be caused by a similar mechanism.

Total brain *SOD1* activity is reduced in FALS patients with *SOD1* mutations but not in sporadic ALS patients or individuals with FALS not associated with *SOD1* mutations. Furthermore, *SOD1* activity is reduced in red blood cells and lymphoblasts selectively in FALS patients with *SOD1* mutations. The mutations appear to render *SOD1* less stable while variably reducing activity levels. Although several lines of evidence point to a possible role for superoxide as a signaling factor in a cascade of events that culminates in programmed cell death of motor neurons, oxidative injury to neurons bearing mutant *SOD1* molecules remains unproven.

Recessive (Juvenile-Onset) Amyotrophic Lateral Sclerosis

Clinical Features. A form of motor neuron disease characterized by chronic slow degeneration of both upper and lower motor neurons occurs in early childhood. It has occurred primarily in highly inbred families and appears to be transmitted as an autosomal recessive trait. The lower motor neuron component causes extensive atrophy of the forelegs and even clubbing of the feet. Marked spasticity is present, and some patients have pseudobulbar disturbances of affect. Cognitive and sensory functions are not affected. Individuals with juvenile ALS may survive for several decades.

Genetic Features. Linkage of the disease to a locus on the long arm of chromosome 2 is described. The gene locus and abnormal gene product are unknown.

Disorders of the Lower Motor Neurons

Spinal Muscular Atrophy

The spinal muscular atrophies (SMAs) are a family of disorders characterized by progressive degeneration of motor neurons in the brain stem and spinal cord. With rare exceptions, the inheritance pattern of the SMAs is autosomal recessive.

CLINICAL FEATURES. The presenting feature of the SMAs is progressive, symmetric weakness, usually with profound wasting due to denervation atrophy. SMAs are divided into four categories. The most fulminant is SMA-I, which begins before 6 months of age and may be clinically evident before birth. Mothers may report diminished fetal movements in the last 2–3 weeks of pregnancy. Newborns with SMA-I are severely hypotonic with feeble sucking, feeding, and crying. They never attain sitting balance and usually survive less than 2 years. SMA-I affects about 1 in 20,000 babies; its carrier frequency is approximately 1 in 80.

SMA-II usually begins before 18 months of age, and affected children may survive into the second decade. SMA-II patients sit but never stand or walk unassisted. SMA-III has a milder phenotype, with onset after 18 months. Affected children stand and walk and may survive into adult life. The onset of SMA-IV is in adult life. Proximal weakness is severe, with greater involvement of the legs than the arms.

GENETIC FEATURES. Most cases of SMA-I, -II, and -III are linked to a locus on the proximal long arm of chromosome 5. It is likely that these disorders all result from mutations within the same gene. Two candidate genes have been identified within this locus. One is the survival motor neuron gene (*SMN*), and the other is the neuronal apoptosis inhibitory protein (*NAIP*). The entire region is normally duplicated and contains two copies of each gene. Moreover, the region has multiple pseudogenes and repeat elements. Initially, the telomeric copy of *SMN* was reported to be defective in virtually all SMA patients but not in healthy controls. *NAIP* is deleted homozygously in many SMA patients but also in some clinically normal parents. Both proteins are widely expressed; both copies of *SMN* may undergo alternate splicing in some tissues.

Adult-Onset Tay-Sachs Disease

See Chapter 6.

X-Linked Spinal Bulbar Muscular Atrophy

X-linked spinal bulbar muscular atrophy (X-SBMA) is also known as *Kennedy's disease.*

Clinical Features. X-SBMA is a slowly progressive, lower motor neuronopathy of adult men. The weakness is accompanied by a variable degree of gynecomastia and testicular atrophy with reduced fertility, suggesting androgen insensitivity.

Genetic Features. X-SBMA is caused by an expansion of a normal CAG repeat within the first exon of the androgen receptor gene. This leads to an expanded polyglutamine tract within the receptor. In general, the larger the tract of repeated CAGs, the more severe the illness. Although the mechanism for the neurotoxicity of the expanded CAG is not clear, several considerations suggest that it is a gain of function mutation.

Disorders of the Upper Motor Neurons

Familial Spastic Paraplegia

Familial spastic paraplegia (FSP) typically is inherited as an autosomal dominant trait characterized by progressive, spastic weakness beginning in the distal legs. Recessive and X-linked inheritance also occurs.

Clinical Features. Two categories of dominant FSP are distinguished on clinical grounds. FSP-I is characterized by onset before age 35 years (mean onset, 13 years). The initial symptom is often motor delay. The progression of motor disturbance is slow, and sensory or sphincter involvement is minor or absent. The onset of FSP-II is after age 35 years (mean onset, 45 years). Weakness is prominent, and abnormalities of sensation (especially vibration), sphincter function, and gait are associated. In both types of FSP, respiration is largely spared, and most patients survive several decades. The major neuropathologic finding is corticospinal tract degeneration, which is more pronounced caudally. FSP corresponding to this clinical description is described as "pure" or "uncomplicated," in contrast to the less common "complicated" FSP associated with amyotrophy, mental retardation, optic atrophy, and sensory neuropathy.

Genetic Features. Extensive genetic heterogeneity exists in dominant FSP, and at least five loci for FSP have been established. An FSP-

I pedigree with spastic gait, relatively little weakness, and a slow disease course was mapped to chromosome 14q. This family included individuals who were asymptomatic although clinically affected. Another large family with uncomplicated FSP-I was linked to chromosome 15q. The 15q family showed greater variability in age of onset and a more rapid course than the 14q family. Families with FSP-I and FSP-II have shown linkage to a locus on chromosome 2p.

A locus for recessively inherited, uncomplicated FSP has been identified on chromosome 8q. X-linked FSP is associated with mutations in the gene-encoding proteolipid protein. Strikingly, different mutations within the same gene causes Pelizaeus-Merzbacher disease. Another X-linked FSP disorder is caused by mutations in the gene encoding the adhesion molecule L1CAM.

Other Inherited Motor Neuron Diseases

Several other rare inherited motor neuron diseases are recognized that may arise as relatively pure motor nerve disorders or, as with FSP, as complex disorders with multisystem degenerations. Fazio-Londe disease, or progressive juvenile bulbar palsy, is a form of motor neuronopathy characterized by onset of relatively focal paralysis of bulbar motor nerves during childhood. The initial features may be respiratory distress with stridor, or symptoms referable to other cranial nerve motor nuclei. The disease may progress to involve limb weakness. Death usually occurs within 2 years. Both autosomal recessive and dominant inheritance patterns have been proposed. Genetic heterogeneity is likely.

The arthrogryposes are a complex set of disorders characterized by the presence of contractures at birth. These contractures may arise as a consequence of motor neuron cell loss. Some are sporadic cases; others are inherited as autosomal recessive, autosomal dominant, or X-linked traits. In many, the contractures are conjoined with non-neurologic features, suggesting the defect affects development in tissues outside the nervous system, as well as motor neurons. Some cases have a prolonged survival and, in one such pedigree, this trait was dominantly inherited. Others have a fulminant, fatal course and are actually a variant of SMA-I with a locus on chromosome 5q.

The scapuloperoneal muscular atrophies are characterized by an unusual focal distribution of neuropathic weakness with onset in the shoulder muscles and in the peroneal groups. One of the best described families had an onset in early to mid-adult life, with an autosomal dominant inheritance pattern. A variant with early laryngeal involvement and evidence of genetic anticipation has been described.

INHERITED DEMYELINATING NEUROPATHIES

Charcot-Marie-Tooth Disease

Charcot-Marie-Tooth (CMT) disease is also called *hereditary motor sensory neuropathy* (HMSN). CMT is a heterogeneous group of inherited diseases of peripheral nerve.

Clinical Features

The onset of most CMT disease is in childhood and its progression is usually slow. Symmetric motor and sensory nerve dysfunction are characterized by distal weakness and atrophy, impaired sensation, and diminished or absent tendon reflexes. Weakness of the intrinsic muscles of the feet and hands causes pes cavus and claw hand deformities. CMT1 is a hypertrophic demyelinating neuropathy with reduced nerve conduction velocities, whereas CMT2 is an axonal neuropathy. Although CMT1 and CMT2 are readily distinguished by electrophysiologic studies, the clinical phenotypes cannot be used to classify patients. The nosologic classification within CMT has been advanced by molecular diagnosis of gene abnormalities. Table 12.1 summarizes a current classification scheme based on recent genetic studies.

Genetic Studies in CMT1

In most CMT1 pedigrees, the mode of inheritance is autosomal dominant. Some show X-linked inheritance, and rare pedigrees show autosomal recessive inheritance. The majority of CMT1 pedigrees show linkage to chromosome 17p11.2–12 and are designated *CMT1A*. Pedigrees with a mutant gene on chromosome 1 with linkage to the Duffy blood group locus are designated *CMT1B*. Autosomal dominant CMT1 pedigrees that do not map to the proximal chromosome 17p or the region of the Duffy locus on chromosome 1q are designated *CMT1C*. The CMT1C locus, or perhaps loci, remains unassigned.

CMT1A is caused by a tandem DNA duplication in chromosome 17p11.2–12. The duplication results from errors in spermatogenesis and is stably inherited. It may also arise de novo, suggesting that many sporadic cases of CMT1A are not due to autosomal recessive inheritance. A small number of patients have total or partial trisomy of 17p, including the region of the DNA duplication in CMT1A patients. The consistent phenotypic features of these patients are mental retardation, micrognathia, hypoplastic low-set ears, and foot deformities. Features consistent with CMT1A were detected in three patients, supporting the hypothesis that the duplication in CMT1A may have phenotypic consequences through

Table 12.1
Charcot-Marie-Tooth neuropathy (hereditary motor and sensory neuropathy) and related disorders.

	Locus	*Gene*	*Mechanism*
Charcot-Marie-Tooth type 1 (HMSNI)			
CMT1A	17p11.2–12	*PMP22*	Duplication/point mutation
CMT1B	1q22–23	P_0	Point mutation
CMT1C	Unknown	Unknown	Unknown
CMTX	Xq13.1	*Cx32*	Point mutation
CMT4	8q	Unknown	Unknown
Charcot-Marie-Tooth type 2 (HMSNII)			
CMT2A	1p36	Unknown	Unknown
CMT2B	3q	Unknown	Unknown
CMT2C	Unknown	Unknown	Unknown
Dejerine-Sottas disease (DSD) (HMSNIII)			
DSDA	17p11.2–12	*PMP22*	Point mutation
DSDB	1q22–23	P_0	Point mutation
Hereditary neuropathy with pressure palsies (HNPP)			
HNPPA	17p11.2–12	*PMP22*	Deletion/point mutation
HNPPB	Unknown	Unknown	Unknown

HMSN = hereditary motor and sensory neuropathy.

a gene dosage effect. The critical gene for CMT1A has been identified as the myelin protein gene *PMP22*. The importance of gene dosage for *PMP22* is demonstrated by a rare individual with four copies of this gene leading to a Dejerine-Sottas disease phenotype (see the section on Dejerine-Sottas Disease). Approximately 75% of patients with a clinical diagnosis of CMT1 carry the 17p11.2–12 duplication. An assay for the duplication provides a powerful marker for screening suspected patients and family members at risk. Clinical studies show uniform slowing of nerve conduction velocities in patients with the 17p11.2–12 duplication.

CMT1B is associated with abnormalities in the myelin protein zero gene (P_0). The P_0 gene was isolated and mapped to chromosome 1q22–q23 in the region of the CMT1B locus. P_0 is the major structural component of peripheral nervous system myelin, approximately 50% by weight and approximately 7% of Schwann cell message. Analysis of P_0 as a candidate gene for CMT1B detected several different point mutations in CMT1B pedigrees.

Dejerine-Sottas Disease

Dejerine-Sottas disease (DSD) is a continuation of the CMT1 phenotypic spectrum. It is also called *HMSNIII.*

Clinical Features

DSD is a severe, hypertrophic demyelinating polyneuropathy of infancy and childhood onset. The clinical features of DSD overlap with those of severe CMT1. The cerebrospinal fluid protein concentration may be elevated. Many cases are sporadic, and autosomal recessive inheritance was assumed.

Genetic Features

Molecular genetic studies show that DSD is associated with point mutations in either the *PMP22* or the P_0 gene. All mutations are heterozygous, suggesting that DSD is actually caused by dominantly acting genetic defects.

Hereditary Neuropathy with Liability to Pressure Palsies

Hereditary neuropathy with liability to pressure palsies (HNPP) is also called *tomaculous neuropathy*.

Clinical Features

HNPP is an autosomal dominant disorder that causes an episodic, recurring demyelinating neuropathy. Peroneal palsies, carpal tunnel syndrome, brachial plexopathy, and other entrapment neuropathies are manifestations of HNPP. Motor and sensory nerve conduction velocities may be reduced in clinically affected patients as well as in asymptomatic gene carriers. Pathologic changes observed in peripheral nerves of HNPP patients include segmental demyelination and, in some pedigrees, tomaculous or sausage-like formations.

Genetic Features

The HNPP locus has been assigned to chromosome 17p11.2–12 and is associated with a 1.5-mb deletion. HNPP probably results from deletion of the *PMP22* gene and underexpression of this locus. De novo deletion of paternal or maternal origin has been detected as a basis for sporadic HNPP. The possibility of genetic heterogeneity in HNPP was raised by the identification of an HNPP pedigree that did not show linkage to the region of 17p11.2–12.

It has been proposed that the deleted chromosome in HNPP and the duplicated chromosome in CMT1A are the reciprocal products of unequal crossing-over, a likely mechanism for generating the DNA duplication and the deletion. The apparent homogeneity for size of the duplication or deletion in unrelated patients and detection of de novo duplication or deletion events suggest that a common mechanism may account for the generation of the duplicated CMT1A chromosome and the deleted HNPP chromosome.

Hereditary Neuralgic Amyotrophy

Hereditary neuralgic amyotrophy with predilection for the brachial plexus (HNA) is also called *familial brachial plexus neuropathy*.

Clinical Features

HNA, like HNPP, is an autosomal dominant disorder that causes recurrent attacks of peripheral neuropathy. The attacks are characterized by pain, muscle weakness, and sensory disturbances in the brachial region. Onset is frequently in childhood. HNPP and HNA share the feature of brachial plexopathy and may be confused clinically, although the plexopathy in HNPP is painless.

Genetic Features

HNPP and HNA are genetically distinct. Markers from the HNPP region do not segregate with HNA, and the HNA gene has been mapped to the distal long arm of chromosome 17 (17q23–25).

X-Linked Charcot-Marie-Tooth Neuropathy

Clinical Features

The clinical features of X-linked CMT (CMTX) include demyelinating neuropathy, absence of male-to-male transmission, and a generally earlier onset and faster rate of progression of illness in males.

Genetic Features

The gene assignment for CMTX is to the region of Xq13–q21, flanked proximally by the phosphoglycerate kinase pseudogene, PGKP1

(Xq11.2), and distally by marker DXS72 (Xq21.1). The CMTX candidate region (*Cx32*) encodes a major component of gap junctions found to be expressed in peripheral nerves. At least 33 different *Cx32* mutations have now been found in 39 CMTX families. *Cx32* has a pattern of expression in peripheral nerves similar to that of other myelin protein genes. Unlike *PMP22* and P_0, which are present in compact myelin, *Cx32* is located at uncompacted folds of Schwann cell cytoplasm around the nodes of Ranvier and at Schmidt-Lanterman incisures.

Autosomal Recessive Neuropathy

Rare autosomal recessive families with motor and sensory neuropathy have been reported, particularly in Tunisian families in which parental consanguinity is present. Both demyelinating and axonal types have been described and given the tentative designation of *CMT4*. One form of autosomal recessive demyelinating neuropathy has been mapped to chromosome 8q (CMT4A). Other families with CMT4 do not show linkage to chromosome 8q; the other chromosomal loci have not yet been determined.

INHERITED AXONAL NEUROPATHIES

The spectrum of disorders that falls within the classification of inherited axonal neuropathies is broad. Most are discussed in other chapters. The diseases considered here are listed in Table 12.2 along with their mode of inheritance and most important clinical features.

Charcot-Marie-Tooth Neuropathy Type 2

CMT2 is also called *hereditary motor and sensory neuropathy type II* (HMSNII). Although males are more often affected than females, the inheritance in most families is autosomal dominant.

Clinical Features

CMT2 is a less common disorder than CMT1 (all forms combined). Generally, CMT2 has a later age of onset, less involvement of the small muscles of the hands, and no palpably enlarged nerves. Extensive demyelination with "onion bulb" formation is not present in CMT2. Motor nerve conduction velocities are normal or only slightly prolonged.

Genetic Features

CMT2 is genetically distinct from all mapped forms of CMT1. A CMT2 locus was assigned by linkage studies to the short arm of chromosome 1 (1p36) and designated *CMT2A*. Other families fulfilling the diagnostic criteria for CMT2 have failed to show linkage to the 1p36 locus. One CMT2 pedigree was found to link to markers from chromosome 3q and is designated *CMT2B*. A syndrome of axonal neuropathy, diaphragm weakness, and vocal cord paralysis is designated *CMT2C*. The CMT2C locus does not map to the regions of the CMT2A or CMT2B genes.

Hereditary Sensory Neuropathies

A classification of the hereditary sensory neuropathies (HSNs) appears in Table 12.3.

Clinical Features

In the dominant form of HSN, the onset of the acral sensory loss is postnatal and progressive. The main features are insidious loss of cutaneous sensation, mainly pain and temperature sensibility with variable degrees of hypoesthesia to touch, predominantly in the feet and lower legs but also later in the hands. In some families, spontaneous, severe lancinations of pain may accompany progression but eventually subside. At times, when distal cutaneous sensations are deficient, proprioception and ankle jerks may still be relatively normal, although the sural nerve trunk at the ankle may show few remaining myelinated fibers. This suggests that the muscle spindle and joint position afferents are affected less severely and later in the course than the smaller cutaneous afferents.

It is probable that neuronal systems more than the sensory system are at risk in hereditary sensory neuropathy type I (HSN-I). Postmortem examination shows extensive cell loss and gliosis in the thalamus, red nuclei, inferior olivary nuclei, and claustrum, all outside the somatosensory and auditory pathways, suggesting a multisystem degeneration of neurons.

In the recessively inherited hereditary sensory neuropathies (HSN-II through HSN-V), the sensory abnormality often seems present from birth, although the secondary changes due to unheeded trauma may not be evident until late infancy or childhood. The neurologic deficit does not appear to be progressive, although the secondary complications may give that appearance. The frequently congenital nature of the neurologic deficit does suggest that a specific and selective failure of neuronal development may have occurred during fetal life.

Table 12.2
Inherited axonal neuropathies considered in this chapter.

Disorder	*Mode of Inheritance*	*Age at Onset*	*Systemic Abnormalities*	*Neurologic Features*
HMSN-II	Autosomal dominant*; some kinships show linkage to chromosome 1p35–p36 or 3q	Third to fifth decades	None that are frequent	Distal, mainly motor findings; insidious progression; variable expression
HSAN-I (see also Table 12.3)	Autosomal dominant	First to third decades	Nerve deafness in some families	Progressive acral anesthesia with centripetal spread; may have lancinations; ataxia unusual; plantar ulcers
HSAN-II through HSAN-V (see also Table 12.3)	Autosomal recessive	Birth to third decade	Many secondary effects such as fractures, osteomyelitis, ulcerations, abscesses, lost digits, corneal damage	More severe and widespread manifestations and earlier onset than dominant form; many cases have congenital onset
Giant axonal neuropathy	Autosomal recessive	First 3 years	Intermediate filament masses in cytoplasm of many cell types, particularly axoplasm	Slowly progressive ataxia, weakness and areflexia; in later stages, leukoencephalopathy and dementia; death by age 30

Hereditary tyrosinemia, type 1	Recessive; abnormal gene cloned and mapped to chromosome 15q23–q25	Infancy	Deficiency of fumary lacetoacetate hydrolase; acute and chronic liver disease; renal failure	Acute episodes of painful weakness with hypotonia, gastrointestinal dysfunction and sometimes encephalopathy
Friedreich's ataxia	Recessive; chromosome 9 linkage	First or second decade	Cardiomyopathy; scoliosis; increased frequency of diabetes	Progressive ataxia of both cerebellar and sensory types; dysarthria; weakness, both upper and lower motor neuron; areflexia early; loss of large primary sensory neurons
Multiple symmetric lipomatosis	Mitochrondriopathy (?)	Fourth to sixth decades	Lipomas, particularly neck; overlap with MERRF	Progressive, late-onset polyneuropathy

HMSN = hereditary motor and sensory neuropathy; HSAN = hereditary sensory neuropathy; MERRF = myoclonus epilepsy with ragged-red fibers.
*Some families are X-linked dominant; see text.

Table 12.3
Hereditary sensory neuropathies, classified by the pattern of axonal loss in sensory nerves.

Pattern of Fiber Loss	*Mode of Inheritance*	*Dyck Classification*	*Neurologic Syndromes and Variants*	*Comments*
Loss of myelinated and unmyelinated fibers	Autosomal dominant	HSAN-I	Progressive, acral cutaneous and deep sensory loss (pain and temperature)	Trophic change is the result of recurrent, unheeded trauma and can be avoided with proper care
			Variants	
			With nerve deafness	
			With nerve deafness and dementia	
			With peroneal muscular atrophy	
			With late-onset ataxia	
			With paraparesis	
	Autosomal recessive	HSAN-II	More severe than dominant form, more likely to be congenital	Mutilated foot in an animal model
			Variants	
			With dysautonomia	
			Without trophic changes	
			With paraparesis	
			With corneal opacification	In Navajo children
Loss of unmyelinated fibers with or without loss of small myelinated fibers	Autosomal recessive	HSAN-III	Riley-Day syndrome (familial dysautonomia)	Autonomic abnormalities affect thermoregulation and sweating
		HSAN-IV	Congenital sensory neuropathy with anhydrosis	Mild mental retardation is usual
			Neurogenic arthropathy	In Navajo children

Loss of small myelinated fibers	Autosomal recessive (presumed)	HSAN-V	Congenital sensory neuropathy	Inheritance uncertain
			Congenital sensory neuropathy	With corneal opacification
			Congenital sensory neuropathy	Dysmorphic; cataracts; growth hormone deficiency
	X-linked recessive		Sensory neuropathy; onset second decade	Classification uncertain
No loss of fibers	Autosomal dominant		Congenital indifference to pain	Clinically normal sensation

HSAN = hereditary sensory neuropathy.

Giant Axonal Neuropathy

Giant axonal neuropathy is a rare disorder of cytoplasmic intermediate filaments.

Clinical Features

Affected children display clumsiness, ataxia, and hyporeflexia beginning at approximately age 3 and progress to wheelchair confinement and death by the end of the third decade. Central nervous system dysfunction, including progressive dementia, cerebellar signs, dysarthria, and long tract signs, appear by age 10 years. Most cases show distinctive tightly curled hair.

Diagnosis of giant axonal neuropathy should be suspected if ataxia and areflexia appear in early childhood, particularly if the child but not the parents has tightly curled hair. Sural nerve biopsy is the usual method of confirming the diagnosis. Many cell types, including fibroblasts, show intracytoplasmic accumulations of intermediate filaments. Sausage-shaped masses of whorled neurofilaments produce discontinuous swellings of peripheral axons. Severe white matter axonal loss and myelin pallor with accumulations of Rosenthal fibers is seen in the brain. Both the peripheral neurofilamentous masses and the Rosenthal fibers are ubiquitin-positive.

Type 1 Hereditary Tyrosinemia

Type 1 hereditary tyrosinemia, a relatively rare, recessively inherited inborn error of metabolism, leads to liver and renal failure due to deficiency of the enzyme fumaryl acetoacetate hydrolase. It occurs mainly in individuals of French-Canadian origin.

Clinical Features

The clinical course in children with the disorder is often punctuated by the occurrence of acute neuropathic episodes with pain, weakness, occasionally self-mutilation, and a high frequency of vomiting or paralytic ileus. Respiratory assistance is sometimes required because of weakness. Electrodiagnostic studies and nerve and muscle biopsies show an axonopathic process.

Biochemical Features

The episodes resemble the crises of the neuropathic porphyrias. A product of the blocked tyrosine pathway, succinylacetone, inhibits porphyrin biosynthesis and causes elevated levels of δ-aminolevulinic acid. Although drugs designed to reduce porphyria precursors have been tried with variable results, good long-term results have been attained with successful orthotopic liver transplantation.

Genetic Features

The gene for the deficient enzyme fumarylacetoacetate hydrolase has been cloned and mapped to chromosome band 15q23–q25. The most common mutation causing hereditary tyrosinemia in French Canada is a guanine-to-adenine intron 12-splice mutation. Most affected individuals are homozygous for the mutation.

Friedreich's Ataxia

See Chapter 7.

Multiple Symmetric Lipomatosis

Multiple symmetric lipomatosis (MSL) is also called *Madelung disease.*

Clinical Features

MSL is an unusual disorder marked by mid-life appearance of lipomas, often massive and collar-like, of the neck, upper torso, proximal arms, and mediastinum. A chronic, often severe motor-sensory axonal neuropathy frequently accompanies MSL, as does chronic alcoholism. Patients with MSL may also have evidence of mitochondrial dysfunction, ragged-red fibers, reduced cytochrome *c* oxidase deficiency, or both (see Chapter 4).

Genetic Features

Overlap of MSL, peripheral neuropathy, sensory-neural hearing loss, mitochondrial dysfunction, myoclonic epilepsy, and an mtDNA point mutation (adenine to guanine) at nucleotide 8,344 has been noted in several cases.

FAMILIAL AMYLOIDOTIC POLYNEUROPATHY

Clinical Features

The clinical presentation of various kindreds with familial amyloidotic polyneuropathy (FAP) provided the basis for a system of classification based on phenotype. In that system, type I referred to the Portuguese variant in which peripheral neuropathy began in the legs and later progressed to the arms; type II referred to cases presenting with upper limb neuropathy, usually a compression neuropathy with carpal tunnel syndrome followed 5–10 years later by the appearance of lower limb neuropathy and vitreous opacities; type III referred to a pedigree with generalized polyneuropathy and a high incidence of nephrotic syndrome secondary to renal amyloidosis; and type IV was characterized by the triad of corneal lattice dystrophy, cranial neuropathy, and cutis laxa. Biochemical advances have rendered this classification obsolete.

The prototype of the FAPs is type I. Systemic amyloidosis with characteristic involvement of the peripheral nerves is a constant feature of the disease. Onset of symptoms usually occurs in the third or fourth decade. In half of cases, the first symptom is a sensory neuropathy (paresthesias, hypoesthesia, and burning or lancinating pain) of the legs followed within a few years by progressive autonomic dysfunction. In one-third of cases, dysautonomia precedes the sensory symptoms. Gastrointestinal disturbances and sexual impotence are common early features. Motor neuropathy appears later, first in the legs and progressing gradually to the arms. Severe weight loss is a common early sign. Disease progression is inexorable, with death due to inanition or intercurrent infection within 15 years.

Biochemical Features

The term *transthyretin* (TTR) is used for a plasma protein formerly known as *prealbumin*, or *thyroxine-binding prealbumin*. The term *prealbumin* is a misnomer because TTR bears no chemical relationship to serum albumin and prealbumin refers only to its electrophoretic migration in gels. Amyloid fibril protein is related immunologically to serum TTR. The two variants designated FAP type I and FAP type II are now known to be associated but with distinct point mutations in the TTR gene, whereas FAP types III and IV involve entirely different amyloid proteins. Different FAP pedigrees are now classified by fibril type and biochemical mutation.

Genetic Features

Partial amino acid identity was identified between amyloid fibril protein and TTR. At present, there are more than 50 known amyloidogenic mutations in the TTR gene. The majority of affected individuals are heterozygous for one mutant and one normal TTR allele. In general, the clinical picture is monomorphic, suggesting that the same mutation is responsible for the disease in different geographic locations. Although the aberrant protein is present in plasma throughout life, onset of clinical symptoms is invariably delayed, ranging from the second to the ninth decades, and asymptomatic heterozygotes are well documented. The phenomenon of genetic anticipation has been described within pedigrees.

Although the majority of FAP patients are heterozygous for one normal and one mutant TTR gene, homozygosity has occasionally been reported. Some individuals homozygous for some mutations have more aggressive disease although others do not.

Gene carrier detection is possible for diagnosis of TTR mutation using DNA analysis. This is relatively simple and rapid, requires only small amounts of blood, may be performed on embedded tissue specimens, and is suitable for prenatal testing. Prenatal diagnosis has been performed successfully in FAP using specimens from chorionic villous biopsy or amniotic fluid cell cultures.

Treatment

Treatments fall into two general categories: those aimed at alleviating the consequences of the disease and those meant to prevent further amyloid deposition. Symptomatic relief must be pursued aggressively even though this is often a frustrating experience. Despite the best supportive care, most patients with FAP eventually die from the combined ravages of infection, myocardial damage, orthostasis, and malnutrition.

Orthotopic liver transplantation has met with considerable success and is now considered the treatment of choice in appropriate patients. This procedure effectively removes the source of mutant plasma TTR from the plasma, although choroid plexus and ocular synthesis are not affected. During follow-up lasting up to 2.5 years, marked and rapid improvements have been reported in general well-being and autonomic dysfunction, including gastrointestinal symptoms, impotence, syncope, neurogenic bladder, and weight loss.

For a more detailed discussion see Wang CH, Carter TA, Gilliam TC. Molecular and Genetic Basis of the Spinal Muscular Atrophies (Chapter 44; pp. 787–795); Brown RH Jr. The Molecular Biology of the Inherited Motor Neuron Diseases: An Overview (Chapter 45; pp. 797–806); Chance PF. Inherited Demyelinating Neuropathy: Charcot-Marie-Tooth Disease and Related Disorders (Chapter 46; pp. 807–816); Scherer SS, Asbury AK. Inherited Axonal Neuropathies and the Molecular Biology of Peripheral Neuropathies (Chapter 47; pp. 817–843); Herbert J.

Familial Amyloidotic Polyneuropathy (Chapter 48; pp. 845–864), in RN Rosenberg, SB Prusiner, S DiMauro, RL Barchi (eds),* The Molecular and Genetic Basis of Neurological Disease *(2nd ed). Boston: Butterworth–Heinemann, 1997.

13

Muscle Disorders

CONGENITAL MYOPATHIES

Central Core Disease

Central core disease (CCD) is the prototype of the congenital myopathies. It was named because of the peculiar well-limited rounded areas (cores) observed in transverse sections of muscle fibers. The cores are devoid of any oxidative staining and correspond on electron microscopy to abnormal regions characterized by myofibrillar compaction with various degrees of sarcomeric disorganization and Z line streaming. The cores extend along the full length of the fibers and selectively affect type I fibers, which usually predominate.

Clinical Features

CCD usually presents with hypotonia at birth, delayed motor development, reduced muscle bulk, and marked hyperextensibility. The weakness is diffuse but more proximal than distal. Hip dislocation, kyphoscoliosis, and pes cavus are common. Facial and oculomotor involvement is rare and slight. CCD has been described as a nonprogressive myopathy, but some cases deteriorate slowly throughout life.

Genetic Features

CCD is transmitted as an autosomal dominant trait with variable expression. Almost asymptomatic affected family members may be detected only by muscle biopsy. Clues to the genetic basis of CCD came from its association with the malignant hyperthermia syndrome (MHS) (see Chapter 10). The locus for MHS is 19q12–13.2, which is the position of the ryanodine receptor gene (*RYRI*). CCD and MHS are allelic disorders. Several mutations of the *RYRI* gene were found in families exhibiting both MHS and CCD. Genetic heterogeneity is established both in MHS and in CCD. Cores are detected in some non–*RYR1*-linked families and cores are also present in families affected by a cardiomyopathy linked to gene abnormalities on chromosome 14.

Nemaline Myopathy

Nemaline myopathy is one of the most frequent and best-characterized congenital myopathies. The cardinal feature is the presence of numerous rods, which either form clusters at the periphery of the muscle fibers or are disseminated throughout the fiber, stain bright red with the modified Gomori trichrome, and selectively involve type I fibers. These rods are lateral polymers of the Z lines and contain actin and tropomyosin.

Clinical Features

Affected children usually present with nonprogressive or slowly progressive weakness, delayed motor milestones, and skeletal deformities, such as elongated face, high-arched palate, pectus excavatum, kyphoscoliosis, and pes cavus. The clinical spectrum, however, encompasses severe neonatal hypotonia requiring ventilation and almost asymptomatic individuals with mild proximal or distal weakness and minor deformities.

Genetic Features

Autosomal dominant transmission is documented in some pedigrees, although recognition of affected persons often requires muscle biopsies. In other families, especially in those with early-onset severe cases, parents are not affected and autosomal recessive inheritance is postulated.

Positive linkage was established at an apolipoprotein A2 (ApoA2) locus at 1q21–q23. The gene for α-tropomyosin (*TPM3*) is assigned to the same region. It is a good candidate for nemaline myopathy because this tropomyosin isoform is expressed predominantly in slow type I fibers. A mutation in exon 1 of *TPM3* segregates with expression of the dominant disease in some families. Other families with dominant disease do not show mutations in the *TPM3* gene. In addition, autosomal recessive nemaline myopathy does not show any linkage with *TPM* loci and maps to chromosome 2q, in a region tentatively assigned to 2q21.2–q22. Mutations in another tropomyosin gene (*TPM1*) affecting the troponin-binding site of the molecule cause a familial hypertrophic cardiomyopathy. A few cases of nemaline myopathy present with severe cardiomyopathy.

Centronuclear or Myotubular Myopathies

The centronuclear or myotubular myopathies are congenital and defined morphologically by the high percentage of centrally located myonuclei.

Clinical Features

At least three different entities are included in the group of centronuclear myopathies:

1. *Autosomal dominant centronuclear myopathies (AD-CNM).* Onset of weakness occurs in adult life and progression is slow. Most patients have limb-girdle symmetric weakness, often with distal muscle involvement; ocular muscles are usually spared.
2. *Autosomal recessive centronuclear myopathies (AR-CNM).* Onset is in infancy or early childhood. Ptosis and limitation of ocular movements are frequently associated with diffuse, progressive muscle weakness. Central nervous system involvement sometimes occurs.
3. *Sex-linked myotubular myopathy (XMTM).* Newborns are severely hypotonic and require respiratory assistance. Neonatal deaths are frequent. Survivors have generalized muscle weakness with facial involvement and ophthalmoplegia. Hip and knee contractures may also occur. Muscle biopsies are characteristic.

Genetic Features

Linkage analysis has not yet been undertaken in AD- or AR-CNM. Several studies in XMTM have shown linkage with an Xq28 locus to a region of approximately 5 Mb (DXS304–DXS497) in Xq28. Positional cloning allowed isolation and characterization of a gene coding for a tyrosine phosphatase in which mutations were detected.

Other Congenital Myopathies

Genetic studies are still preliminary or not yet undertaken for congenital myopathies that are extremely rare or lack defined diagnostic criteria. This is the case in multicore disease, which has been associated with different modes of inheritance; congenital fiber type disproportion, which is not a defined entity; and the congenital myopathies defined by the presence of intrasarcoplasmic inclusion bodies (fingerprint body myopathy, reducing body myopathy, cytoplasmic body myopathy, and hyaline body myopathy).

Congenital Muscular Dystrophies

Congenital muscular dystrophies (CMDs) differ from the congenital myopathies in that the muscle histology is similar to other dystrophies.

Clinical Features

At least three different entities are included in the group of CMDs:

1. *Fukuyama CMD (FCMD).* FCMD is the most common dystrophy in Japan. Affected children appear normal at birth and then develop features of brain disease and muscle disease, either of which may present first. The brain disease is caused by migrational disorders. The children have mental retardation and frequent epileptic seizures. The myopathy is very severe.
2. *Muscle-eye-brain disease (MEBD).* This may be the same as the Walker-Warburg syndrome. This disorder occurs in European children. A muscular dystrophy is present from birth and is associated with lissencephaly and ocular malformations. The disorder is lethal.
3. *Congenital muscular dystrophy.* In Western countries, CMD usually presents as pure myopathy. Many affected newborns have arthrogryposis. Some have a nonprogressive muscle disease and others have a progressive fatal disease. Magnetic resonance imaging (MRI) shows white matter alterations without major cortical abnormalities in some infants with both the mild and severe varieties.

Genetic Features

In Western countries, most cases are sporadic, and only a few pedigrees suggest autosomal recessive inheritance. FCMD and MEBD are transmitted as autosomal recessive traits. A child affected with both FCMD and xeroderma pigmentosum, which had already been localized to the long arm of chromosome 9, led investigators to this locus, where significant linkage with *FCMD* on chromosome 9q31–33 was found.

Analysis of patients with typical CMDs showed that one laminin variant, named *merosin,* was deficient in approximately half of affected children. Merosin anchors the dystroglycan complex to the extracellular matrix. The merosin-deficient CMD group almost invariably showed white matter changes by MRI. The location of the gene encoding laminin M (α_2) chain was known to be chromosome 6q2 and allowed localization of the CMD gene to the 6q2 locus. Mutations (splice site and nonsense) in the laminin α_2-chain gene (*LAMA2*) were found in two families. The genetic basis of the non–merosin-deficient CMD cases is unknown.

THE MUSCULAR DYSTROPHIES

Dystrophinopathies

Clinical Features

Duchenne muscular dystrophy (DMD) is the most common and devastating of the muscular dystrophies; a milder variant is Becker muscular dystrophy (BMD). DMD is one of the most common inherited lethal disorders of humans (1 in 3,500 males). Many cases are sporadic, although when inherited, the disease shows an X-linked recessive pattern. The typical age of onset is younger than 5 years. Affected boys show proximal muscle weakness, toe walking, and calf hypertrophy. Earlier detection is possible due to delay in motor milestones, calf hypertrophy, and elevated muscle enzyme concentrations in serum. The progression of the disorder is relatively constant, with increasing difficulty ambulating and wheelchair confinement usually after age 10 years. The heart muscle is affected and shows a dilated cardiomyopathy, with progressive fibrotic replacement. Approximately 30% of patients show nonprogressive mental retardation that affects verbal more than other functions. All boys have serum creatine kinase (CK) concentrations that are more than 50 times the upper limit of normal at birth.

Muscle biopsy shows features consistent with a dystrophic myopathy, including fiber size variation, eosinophilic hypercontracted fibers, increased endomysial connective tissue (fibrosis), and occasional areas of overt necrosis with macrophage infiltration. No histopathologic feature is diagnostic for DMD, but muscle specimens show absence, or near absence, of dystrophin.

The age of onset of BMD is usually older than 5 years. The phenotype is similar to DMD except the progression of weakness is very slow, and survival to adult life is expected. The disease is often compatible with reproduction, and all daughters of an affected male are carriers of the disease. Dystrophin is reduced in molecular weight or quantity, or both.

Females in families segregating DMD or BMD are at risk of being carriers. Carriers only rarely show clinical symptoms, and if they do, it is the result of skewed X inactivation. The clinical presentation in isolated female dystrophinopathy patients is as varied as BMD.

Genetic Features

DMD was the first human inherited disorder to be discovered at the molecular level by positional cloning, with no prior knowledge of the biochemical defect. The causative gene at the Xp21 site is the largest gene identified to date in any species. The gene product, *dystrophin*, is a large, relatively low-abundance, membrane-associated protein in skeletal muscle, heart, smooth muscle, and some neurons. It is completely absent in muscle biopsies from DMD and present but abnormal in BMD. The most common type of gene mutation in both disorders is a deletion encompassing one or more exons of the enormous gene. Two deletion hot spots are identified, one in the region of exons 44–50, and a second near the beginning of the gene (exons 2–13). In-frame deletion mutations produce BMD, whereas out-of-frame deletions cause DMD. Approximately 8% of deletion mutations are exceptions to the reading frame rule. If the boundaries of a deletion mutation can be precisely identified, there is a 92% accuracy for distinguishing DMD from BMD.

Approximately 45% of DMD patients and 30% of BMD patients do not have deletion mutations and instead have duplications or point mutations. Duplications follow the same in-frame/out-of-frame rule as deletion mutations, and approximately 5% of DMD or BMD patients show this type of mutation.

Biochemical Features

Dystrophin, like other cytoskeletal proteins (spectrin and α-actin), has an amino-terminal actin binding domain, a large central rod domain, a cysteine-rich penultimate domain, and a carboxyl-terminal globular domain. Dystrophin forms a complex with a series of intracellular, transmembrane, and extracellular proteins to form a cytoskeleton that attaches the intracellular actin cytoskeleton to the extracellular basal lamina. A series of components of the myofiber membrane cytoskeleton are recognized and have been divided into three subcomplexes: the dystroglycan complex, the syntrophin complex, and the sarcoglycan complex. The dystroglycan complex consists of two proteins: α-dystroglycan and β-dystroglycan. The extracellular α-dystroglycan interacts directly with merosin, and the transmembrane β-dystroglycan binds to dystrophin. No disease has been associated with the dystroglycan complex.

The sarcoglycan complex is described in the section on Sarcoglycanopathies.

Molecular Diagnostic Testing

The most commonly used test is the dystrophin gene deletion test using 18 exon multiplex polymerase chain reaction (PCR). It tests for the presence or absence of 18 exons of the dystrophin gene. Only 0.5 ml of blood is needed, turnaround is usually quite fast, and the cost is relatively low. Due to the frequently deleted hot spots in the dystrophin genes, 98% of deletions are detected by the 18-exon assay. This test is most frequently used for male probands. If the test is positive (one or more exons of the gene are missing), the patient definitely has a primary dystrophinopathy. Prenatal diagnosis is usually done using DNA testing of amniocytes or chorionic villus samples. A male fetus can be clearly defined as normal or affected if there is a deletion mutation.

Dystrophin Protein Testing

Dystrophin protein analysis of a muscle biopsy, either by immunohistochemistry or by Western blot analysis, is usually able to determine if a patient has a primary dystrophinopathy and can further differentiate DMD from BMD.

Treatment

No cure is available for DMD, but corticosteroids can slow the progress of the disease, and physical therapy and surgical procedures can be used to treat contractures. Surgery is also available for scoliosis. Gene therapy is the hope for a true cure. This would be accomplished by delivering the dystrophin gene to muscle fibers.

Sarcoglycanopathies

The sarcoglycan complex consists of at least four proteins: β-sarcoglycan, α-sarcoglycan, γ-sarcoglycan, and δ-sarcoglycan. Each is a transmembrane dystrophin-associated protein. The sarcoglycan proteins purify as a single complex and are probably directly associated with each other.

Clinical Features

The sarcoglycan complex, like dystrophin, must impart structural integrity to the plasma membrane because phenotypes similar to DMD or BMD result when any component of this complex is missing. Many female cases of DMD are now recognized as sarcoglycan disorders.

Genetic Features

Many muscular dystrophy patients with primarily proximal muscle weakness in both limb girdles show normal dystrophin findings. The majority are considered consistent with an autosomal recessive inheritance pattern. Whereas previous clinical studies have often grouped muscular dystrophy patients by age of onset (congenital muscular dystrophy, severe childhood autosomal recessive muscular dystrophy [SCARMD], and adult-onset muscular dystrophy), genetic linkage studies suggest that all childhood- and adult-onset dystrophies should be called *limb-girdle muscular dystrophy* (LGMD), with more specific etiology determined by distinct gene loci. LGMD 1A is the only dominantly inherited dystrophy genetically mapped to 5q. All recessively inherited loci have been designated *LGMD 2*, with letters indicating specific loci: LGMD 2A (15q), LGMD 2B (2p), LGMD 2C (13q12), LGMD 2D (17q21), and LGMD 2E (4q12). Mutation studies of candidate genes have identified the specific gene and protein corresponding to four of these five genetically mapped loci: LGMD 2A is caused by calpain 3 deficiency, LGMD 2C by γ-sarcoglycan deficiency, LGMD 2D by α-sarcoglycan deficiency, and LGMD 2E by β-sarcoglycan deficiency.

Emery-Dreifuss Muscular Dystrophy

Emery-Dreifuss muscular dystrophy (EDMD), an X-linked disorder, is characterized by early tendon contractures and cardiac arrythmias.

Clinical Features

Contraction deformities of the elbows, ankle tendons, and postcervical muscles begin in childhood. Progression is very slow. Cardiac conduction problems occur in all patients (atrial ventricular block).

Genetic Features

Early genetic studies showed EDMD to be linked with deutan color blindness. This study was followed by molecular genetic linkage analysis showing close linkage between the factor VIII gene and the EDMD gene at Xq28. A map of the EDMD gene region identified 8 transcribed genes in the cloned DNA, which were expressed in skeletal muscle, heart, or brain. One of these showed loss-of-function mutations in all EDMD patients, and the novel serine-rich protein encoded by the gene was called *emerin*. Emerin is a transmembrane protein that is mainly found in connective tissue.

Treatment

For every patient with the disorder, a cardiac pacemaker is needed to prevent sudden death.

Autosomal Recessive Dystrophy Caused by Calpain 3 Mutations

Calpain 3 is a protease. It is not clear why a deficiency of a muscle protease would lead to a progressive muscular dystrophy.

Clinical Features

The disease mainly occurs in isolated populations. It is a progressive limb-girdle dystrophy with onset in childhood.

Genetic Features

The gene for calpain deficiency maps to 15q15 and the locus was subsequently named *LGMD2A*. Pathogenic mutations are found on both alleles, consistent with the expected autosomal recessive inheritance pattern.

MYOTONIC DYSTROPHY

Myotonic dystrophy (MyD) is the most common muscular dystrophy affecting adults and children. It is transmitted as an autosomal dominant trait.

Clinical Features

The most constant feature of MyD is variable expressivity. Despite several readily recognizable features, only 25% of affected individuals are recognizable as gene carriers. During the course of disease, the proportion of recognizable patients increases to approximately 50%.

Multiple organ systems are involved. Myotonia is neither severe nor disabling. The characteristic facies includes a hatchet-like shape of the head associated with balding, slack eyes with obvious ptosis, flat smile with facial and jaw weakness, and a slightly forward carriage of the head due to neck muscle weakness. A low-normal intellectual level with a peculiar hostile, reticent, suspicious, uncooperative personality is common. Affected children are often identified because of mental retardation or severe behavioral problems. Skeletal muscle weakness first involves the distal limb muscles. A potentially life-threatening problem is cardiac involvement. Sudden death may be the first and only feature of MyD. Characteristic cataracts are located in the posterior capsular area and can appear dust-like, scintillating, and iridescent. They do not interfere with vision. Dilatation and hypomotility of the esophagus or bowel can be clinically troublesome but are not usually life-threatening. Testicular and ovarian atrophy is common.

Congenital Myotonic Dystrophy

Congenital myotonic dystrophy (CMyD) occurs in some children of affected mothers. The mother may be asymptomatic at the time of delivery. If a mother bears a child with CMyD, the chance of a subsequent affected child is 80%. Affected newborns have hypotonia, respiratory distress, poor suck, and dysmorphic features. If the child survives the neonatal period, muscle tone increases, although motor development is usually delayed. Mental retardation is common but not progressive. Myotonia is the sustained contraction of skeletal muscle, usually in response to voluntary contraction, percussion, or electrical stimulation. Myotonia develops during the first decade as the apparent inability to release hand grip or jaw clench.

Genetic Features

The MyD locus is on the proximal long arm of chromosome 19 (19q13.3). Within that region of DNA is a variable trinucleotide repeat insert consisting of 50 to several thousand CTG repeats. Normal individuals have approximately 36–40 repeats. The inheritance of the inserted element, designated *$(CTG)_n$ repeat,* is a dynamic mutation that does not remain of constant size in individuals within a pedigree The length of the $(CTG)_n$ repeat usually increases in subsequent generations, but it can contract as well. Each tissue of an individual can have different-size repeat sequences, suggesting an early embryologic effect. The length of the repeat in blood DNA appears to increase in CMyD patients compared with their mothers. The repeat length in multiple CMyD tissues is generally similar in size to the enlarged repeat sequences found in their blood DNA. The site of the dynamic mutation interrupts the 3' untranslated region of a protein kinase gene that has been named *myotonin protein kinase*. It is still unclear how the expansion of the $(CTG)_n$ repeat in the 3' untranslated region of the myotonin protein kinase is related to the pathogenesis of the disease in muscle or any of the other organ systems affected by MyD.

MyD appears to start earlier and be more severe in successive generations (anticipation). The discovery that trinucleotide repeats get larger in successive generations explains the phenomenon of anticipation.

FACIOSCAPULOHUMERAL MUSCULAR DYSTROPHY

Facioscapulohumeral muscular dystrophy (FSHD) is transmitted as an autosomal dominant trait with variable expression.

Clinical Features

FSHD has a characteristic distribution of weakness. The face and shoulder girdle muscles are affected first, followed by involvement of the peroneal or hip girdle muscles. Patients often give a history of long-standing difficulties in keeping up with peers, climbing stairs, whistling, and drinking through a straw. Progression is usually slow. Eventually, 20% of patients are wheelchair-confined. An infantile-onset form is characterized by rapid progression and severe disability at an early age. The most common initial feature is scapular winging from weakness of the serratus, rhomboid, supraspinatus, and infraspinatus muscles. The pectoral muscles, the biceps, and the triceps muscles are atrophied and the deltoid muscles spared. Facial weakness is always present but without perceived symptoms. Facial expression is decreased, but extraocular, eyelid, and bulbar muscles are spared. The peroneal muscles are involved and the calf muscles spared. Some patients have more severe weakness in proximal than distal leg muscles. Tendon reflexes are often reduced.

The only definite extramuscular manifestations of FSHD are sensorineural hearing loss and retinal telangiectasias. Peripheral retinal telangiectasias are usually asymptomatic but can result in exudative retinal detachment (Coats' disease). Symptomatic cardiac involvement has not been clearly documented.

Genetic Features

The gene locus of FSHD is distal to 4q35. A small *Eco*RI fragment cosegregates with FSHD in the subtelomeric region of 4q. This DNA rearrangement is a deletion of variable size in a 3.3-kb repetitive element. Sequences with homology to homeobox genes within the 3.3-kb repeat elements led to speculation that a defective homeobox gene may be responsible for FSHD. No transcriptional units have been identified within the repeat elements. Several affected individuals from families with the FSHD-associated small *Eco*RI fragment show recombination proximal to the deletion, which raises the possibility that the FSHD gene may be more centromeric than the 3.3-kb repeats. This finding has led to the hypothesis that the deletion within the 3.3-kb repeat elements brings the FSHD gene closer to heterochromatic telomeric DNA, thus interfering with gene expression, a mechanism referred to as *position effect variegation*.

The size of the 4q35 deletion varies from kindred to kindred but is stable within members of the same kindred. A significant correlation exists between fragment size and disease severity in sporadic FSHD cases. Disease severity is the same whether FSHD is maternally or paternally inherited.

The use of DNA testing to confirm the diagnosis of FSHD or to perform prenatal diagnosis is limited to certain specific situations. FSHD will remain a clinical diagnosis until specific mutations can be detected.

Treatment

Treatment remains supportive. Ankle-foot orthoses are useful for footdrop, and surgical scapular fixation can improve arm mobility. Pharmacologic treatments aimed at slowing disease progression have not been successful. An open, natural history–controlled trial of prednisone in eight patients showed no improvement.

DISEASES ASSOCIATED WITH DEFECTS OF BETA-OXIDATION

Mitochondrial β-oxidation of the long-chain fatty acids is crucial for energy production in the skeletal muscle and the heart and is essential for the synthesis of ketone bodies in the liver. Genetic diseases of fatty acid mitochondrial β-oxidation are autosomal recessive disorders of infancy and childhood, although some patients present later in life. Although these disorders are multisystemic, the presenting symptoms tend to be homogeneous, and in only a few diseases is the diagnosis suggested by the clinical features alone (Table 13.1).

Plasma free fatty acids are the main lipid fuel for peripheral organs. Once delivered into the cytosol, free fatty acids must undergo a series of enzymatic reactions to enter the mitochondrial matrix, where β-oxidation occurs. First, long-chain acyl coenzyme A (acyl-CoA) esters are synthesized, from the corresponding long-chain fatty acids and the cytosolic free coenzyme A pool, by the long-chain acyl-CoA synthetase of the outer mitochondrial membrane. Because the inner mitochondrial membrane is impermeable to acyl-CoA esters, the acyl groups are transferred into mitochondria as acyl-carnitine esters. L-Carnitine; two carnitine palmitoyltransferases (CPT), located to the inner aspect of the outer mitochondrial membrane (CPT I) and to the matrix side of the inner mitochondrial membrane (CPT II); and a carnitine-acylcarnitine translocase (CT), embedded in the inner mitochondrial membrane, are required in mammalian tissues to transfer long-chain acyl-CoAs across the inner membrane. To generate acetyl CoA, fatty acyl-CoA esters undergo a process characterized by repeated cycles of four concerted reactions involving flavin adenine dinucleotide (FAD)–dependent dehydrogenation of acyl-CoAs, hydration of 2-enoyl CoAs, nicotinamide adenine dinucleotide

Table 13.1
Clinical features in diseases of mitochondrial β-oxidation.

Hepatic signs
- Hypoglycemia associated with low ketones (hypoketotic hypoglycemia)
- Reye's-like syndrome
- Steatosis
- Acute hepatic failure
- Sudden infant death syndrome

Muscle signs
- Hypotonia
- Weakness and wasting
- Proximal myopathy with lipid storage
- Exercise intolerance and muscle pain with increased levels of creatine kinase
- Episodic rhabdomyolysis (with occasional paroxystic myoglobinuria)

Cardiac signs
- Hypertrophic and dilated cardiomyopathy
- Progressive heart failure
- Arrhythmias
- Cardiac arrest
- Sudden infant death syndrome

Nervous system signs
- Permanent brain damage due to hypoglycemia, arrhythmias, or cardiac arrest
- Microgyria, cortical atrophy, and neuronal heterotopia
- Pigmentary retinopathy
- Peripheral sensorimotor neuropathy

Malformations
- Renal dysplasia and nephromegaly*
- Polycystic kidney
- Facial dysmorphism
- Brain malformations

*Proximal and distal tubulopathy is observed in carnitine palmitoyltransferase I deficiency.

(NAD)–dependent oxidation of 3-hydroxyacyl-CoAs, and coenzyme A (CoA-SH)–dependent thiolysis of 3-ketoacyl-CoAs. The first step of the β-oxidation spiral is catalyzed by FAD-dependent dehydrogenases, the fatty acyl-CoA dehydrogenases, which are present in mammalian mitochondria in three molecular forms: the very-long-chain acyl-CoA dehydrogenase (VLCAD) of the inner mitochondrial membrane; the long-chain, medium-chain, and short-chain acyl-CoA dehydrogenase (LCAD, MCAD, and SCAD) of the mitochondrial matrix; and trifunctional protein (TP), a multifunctional protein that exibits long-chain 3-hydroxyacyl-CoA dehydrogenase (LCAD) activity in addition to enoyl CoA hydrase and 3-oxoacyl-CoA thiolase activities. During fatty acid oxidation the electrons are transferred to the respiratory chain (see Chapter 4).

Defects of Long-Chain Fatty Acid Transport

Classification of diseases of long-chain fatty acid transport is based on knowledge of the fundamental biochemical defects (Tables 13.2 and 13.3). L-Carnitine has an essential role in the transport of long-chain fatty acids into mitochondria for β-oxidation, and must, itself, be actively transported from the blood into fatty acid–metabolizing organs.

Primary Carnitine Deficiency with Cardiomyopathy

Clinical Features. Primary carnitine deficiency with cardiomyopathy presents in familial form, suggesting autosomal recessive inheritance. It is characterized by the combination of cardiomyopathy, hypoglycemia attacks, systemic carnitine deficiency, and defective carnitine transport. Half of patients present with a progressive dilated cardiomyopathy and half with hypoglycemia and hypoketonemia; a few start with myopathic symptoms. Carnitine content is low in muscle, heart, liver, and plasma. Plasma total and free carnitines are less than 10% of normal, but carnitine esters are not increased. Total carnitine is reduced to 1–2% of the normal mean in skeletal muscle; it is also low in heart. Morphologic features include lipid storage in type I skeletal muscle fibers, heart, and liver. Carnitine supplementation (usually 2–6 g/day of oral L-carnitine) allows heart function and muscle strength to progressively return to normal, and attacks of hypoglycemia tend to disappear.

Genetic Features. Carnitine transport across the cell membrane is defective. Autosomal recessive inheritance is suspected. Patients homozygous for the putative mutation lack functionally active plasma-membrane high-affinity carnitine receptors, whereas heterozygotes retain approximately 50% of the receptor pool.

Carnitine Palmitoyltransferase I Deficiency

Clinical Features. Infants with CPT I deficiency have recurrent attacks of fasting-induced life-threatening hypoketotic hypoglycemia. Hypoglycemia attacks may be associated with lethargy, coma, and seizures. They may cause death or result in psychomotor developmental delay, hemiplegia, or generalized epilepsy. Hepatomegaly and

Table 13.2
Defects of fatty acid transport.

	Phenotype			
Enzyme/Cofactor	*Myopathy/ Hypotonia*	*Cardiomyopathy*	*Myoglobinuria*	*Hypoglycemia Hypoketonemia*
Carnitine	+	++	–	++
Carnitine palmitoyltransferase I	±	±	–	++
Carnitine palmitoyltransferase II*	–	++	++	++
Carnitine acylcarnitine translocase	±	+	+	+

++ = present; + = sometimes present; ± = rarely observed; – = absent.
*Neonatal forms with multiple organ malformations.

Table 13.3
Defects of enzymes of the β-oxidation spiral.

	Phenotype			
Enzyme/Cofactor	*Myopathy/ Hypotonia*	*Cardiomyopathy*	*Myoglobinuria*	*Hypoglycemia Hypoketonemia*
Very long-chain acyl-CoA dehydrogenase	+	++	++	+
Long-chain 3-hydroxyacyl-CoA dehydrogenase; trifunctional protein[a]	++	++	+	++
Long-chain acyl-CoA dehydrogenase[b]	+	++	–	++
Medium-chain acyl-CoA dehydrogenase	±	±	±	++
Short-chain acyl-CoA dehydrogenase	+	±	–	+
Short-chain 3-hydroxyacyl-CoA dehydrogenase	+	++	++	++
2-4 dienoyl CoA reductase	+	–	–	–

++ = present; + = sometimes present; ± = rarely observed; – = absent.
[a]Peripheral neuropathy and pigmentary retinopathy is present in a subgroup of patients.
[b]The very existence of this disease has not yet been proved.

liver steatosis are typical. Plasma carnitine levels tend to be increased rather than low, as in most defects of β-oxidation.

Carnitine Palmitoyltransferase II Deficiency

CLINICAL FEATURES. In the neonatal–early infantile form of CPT II deficiency, affected newborns have severe hypoketotic hypoglycemia and generalized steatosis. Death usually occurs within a few days. Patients often show multiple organ malformations, including renal cystic dysplasia, nephromegaly, microgyria, subarachnoid hemorrhages, neuronal heterotopia in the brain, and facial dysmorphism.

CPT II enzyme activity is either barely detectable or reduced to less than 10% of normal. The infantile hepatomuscular phenotype is similar to CPT I deficiency: acute episodes of fasting hypoglycemia with inappropriate levels of blood ketones leading to lethargy, coma, and death. CPT I activity is normal, but CPT II activity is reduced to less than 10% of normal. Cells lack CPT II protein, as in patients with the adult muscular phenotype.

The adult muscular phenotype is characterized by exercise-induced myoglobinuria in a young adult. The disease is inherited as an autosomal recessive trait but occurs most frequently in young adult males, probably because environmental and hormonal factors influence the expression of the defect. In typical patients, the attacks are triggered by prolonged exercise in fasting conditions and consist of pain, stiffness, and discomfort of skeletal muscles, without clinical and neurophysiologic evidence of cramps. Sometimes, these metabolic attacks end in massive rhabdomyolysis with myoglobinuria, evidenced by dark urine, and often resulting in acute renal failure. Typically, serum CK concentrations may peak up to 100,000 mU/liter. Between episodes, the serum CK concentration is either normal or only slightly elevated.

BIOCHEMISTRY AND GENETIC FEATURES. CPT II is a homotetrameric enzyme of 68-kd subunits. A 2.2-kb cDNA encoding the full-length CPT II subunit of 658 amino acids was cloned. The corresponding gene (*CPT1*) has been mapped to human chromosome 1p32. Studies of the CPT II promoter region suggest that the gene expression might be hormonally regulated. The first mutation in the CPT II gene was described in the hepatomuscular form: It consisted of a C-to-T transition at nucleotide 1,992, causing an arginine-to-cysteine substitution at codon 631 (R631C). A different missense mutation in the carboxy-terminal of CPT II was reported later in another patient with the same phenotype. In patients with the adult muscular presentation, the prevalent mutation is a C-to-T transition at nucleotide 439, changing a highly conserved serine into leucine (S113L). Subsequently, other mutations were shown to segregate with the adult muscular form of CPT II deficiency, including a C-to-A transversion at nucleotide 665 in exon 1, resulting in a proline to histidine substitution at residue 50 of the protein (P50H).

For a more detailed discussion see Fardeau M, Tomé FMS, Samson F, Romero N, Helbling-Leclerc A. Congenital Myopathies (Chapter 49; pp. 867–876); Hoffman EP. The Muscular Dystrophies (Chapter 50; pp. 877–912); Roses AD. Myotonic Dystrophy (Chapter 51; pp. 913–930); Tawil R, Griggs RC. Facioscapulohumeral Muscular Dystrophy (Chapter 52; pp. 931–937); Di Donato S. Diseases Associated with Defects of Beta-Oxidation (Chapter 53; pp. 939–956), in RN Rosenberg, SB Prusiner, S DiMauro, RL Barchi (eds), **The Molecular and Genetic Basis of Neurological Disease** ***(2nd ed). Boston: Butterworth–Heinemann, 1997.***

14

The Phakomatoses: Disorders of Skin and Brain

The neurofibromatoses and von Hippel-Lindau disease are discussed in Chapter 9.

XERODERMA PIGMENTOSUM

Xeroderma pigmentosum (XP), a rare, recessively inherited disorder, is one of a family of conditions involving cellular defects in the ability to process DNA damage. DNA damage and permanent mutations occur continuously in all cells.

Clinical Features

All cell types examined from patients with XP exhibit a similar defect in unscheduled DNA repair. These include intact or dissociated epidermal cells, dermal fibroblasts, lymphocytes, conjunctival cells, corneal cells, vascular endothelium, smooth muscle cells, liver cells, and basal cell carcinoma cells. Amniotic fluid cells obtained during pregnancy can show defective DNA repair after ultraviolet (UV) irradiation and have been used for prenatal diagnosis of XP.

The cutaneous manifestations occur by 18 months of age in 50% of patients, by 4 years in 75%, and by 15 years in 95%. The first sign is sunburn, due to acute sensitivity to sunlight (photodermatoses), then excessive freckling (solar lentigenes), and finally skin atrophy and telangiectasia of exposed areas. Even the tip of the tongue, gingivae, and palate may be affected. Irregular pigmented and depigmented areas of skin occur because of local multiplication of a mutant clone of melanocytes. Premalignant actinic keratoses cause the mouth to tighten from scarring. Half of children have skin cancer by age 14 years. Eye damage usually occurs by age 4 years; loss of eye protection causes exposure keratitis and corneal scarring, and squamous cell and basal cell carcinoma occur on the conjunctiva or cornea.

Approximately 20% of XP patients have neurologic manifestations. They are divided into three groups by age of onset (Table 14.1). The initial feature is psychomotor retardation followed by progressive neurologic deterioration, abnormal ocular motility, ataxia, choreoathetosis, spasticity, dementia, sensorineural deafness, and microcephaly.

Neuroimaging studies show loss of brain volume with a thickened calvarium, ventricular dilatation, and enlarging subarachnoid spaces. Atrophic changes in brain stem and cerebellum suggest olivopontocerebellar degeneration.

Genetic Features

XP is a recessive disorder with increased consanguinity in parents. Subtypes of XP may predominate in particular regions and explain the over-representation of XP neurologic patients in Japan, as a majority of Japanese patients belong to complementation group A. A family in Scotland is reported with a dominant pattern of inheritance.

Human DNA is constantly being damaged, both spontaneously (endogenously) and after exposure to environmental agents (exogenously), such as radiation from UV light, smoking, and chemotherapeutic agents. Damaged mammalian DNA is repaired by mismatch mechanisms involving specific glycosylases or by nucleotide excision repair (NER). For example, damage to a specific nucleotide can be repaired (mismatch repair) by a pathway of glycolytic cleavage of the abnormal base, with subsequent processing by an endonuclease or exonuclease, DNA polymerase, and ligase. Gene defects localized to chromosomes 2, 9, 10, 13, and 19 and their respective gene products are involved in NER mechanisms and XP.

In NER, an enzyme system hydrolyzes two phosphodiester bonds, one on either side of the DNA lesion, and the oligonucleotide carrying the damage is released from the duplex. The resulting gap is filled in with complementary DNA (cDNA) and ligated to complete the repair process. Approximately one dozen enzymes are involved in this repair system.

The relationship between defective DNA repair and the neuronal degeneration is not established, because UV light cannot penetrate to the brain. An intrinsic accumulation of damaged neuronal DNA, leading eventually to an inability to maintain normal neuronal function and early onset of cell death, is proposed. DNA damage could be due to spontaneous physicochemical changes affecting cellular DNA, accumulation of normal intraneuronal metabolites, or extracellular substances entering the neurons and interacting with the DNA. Selective vulnerability of neurons to endogenous damage from oxidative stress

Table 14.1
Xeroderma pigmentosum with neurologic abnormalities.

Classification	*Symptomatic Onset (Age in Years)*	*Complementation Group*
Juvenile-onset		
Early-onset (De Sanctis-Cacchione)	<7	A
Intermediate-onset (Neisser)	7–12	D (G)
Late-onset	13–20	A
Adult-onset	>21	C
XP-Cockayne's syndrome	<7	B, D, G
XP-trichothiodystrophy	<7	B, D, G

XP = xeroderma pigmentosum.
Source: Adapted from JE Cleaver, KH Kraemer. Xeroderma Pigmentosum and Cockayne Syndrome. In CR Scriver, AL Beaudet, WS Sly, D Valle (eds), The Metabolic and Molecular Bases of Inherited Disease (7th ed). New York: McGraw-Hill, 1995;4393; KH Kraemer, H Slor. Xeroderma pigmentosum. Clin Dermatol 1985;3:33; and JH Robbins. A childhood neurodegeneration due to defective DNA repair: a novel concept of disease based on studies of xeroderma pigmentosum. J Child Neurol 1989;4:143.

reactions (free radicals) and normal metabolites could depend on specific and different functions of neuronal populations.

Treatment

Treatment is directed at early diagnosis of XP so that abnormally sensitive skin can be protected from harmful UV radiation in sunlight and other sources, such as germicidal lamps and artificial sun lamps. Protective clothing, glasses, and headgear together with sunblock applications to exposed skin surfaces have been successful in avoiding acute and chronic skin changes to UV light. Unfortunately, no specific treatment to prevent the progressive neurologic disease is available.

TUBEROUS SCLEROSIS

Tuberous sclerosis complex (TSC) is a disorder of cellular differentiation and proliferation.

Clinical Features

Many of the clinical features result from hamartomatous malformations in the affected organs, and abnormal neuronal migration is a major factor in neurologic dysfunction. The skin lesions of TSC are important in establishing the diagnosis. These include hypomelanotic macules, the shagreen patch, ungual fibromas, and facial angiofibromas. Almost all patients with TSC have at least one cutaneous lesion. Hypomelanotic macules (ash leaf spots) are found in at least 90% of patients. One or two hypomelanotic macules are commonly found in normal individuals and are not specific for TSC. Facial angiofibromas (adenoma sebaceum) are hamartomatous nodules of vascular and connective tissue elements. Although considered specific for TSC, they occur in only three-fourths of patients and do not become apparent for several years after birth. The shagreen patch, usually found on the back or flank area, is an irregularly shaped, slightly raised or textured skin lesion. Ungual fibromas are nodular or fleshy lesions that arise adjacent to or from underneath the nails.

Retinal hamartomas are relatively frequent when pupillary dilatation and indirect ophthalmoscopy are used for examination. Pigmentary iris defects are not as common as retinal lesions.

Epileptic seizures and mental retardation are the most important neurologic problems. Seizures occur in 80–90% of patients. Infantile spasms and tonic-clonic seizures are particularly common, but tonic, akinetic, myoclonic, and atypical absence seizures also occur. Epileptic foci tend to arise near the larger cerebral lesions as seen on magnetic resonance imaging (MRI). Some children develop normally until the onset of seizures, after which their progress slows and developmental regression may occur. Children whose seizures begin early in life are more likely to also have intellectual impairment, and children whose seizures are uncontrolled probably have an even higher likelihood of intellectual impairment.

Giant cell astrocytomas develop in up to 15% of TSC patients. The initial feature may be a focal neurologic deficit, increased intracranial pressure, unexplained behavior change, or deterioration of seizure control. Acute or subacute onset of neurologic dysfunction may result from sudden obstruction of the ventricular system by an intraventricular portion of the tumor or by hemorrhage within the tumor itself. Giant cell astrocytomas most often occur in the anterior horn of the lateral ventricle. Calcified subependymal nodules are a characteristic feature on neuroimaging studies. MRI lesions in the cortex and subcortical white matter probably correspond to the hamartomas, gliotic areas, and neuronal migration defects. Both CT and MRI are recommended as a means of identifying TSC in family members with few other signs.

Cardiac rhabdomyomata occur in more than half of patients, but few become symptomatic. Like most other tumors associated with TSC, they are considered hamartomas. Occasionally, patients develop cerebral thromboembolism, probably because an intracardiac tumor pro-

Table 14.2
Diagnostic criteria for tuberous sclerosis.[a]

A. Primary features
1. Facial angiofibromas[b]
2. Multiple ungual fibromas[b]
3. Cortical tuber (histologically confirmed)
4. Subependymal nodule or giant cell astrocytoma (histologically confirmed)
5. Multiple calcified subependymal nodules protruding into the ventricle (radiographic evidence)
6. Multiple retinal astrocytomas[b]

B. Secondary features
1. Affected first-degree relative
2. Cardiac rhabdomyoma (histologic or radiographic confirmation)
3. Other retinal hamartoma or achromic patch[b]
4. Cerebral tubers (radiographic confirmation)
5. Noncalcified subependymal nodules (radiographic confirmation)
6. Shagreen patch[b]
7. Forehead plaque[b]
8. Pulmonary lymphangiomyomatosis (histologic confirmation)
9. Renal angiomyolipoma (radiographic or histologic confirmation)
10. Renal cysts (histologic confirmation)

C. Tertiary features
1. Hypomelanotic macules[b]
2. "Confetti" skin lesions[b]
3. Renal cysts (radiographic evidence)
4. Randomly distributed enamel pits in deciduous or permanent teeth
5. Hamartomatous rectal polyps (histologic confirmation)
6. Bone cysts (radiographic evidence)
7. Pulmonary lymphangiomyomatosis (radiographic evidence)
8. Cerebral white matter "migration tracts" or heterotopias (radiographic evidence)
9. Gingival fibromas[b]
10. Hamartoma of other organs (histologic confirmation)
11. Infantile spasms

[a]Definite TSC: one primary feature, two secondary features, or one secondary feature plus two tertiary features; probable TSC: either one secondary feature plus one tertiary feature or three tertiary features; suspect TSC: either one secondary feature or two tertiary features.
[b]Histologic confirmation is not required if the lesion is clinically obvious.
Source: Reprinted with permission from ES Roach, M Smith, P Huttenlocher, et al. Report of the diagnostic criteria committee of the National Tuberous Sclerosis Association. J Child Neurol 1992;7:221.

motes thrombus formation, rather than tumor embolization. Renal angiomyolipomas occur in approximately two-thirds of patients and are probably the leading cause of death in adults with TSC.

The diagnostic criteria of TSC are listed in Table 14.2.

Genetic Features

TSC is inherited as an autosomal dominant trait with variable penetrance. Estimates of the rate of spontaneous mutation vary from 56% to 86%. The clinical pattern of TSC is variable even among affected members of the same family. Linkage between TSC and the ABO blood group locus assigned TSC to the distal long arm of chromosome 9 at q34. The gene on chromosome 9 is called *TSC1*, and has been narrowed to the 9q34.1 region. Linkage to chromosome 9 occurs in only one-third to one-half of families.

The gene for adult polycystic kidney disease is on chromosome 16. The frequent occurrence of renal cysts in TSC led to the identification of a TSC locus on chromosome 16 called the *TSC2* gene. The *TSC2* gene encodes a 198-kd protein (tuberin). This gene accounts for at least one-half of the patients with TSC. Therefore, at least two different genes cause TSC, but evidently neither produces a distinct phenotype. It is postulated that both *TSC1* and *TSC2* function as tumor suppressor genes and that a tumor occurs if both genes dysfunction. An individual with an existing mutation, either spontaneous or inherited, develops a tumor after a second somatic mutation occurs in the other allele. A reliable means of carrier detection or antenatal diagnosis is not available.

STURGE-WEBER SYNDROME

The Sturge-Weber (SW) syndrome is a sporadic disorder consisting of a malformation of the capillaries and venules of the leptomeninges and the ipsilateral face in the distribution of the first branch of the trigeminal nerve.

Clinical Features

The facial vascular malformation is congenital and usually evident at birth as a pink macule. It is ipsilateral to the leptomeningeal malformation, but of patients with bilateral facial nevus, only one-half have bilateral cerebral involvement. Unilateral facial involvement is the rule. The facial angioma almost always involves the eyelids. Many patients with a port-wine stain in the distribution of the first branch of the trigeminal nerve do not have SW syndrome. The pink macules of infancy darken with age to red or purple. The affected skin may become roughened and bleed after minor trauma.

Ocular involvement occurs in 40% of patients. The vascular lesion may involve the conjunctiva or the choroid. The choroidal lesion may displace the retina, resulting in refractive error or cystoid degeneration. Glaucoma occurs ipsilateral to the port-wine stain in up to 45% of patients.

Seizures may be the first sign of neurologic involvement. The mean age of onset is 24 months in those with unilateral brain involvement and 6 months in those with bilateral involvement. Patients usually are neurologically normal at birth. Intractable seizures in the first year of life may lead to mental retardation. Clinical status correlates with the extent of brain involvement and parenchymal atrophy as demonstrated by MRI.

Genetic Features

Family history is almost always negative for SW syndrome, and the disorder has been reported in one of identical twins.

Treatment

Treatment of the port-wine stain by radiation, cryotherapy, dermabrasion, or tattooing has been unsuccessful. The argon laser is successful for 80% of adults; however, slight sclerosis and erythema are common. Ninety-four percent of children treated with the flash lamp-pulsed tunable dye laser have normal skin texture and color. Seizures can be controlled by anticonvulsants in at least 50% of patients, which results in improved intellectual function. Hemispherectomy should be considered to control seizures that are refractory to medical management.

INCONTINENTIA PIGMENTI

Incontinentia pigmenti (IP) is a generalized ectodermal and mesodermal dysplasia that most visibly affects the skin but has potential impact on multiple organ systems.

Clinical Features

The first stage usually begins at birth or within the first month of life. The inflammatory phase occurs in a linear, whorled, or splashlike distribution, sparing the face but involving the scalp, trunk, and especially the proximal and flexor surfaces of the limbs. The lesions are primarily vesicular but may be macules, papules, bullae, and rarely, pustules. Blood eosinophilia ranges up to 65% with an associated peripheral leukocytosis. Affected children appear well, which helps to discriminate IP from other disorders such as disseminated herpes. The rash resolves spontaneously without sequelae. The second (verrucous or lichenoid) stage, seen in approximately 30% of patients, peaks between 2 and 6 weeks of age but often recurs during infancy. The eruptions are distributed as before but are linear with acanthotic, dyskeratotic, hyperkeratotic, or papular lesions. The verrucous lesions are particularly prominent on the dorsal surfaces of the hands and feet. Resolution of most of the lesions occurs after a few months; mild atrophic changes may remain. In the third, or pigmented, stage, melanin is deposited outside as well as within melanophores in the upper dermis. This peaks between the twelfth and twenty-sixth weeks of life. Striking skin changes, with tan, gray, or brown pigment distributed in streaks, whorls, speckles, and even bizarre patterns such as zebra stripes or veins in marble, are seen primarily on the lateral trunk and proximal extremities. These lesions often occur in areas not previously involved. They do not follow nerve, vessel, or cleavage lines. This pigmented phase is the longest in duration and the one most commonly recognized with the diagnosis. These lesions often fade in the second or third decades. A fourth cutaneous stage is best seen in adolescents and adults. It is often missed because the hypopigmented, hairless, atrophic patches or streaks are not easily appreciated. Depigmented lesions, particularly linear streaks on the posterior aspects of the calves, may represent the only expression in an adult of the obligate carrier state.

Dental anomalies in conjunction with strabismus are the most common extradermatologic findings. Sixty-five percent of patients have abnormal deciduous dentition. Alterations of dental structures have included delayed tooth eruptions, pegged teeth, missing teeth, and conical formation of the crowns, which is similar to that observed in the anhidrotic form of ectodermal dysplasia. The incidence of ocular abnormalities is estimated to be approximately 35%. They range from strabismus and nystagmus to complete blindness.

One-third of patients have disorders of the central nervous system, with seizures being most common. Spastic paralysis, mental retardation, and slow motor development follow in frequency. An acute encephalopathy may occur that primarily involves the white matter and is associated with remittent bouts of focal edema and probable hemorrhagic necrosis. The result is focal necrosis, white matter cavitation, and neuronal loss.

Genetic Features

Family history is positive in half of cases, and a female predominance (37:1) exists. The current thought is that IP represents an X-linked dominant disorder with male hemizygote lethality. Two loci, Xp11.21

and Xq28, have been identified and named *IP1* and *IP2*. IP1 does not consistently demonstrate the associated clinical findings and is sometimes designated *X-autosome translocation associated with pigmentary abnormality*. IP2 is believed to represent what was originally defined as IP.

Treatment

Bone and dental anomalies are treated symptomatically. The dermatologic involvement defies treatment. Photocoagulation cryotherapy and vitreous surgery are occasionally used for the neovascularization in the ocular lesions. Seizures are treated with anticonvulsants appropriate to clinical and electroencephalographic typing.

For a more detailed discussion see Butler IJ. Xeroderma Pigmentosum (Chapter 54; pp. 959–967); Roach ES. Tuberous Sclerosis (Chapter 55; pp. 969–980); Michels VV. Von Hippel–Lindau Disease (Chapter 56A; pp. 981–988); Michels VV. Sturge-Weber Syndrome (Chapter 56B; pp. 989–994); Tilton AH, Willis JK II. Incontinentia Pigmenti (Chapter 57; pp. 995–1000), in RN Rosenberg, SB Prusiner, S DiMauro, RL Barchi (eds), **The Molecular and Genetic Basis of Neurological Disease** ***(2nd ed). Boston: Butterworth–Heinemann, 1997.***

15

Lipoprotein Disorders

The system of lipoproteins that transports lipids in plasma also interacts with neural tissue. The transport of antioxidant tocopherols is critically dependent on lipoproteins of intestinal and hepatic origin that contain the B apolipoproteins (apo B). Severe impairment of absorption of tocopherols by the intestine occurs in disorders in which intestinal apo B-48 cannot be secreted normally, including abetalipoproteinemia (ABL) and chylomicron retention disease. The second phase of tocopherol transport, from liver to peripheral tissues, is impaired in those disorders in which hepatic secretion of apo B-100 is defective. The neuropathologic features common to all these disorders are attributable to the accumulation of oxidized lipids in myelin, leading to peripheral neuropathy and degeneration of posterior columns and spinocerebellar tracts.

Several apolipoproteins are synthesized in the central nervous system, and others distribute there passively. Some of these appear to play important roles in the sequestration and retrieval of lipids during the regeneration of injured neural tissue. The relationships so far identified between disorders of lipoprotein metabolism and dysfunction of nerve tissue are chiefly the consequences of alterations in lipid constituents of the neuron and its intimate environment. It is now appreciated that several apolipoproteins and the LP(a) protein are found in central nervous system tissue or in cerebrospinal fluid. At least two apolipoproteins, E and D, are expressed there in substantial quantities and appear to play important roles in the response of nerve tissue to injury. Several others that enter the central nervous system passively may also contribute to regeneration or remyelination of nerves.

DISORDERS OF LIPOPROTEINS CONTAINING APOLIPOPROTEIN B

Abetalipoproteinemia

ABL is transmitted as an autosomal recessive disorder.

Clinical Features

The absence of plasma lipoproteins that contain apo B cause fat malabsorption, acanthocytosis, retinopathy, and progressive neurologic disease. These features develop over time. Malabsorption of fat may start in the neonatal period with diarrhea, vomiting, and failure to gain weight, followed by failure to thrive. The malabsorption results from the failure of the intestinal cells to secrete lipids in chylomicrons. Endoscopy shows yellowish discoloration of the duodenal mucosa and biopsy specimens reveal normally formed villi that are engorged with lipids. Although stool loss of fatty acids may be as little as 20% of the ingested amount, this is enough to induce oxalate urolithiasis in adults with ABL.

Deficiencies of the fat-soluble vitamins A, E, and K result from the malabsorption of lipids. Low levels of vitamin K in plasma result in prothrombin deficiency. Vitamin D has its own transport protein, and hence its absorption is unimpaired. Normal plasma concentration levels of vitamins A and K are achieved when supplemental vitamin is given; however, even massive doses of vitamin E do not raise plasma levels to the normal range in some patients.

Acanthocytes account for 50% to nearly 100% of circulating erythrocytes in patients with ABL but are not seen in bone marrow. Erythrocyte sedimentation rates are low because rouleau formation is inhibited. Erythroid hyperplasia, reticulocytosis, hyperbilirubinemia, and decreased red cell survival occur. Severe anemia in children with ABL probably reflects deficiencies of iron, folate, and vitamin E secondary to fat malabsorption.

Pigmentary retinal degeneration resembling retinitis pigmentosa, which is not associated with lipoprotein deficiency, is a prominent feature of ABL. The most severe degeneration occurs in patients with severe neurologic symptoms, suggesting a common mechanism. The retinopathy of ABL may be related to deficiency of vitamin A, because some improvement occurs when vitamin A supplements are given, but it is not the key factor. Loss of night vision is frequently the earliest symptom. Decreased tendon reflexes may appear in the first decade, probably reflecting the loss of function in posterior columns and spinocerebellar pathways. Ataxic gait and loss of proprioception and vibratory sense are usually progressive. Before the advent of vitamin E therapy, patients were frequently unable to stand by the third decade, and dysmetric movements and dysarthria became severe. Muscle contractures result in equinovarus, pes cavus, and kyphoscoliosis. Mental retardation is a feature in some cases but cannot be attributed to the basic metabolic defect of ABL.

Genetic Features

The genes for apo B-100 appear to have grossly normal structure. The concentration of apo B-100 mRNA is increased compared with normal subjects, and a B-100–like protein has been detected. These findings indicate that the defect involves the posttranslational modification of apo B-100 or its incorporation into lipoproteins and secretion into plasma. Mutations in the microsomal triglyceride transport protein (MTP) explain recessive ABL in a number of cases. It is likely that the majority of cases involve defects in the heterodimeric protein MTP–protein disulfide isomerase or other elements required for lipidation of nascent apo B. Failure to detect apo B in some cases may reflect heterogeneity of the genetic mechanisms underlying this disorder.

Hypobetalipoproteinemia

Hypobetalipoproteinemia (HBL) is characterized by very low levels of apo B and low-density lipoprotein (LDL) cholesterol in plasma.

Clinical Features

Patients heterozygous for familial HBL are usually asymptomatic. Plasma cholesterol concentrations range from 40 to 180 mg/dl and triglycerides from 15 mg/dl up to the normal range. Lipid composition of the lipoproteins is normal. One patient with heterozygous familial HBL had neurologic findings that resembled olivopontocerebellar atrophy.

Homozygous patients resemble those with ABL and generally have no detectable apo B–containing lipoproteins. Chylomicrons do not appear after consumption of foods with high fat content. The acanthocytosis, gastrointestinal features, retinitis, and neuromuscular manifestations described in ABL are usually present.

Genetic Features

HBL is caused by mutations in the apo B gene that interfere with translation of complete apo B-100, or apo B alleles are present that produce reduced amounts of normal apo B-100. Several mutations leading to truncations of apo B protein have been identified. Truncated B proteins shorter than B-31 apparently cannot be secreted from hepatocytes or enterocytes. Longer B proteins are secreted in lipoproteins. Because the ability to incorporate lipids into lipoprotein complexes is a monotonic function of the length of the apo B chain, many of the secreted lipoproteins have abnormal densities. Apo B chains longer than B-50 are able to organize triglyceride-rich, very low-density lipoprotein (VLDL)-like particles, whereas shorter products may appear as hyperdense LDL or may even be found in the high-density lipoprotein (HDL) density interval. All of the truncations described to date involve the deletion of linear sequence from the carboxyl end of the protein and are attributable to mutations leading to the formation of premature stop codons. Truncated proteins shorter than B-70 would be expected to lack the ligand domain for the LDL receptor. In addition, HBL that cosegregates with the apo B locus but that is not associated with truncations has been observed. These mutations may involve regulatory elements for the gene. An additional, distinct mechanism for HBL is suggested by a kindred in which the B-48 protein is secreted into plasma but no B-100 is found. Haplotyping studies have established that, unlike most cases of HBL, the disorder in this family is not linked to the apo B gene locus. It is possible that this represents a tissue-specific defect in B-100 secretion, or perhaps complete editing of B-100 mRNA in liver and intestine.

Chylomicron Retention Disease

Clinical Features

The age of onset of chylomicron retention disease is in infancy. Fat malabsorption, fat-laden intestinal epithelial cells, and low levels of LDL, HDL, and fat-soluble vitamins are the main features. Postprandial chylomicronemia is absent. Growth retardation follows. One patient had mild acanthocytosis, and three developed neurologic symptoms in the second decade that included diminished tendon reflexes and vibratory sense, low or low-normal intelligence, and mildly abnormal retinal function. Apo B-48 synthesis is normal, but formation and secretion of chylomicrons are impaired.

Genetic Features

The absence of vertical transmission, its frequency among siblings, and consanguineous relationships in families of affected persons suggest an autosomal recessive inheritance. Abnormalities of the apo B gene locus have been excluded as a cause of this disorder.

Treatment

The intestinal symptoms of ABL and the homozygous form of familial HBL correlate with the amount of dietary fat. Restriction of triglycerides containing long-chain fatty acids is a key factor in management of these patients and in those heterozygous for familial HBL who have evidence of any malabsorption or oxalate urolithiasis. Medium-chain triglycerides should be used sparingly, if at all, because cirrhosis of the liver occurs after prolonged use. Supplementation with tocopherol inhibits progression of neurologic sequelae and should be instituted as soon as the diagnosis of ABL or familial HBL is made. Retinopathy and myopathy may be prevented or stabilized if vitamin E is given early. Very large doses are well tolerated, and concentrated preparations allow convenient dosage of 1,000–2,000 mg/day for infants and up to as much as 10,000–20,000 mg/day for older children or adults. Supplementation with water-soluble preparations of vitamin A is also indicated whenever plasma levels are low. Vitamin K should be given if the patient exhibits bleeding or hypoprothrombinemia. Treatment of patients with chylomicron retention disease should include restriction of dietary fat and supplementation with vitamin E and perhaps also vitamin A.

DISORDERS OF HIGH-DENSITY LIPOPROTEINS

Tangier Disease

Tangier disease is associated with very low levels of HDL and of apo A-I and apo A-II in plasma.

Clinical Features

Enlarged, orange-colored tonsils and orange pigment in the rectal mucosa are the clinical hallmarks of this disorder, but lipid deposits are also observed in the cornea, Schwann cells, spinal ganglia, and smooth muscle cells of the intestine. Lymphadenopathy and splenomegaly are common. The latter is associated with thrombocytopenia and increased hemolysis in some patients. Cholesteryl ester–laden histiocytes (foam cells) may occur in the thymus, ureters, heart valves, bone marrow, and pulmonary artery. Diffuse corneal infiltrates occur in one-fourth of patients.

The main neurologic features are relapsing multiple mononeuropathies or a syringomyelia-like disorder involving loss of pain and temperature sense. Acute, disabling sensorimotor polyneuropathy is described. Loss of corneal sensation and orbicular muscle weakness may lead to ectropion. No specific treatment is known.

Genetic Features

Total plasma cholesterol levels average approximately 70 mg/dl in homozygotes and 160 mg/dl in heterozygotes; however, triglyceride plasma concentrations tend to be elevated. Fasting chylomicronemia is also frequent. The content of C proteins in VLDL is high, possibly reflecting the lack of acceptor HDL particles. Although the levels of apo A-I and apo A-II are very low, often 1–2 mg/dl, the sequences of those proteins and their precursors are normal, as are their production rates; however, the catabolic rate of these apolipoproteins is abnormally rapid. The activity of lecithin:cholesterol acyl transferase (LCAT) is normal in Tangier disease if the content of substrate lipoproteins is considered. The underlying biochemical mechanism is unknown, but the HDL pathway that normally assists in the removal of cellular cholesterol via endocytosis and retroendocytosis may be abnormal.

Familial Lecithin:Cholesterol Acyl Transferase Deficiency

Clinical Features

Familial LCAT deficiency causes an increased incidence of premature atherosclerosis, suggesting that the abnormal lipoproteins may be atherogenic. Overt neurologic symptoms are rare. Two siblings known to be homozygous for a sequence anomaly in the structural gene had mild peripheral neuropathy, however. Both were also unusual in that they had cutaneous xanthomas.

Genetic Features

In specific cases, mutations of the structural gene for the enzyme have been identified. The content of unesterified cholesterol in plasma and all lipoprotein classes is very high, and conversely, that of cholesteryl esters is low, with a preponderance of palmityl and oleyl esters. VLDL are relatively deficient in C apolipoproteins. Cholesterol-rich lipoproteins with multilamellar and discoidal structures are found in the LDL density interval. Some very large spherical particles appear to be modified chylomicrons. Most of these abnormal particles contain little or no apo B-100. Foam cells may be found in bone marrow, presumably reflecting the phagocytosis of abnormal lipoproteins.

Treatment

Treatment of LCAT deficiency involves minimizing the dietary fat intake to reduce the production of lamellar lipoproteins, which are derived from chylomicrons.

APOLIPOPROTEIN E AND ALZHEIMER'S DISEASE

A clinical overview of Alzheimer's disease (AD) is summarized in Chapter 7. This chapter summarizes the major genetic causes of AD

Table 15.1
Genetic classification of the Alzheimer's diseases.

Gene Locus	*Clinical Type*	*Gene*
AD1 (chromosome 21)	Early-onset autosomal dominant; <20 known families	Amyloid precursor protein (APP)
AD2 (chromosome 19)	Late-onset familial and sporadic; susceptibility factor present in >60% of common forms of Alzheimer's disease	Apoliprotein E (*APOE*)
AD3 (chromosome 14)	Early-onset autosomal dominant; 80–90% of *AD1, AD3,* and *AD4*	Presenilin 1 (*PS1; S182*)
AD4 (chromosome 1)	Early-onset autosomal dominant; two known families	Presenilin 2 (*PS2; E5.1; STM2*)
Next loci	Rare autosomal dominant families that are not linked to chromosomes 21, 14, or 1	
Next loci	Other late-onset susceptibility genes; probably several that affect risk and age of onset	

with special reference to the role of the apoE locus as a major susceptibility gene for the common form of late-onset AD. ApoE plays a key role in both lipid metabolism and neurobiology. A major function of apoE is to mediate the binding of lipoproteins or lipid complexes in the plasma or interstitial fluids to specific cell-surface receptors (the LDL receptor family). Therefore, apoE participates in the distribution of lipids among various cells of the body. In addition, direct intracellular effects of apoE may modulate various cellular processes, including cytoskeletal assembly and stability. Elucidation of the structure and function of the three major isoforms of apoE (apoE-ε2, -ε3, and -ε4) has helped to unravel the role of apoE-ε4 in the pathogenesis of AD.

Genetics of Early-Onset Alzheimer's Disease

Each of the genetic causes leads to virtually identical clinical and pathologic pictures (Table 15.1). It is not known whether the pathogeneses are identical for the early-onset mendelian and late-onset forms of AD. Early-onset AD is defined by an onset before 65 years of age. Genetic loci were identified for the three known early-onset autosomal dominant forms of AD. These loci represent less than 1% of all AD. The frequency of mutations was measured in early-onset AD patients and apoE ε4/ε4 was found in approximately 20–30%.

AD3 is the most common of the three autosomal dominant forms. It is associated with missense mutations at the presenilin 1 locus on chromosome 14. Fewer than 20 families have *AD1*, which is associated with amyloid precursor protein (APP) missense mutations on chromosome 21. The most recently discovered locus, *AD4*, with presenilin 2 missense mutations on chromosome 1, is analogous to *PS1*. More early-onset disease patients are associated with the inheritance of apoE-ε4 alleles at the *AD2* susceptibility locus than with mendelian mutations. It is also apparent that other, as yet undefined, late-onset susceptibility loci contribute to the risk and age of onset of AD.

The function of the presenilins is unknown, but their predicted structure suggests that they may be ion channels or G-coupled receptors, or interact with the metabolism of APP or amyloid β (Aβ) peptide, or both. The predicted sequence of *PS2*, the gene causing AD in three known families, was a 95% match with the gene selected for involvement in mouse T-cell hybridoma apoptosis. This suggests a role in programmed cell death. To date, preliminary immunocytochemistry data suggest that the presenilins and APP are localized to internal membranes in the endoplasmic reticulum, endosomes, and other small membranous organelles.

Genetics of Apolipoprotein E and Late-Onset Alzheimer's Disease

The three common alleles coded at the apoE locus are apoE-ε2, -ε3, and -ε4. Because each individual inherits two alleles, one from each parent, there are six possible genotypes. The proportion of each allele in the white American and most white European populations is approximately: ε3, 78%; ε4, 15%; and ε2, 7%. In Japan, where the allele frequency of ε4 is approximately 7–10% and the ε2 allele frequency is also less than in white populations, the ε4/ε4 genotype is less than 1%, compared with 2–3% in Europeans. These differences in apoE allele frequency contribute to the demographics of AD in each population. With fewer ε4/ε4 individuals in the population, the mean age of onset of AD in Japan is older, and AD is less prevalent.

Epidemiologic studies confirm that few ε4/ε4 homozygotes live into their 80s without the onset of AD. Individuals with the ε4/ε4 genotype who reach their 90s without the onset of AD are quite rare, especially considering that approximately 2–3% of the younger population were found to have that genotype. Decreased ε2 allele frequency in AD has also been widely confirmed. In centenarians, the ε4 allele frequency is reduced by half, and the ε2 allele frequency doubled. In addition, patients believed to have AD are not statistically associated with the ε4 allele because virtually all ε4/ε4 genotypes and a large proportion of ε3/ε4 genotypes have already died.

Use of Apolipoprotein E Genotyping in Clinical Practice

An important caveat of most of the epidemiologic studies is the lack of autopsy confirmation. Thus, the true prevalence of AD within the dementia assessments of most epidemiologic studies is unknown. Particularly in nonfamilial studies, the diagnosis of AD is not synonymous with demented patients ascertained by clinical studies in the field. Until there is clarification of age-specific predictive values for each apoE genotype for autopsy-confirmed AD, clinical and epidemiologic studies that equate dementia with AD must be interpreted appropriately with autopsy-confirmed data.

Genetic testing is an imprecise and potentially confusing term to use because it lumps predictive testing of healthy individuals with diagnostic testing of patients. The term confuses the public as well as nonclinical scientists. At the present time, without additional confirmed susceptibility genes, the age of onset of AD for any healthy individual with any apoE genotype cannot be predicted. Therefore, accurate prediction of disease onset for any cognitively intact individual, whether in a family with AD or not, cannot be recommended as a "genetic test."

Using Apolipoprotein E Genotyping as a Diagnostic Adjunct

The ε4 allele is associated with increased risk and earlier age of onset of AD in virtually every population tested throughout the world. A distinction must be made between the differences in the prevalence of AD in the general population and the prevalence of AD among patients with dementia. Autopsy confirmation of clinically diagnosed series of probable AD patients rarely exceeds 85%. Prevalence of postmortem confirmed AD has provided the best estimates of correct diagnoses for all tests used over the entire period of illness. Whether apoE genotyping increases the diagnostic accuracy in prospectively ascertained autopsy-confirmed series focuses on its use as a diagnostic adjunct.

All patients with the ε4/ε4, ε3/ε4, or ε2/ε4 genotypes have pathologically confirmed AD, but not having an ε4 allele does not preclude the presence of AD. Thus, using apoE genotyping as a diagnostic adjunct is extremely promising. If an individual younger than 50 years presents with early dementia and has an otherwise normal, reliable, neurologic physical examination, the chance that the final diagnosis will be AD ranges from 60–70% in most specialty clinics. The positive predictive value of the ε4/ε4 genotype (approximately 15–20% of cases) increases the accuracy to 100%. Genotyping using apoE is the first specific test that adds positive predictive value to the diagnostic evaluation, rather than using it only to rule out other causes of dementia.

Relationship of Apolipoprotein E Genotypes to Characteristic Pathology

Many believe that the deposition of fibrillary Aβ peptide and the formation of amyloid plaques initiate a cascade of events leading to AD. The evidence used to support a pathogenic role for Aβ deposition is the missense mutations of APP, even though APP mutations account for early-onset AD in fewer than 20 families. The initial identification of apoE as a relevant gene in AD resulted from Aβ binding studies. In fact, ε4 binds Aβ more avidly than ε3 in vitro when delipidated apoE is used. It appears that differences in amyloid load are not associated with more rapid disease progression but may simply be consequences of the differences in Aβ binding to the inherited isoforms of apoE that are bound to apoE receptors on neuron membranes. In this formulation, Aβ deposition is explained as a consequence of neuritic degeneration rather than as a cause.

The other major etiologic hypotheses involve the formation of neurofibrillary tangles. One hypothesis relates apoE isoform–specific protein binding to both microtubule-associated proteins, tau and MAP2. The neurofibrillary changes can be viewed as a final stage of altered metabolism that occurs gradually in many neurons affected by AD, rather than as the structural element that kills cells. The ε3 isoform binds to both microtubule-associated proteins, tau and MAP2, better than the ε4 isoform. ε3 (and ε2) may protect and sequester the MAP proteins better than ε4, reducing the ability of tau to bind to itself to form paired helical filaments (an early stage of neurofibrillary change). The function of ε3 binding may be to facilitate the rapid mobilization of microtubule-associated proteins for efficient microtubule response to stress and stabilization. Thus, ε3 and ε2 may be better than ε4 for neuronal responses to stress and aging.

Alzheimer's Disease as a Model of Complex Late-Onset Diseases

The major causal factor for late-onset AD is the combination of normally occurring polymorphisms inherited at the apoE locus. The same polymorphisms also act as risk factors for other competing risks, such as death from myocardial infarctions or recovery from head injury, stroke, or cardiopulmonary bypass/anesthesia. Over the life span, the genotype at the apoE locus provides a demonstrable factor involved in the competing risks of disease and responses to environmental stresses. ApoE is not the only genetic risk factor for AD, and other polymorphisms of common genes have been suggested as contributing to the rate of disease development. Although confirmations of other factors remain to be established, multigenic influences on AD are now a widely accepted concept. The apoE locus was the first major susceptibility locus found using positional cloning strategies for a common, apparently "sporadic" disease. This model can be used for the investigation of other age-related common diseases.

CEREBROTENDINOUS XANTHOMATOSIS

Cerebrotendinous xanthomatosis is a rare, recessively inherited lipid storage disease caused by defective bile acid synthesis. It is discussed in Chapter 7.

For a more detailed discussion see Malloy MJ, Kane JP. Disorders of Lipoproteins (Chapter 58; pp. 1003–1018); Roses AD. Apolipoprotein E and Alzheimer's Disease (Chapter 59; pp. 1019–1035); Mahley RW. Apolipoprotein E: Structure and Function in Lipid Metabolism and Neurobiology (Chapter 60; pp. 1037–1049); Bergíner VM, Salen G, Shefer S. Cerebrotendinous Xanthomatosis (Chapter 61; pp. 1051–1064), in RN Rosenberg, SB Prusiner, S DiMauro, RL Barchi (eds), **The Molecular and Genetic Basis of Neurological Disease** ***(2nd ed). Boston: Butterworth–Heinemann, 1997.***

16

Carbohydrate Disorders

GLYCOGEN STORAGE DISORDERS

This section deals only with those glycogenoses in which the biochemical defect is expressed in muscle and in the central or peripheral nervous system.

Glycogen as Fuel

The concentration of glycogen in skeletal muscle (approximately 1 g/100 g of fresh tissue) is second only to that of the liver (up to 6 g/100 g), but whereas liver glycogen serves mainly to keep blood glucose constant, muscle glycogen is a major source of energy for contraction. The immediate source of energy for contraction and relaxation derives from adenosine triphosphate (ATP) hydrolysis, but ATP stores are extremely limited, and ATP resynthesis depends on four metabolic processes: (1) oxidative phosphorylation; (2) anaerobic glycolysis; (3) the creatine kinase (CK) reaction, converting phosphocreatine (PCr) to ATP; and (4) the adenylate kinase reaction, which catalyzes the conversion of two molecules of adenosine diphosphate to one molecule of ATP and one of adenosine monophosphate (AMP); this reaction is coupled to the adenylate deaminase reaction converting AMP to inosine monophosphate (IMP).

Oxidative phosphorylation is the most important source of energy. Anaerobic glycolysis plays a relatively minor role in energy production, essentially limited to sustained isometric contraction (such as lifting weights, pushing a stalled car, or water-skiing), in which muscle blood flow and oxygen delivery are drastically reduced. On the other hand, aerobic glycolysis is an important source of energy, especially during the more common, dynamic forms of exercise, such as walking, running, or bicycle riding. Impairment of anaerobic glycolysis is often considered the main deleterious consequence of glycogenoses such as myophosphorylase or phosphofructokinase deficiency, whereas in fact the block of aerobic glycolysis is pathophysiologically much more important in both conditions.

The concentration of glycogen in the brain is only approximately one-tenth that in muscle, rendering it vulnerable to injury within minutes of onset of hypoglycemia or hypoxia. It is generally assumed that glycogen in the brain functions as a reserve of readily mobilizable energy to be tapped in conditions of glucose depletion.

Control of Glycogen Synthesis and Breakdown

Despite an active turnover in both brain and muscle, the concentration of glycogen varies within a narrow range in each tissue, suggesting a delicate feedback control. The two main enzymes involved in glycogen synthesis and degradation, glycogen synthetase and phosphorylase, both exist in two interconvertible forms. Conversion of phosphorylase from the less active (b) form to the more active (a) form is accompanied by conversion of glycogen synthetase from a more active, dephosphorylated form (I, glucose-6-phosphate–independent) to a less active, phosphorylated form (D, glucose-6-phosphate–dependent), so that when glycogen degradation is turned on, glycogen synthesis is turned off, and vice versa. The reciprocity of this control mechanism is facilitated by the fact that synthetase and phosphorylase share some of the interconverting enzymes: Phosphorylase b kinase both activates phosphorylase b and inactivates synthetase I, and the same phosphatase converts phosphorylase a to b and synthetase D to I. Phosphorylase kinase is itself activated through phosphorylation by an epinephrine-sensitive, cyclic AMP–activated protein kinase. In addition, phosphorylase kinase can be activated directly by an increase of cytoplasmic calcium concentration, which occurs during muscle contraction. Also, physiologic control of glycogenolysis during muscle contraction is exerted by changes in the concentration of crucial metabolites, such as AMP, ATP, IMP, inorganic phosphate, and PCr.

Enzyme Defects and Clinical Syndromes

There are nine documented enzyme defects affecting muscle alone or in conjunction with brain and peripheral nerve (Figure 16.1). One (branching enzyme deficiency) involves the glycogenosynthetic pathway. Another (acid maltase deficiency [AMD]) involves the intralysosomal glycogen degradation. The remaining seven defects involve cytoplasmic enzymes acting at different levels in glycogen breakdown and glycolysis.

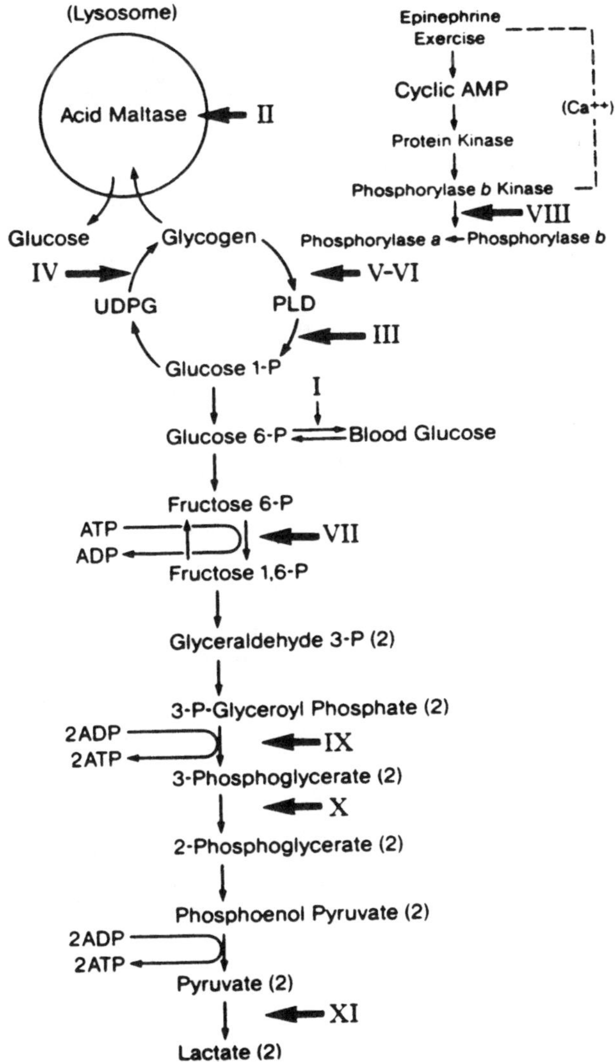

Figure 16.1 Scheme of glycogen metabolism and glycolysis. Roman numerals refer to glycogen storage diseases resulting from deficiencies of the following enzymes: I, glucose-6-phosphatase; II, acid maltase; III, debrancher; IV, brancher; V, muscle phosphorylase; VI, liver phosphorylase; VII, muscle phosphofructokinase; VIII, phosphorylase b kinase; IX, phosphoglycerate kinase; X, phosphoglycerate mutase; XI, lactate dehydrogenase. (From S DiMauro, AF Miranda, S Sakoda, et al. Metabolic myopathies. Am J Med Genet 1986;25:635, with permission.)

Disorders of glycogen metabolism cause two main clinical syndromes: (1) progressive weakness involving limb and trunk muscles but usually sparing extraocular and facial muscles, and (2) exercise intolerance, with cramps followed sometimes by acute muscle necrosis and myoglobinuria. In general, the acute, recurrent, and reversible syndrome of cramps and myoglobinuria is associated with defects in the energy-yielding pathways of cytosolic glycogen degradation (phosphorylase kinase and phosphorylase deficiencies) and glycolysis (phosphofructokinase, phosphoglycerate kinase, phosphoglycerate mutase, and lactate dehydrogenase [LDH] deficiencies). Weakness is characteristic of defects in the glycogenosynthetic pathway (branching enzyme deficiency) or in the lysosomal glycogenolytic system (AMD). There are exceptions, however: (1) Defects of the debrancher, an enzyme that acts "hand in hand" with phosphorylase in the breakdown of glycogen, cause weakness rather than cramps and myoglobinuria; (2) fixed weakness often develops later in life in patients with typical clinical features of phosphorylase or phosphofructokinase deficiency; and (3) weakness without cramps or myoglobinuria characterizes the clinical picture in some patients with phosphorylase or phosphofructokinase deficiency. The genes for the enzymes (or subunits) whose defects cause glycogenoses of muscle or brain have been isolated, sequenced, and assigned to chromosomes (Table 16.1).

Acid Maltase Deficiency

Clinical Features

AMD (glycogenosis type II) causes two major syndromes, a severe and generalized disease of infancy or a myopathy with onset in childhood or in adult life.

Infantile AMD (Pompe's disease) manifests in the first weeks or months of life with diffuse hypotonia and weakness, although muscle bulk may be increased, and macroglossia is common. Cardiomegaly is prominent, but hepatomegaly is not. Affected infants are alert. Respiratory insufficiency leads to pulmonary infections and death before age 2 years.

Childhood AMD manifests in infancy or early childhood as slowly progressive truncal and proximal limb weakness. Motor milestones are delayed, and calf enlargement is common. The phenotype in boys resembles Duchenne's muscular dystrophy. Respiratory insufficiency causes death within the second or third decade. Aside from the milder clinical course, lack of cardiomegaly is the main feature distinguishing the childhood from the infantile form.

Adult AMD is characterized by a slowly progressive myopathy starting in the third or fourth decade or later. The phenotype suggests a

Table 16.1
Chromosomal assignment of human genes encoding enzymes of glycogen metabolism and glycolysis.

Enzyme	*Subunit or Isozyme*	*Chromosome*
Acid maltase	—	17 (q23→q28)
Brancher	—	3
Phosphorylase b kinase	Alpha M	Xq12→q13
	Alpha L	Xp22
	Beta	16q12→q13
	Gamma	7p12→q21
Phosphorylase	M	11q13
	L	14
	B	10, 20
Debrancher	—	1p21
Phosphofructokinase	M	1(cen→q32)
	P	10(p)
	L	21(q22.3)
Phosphoglycerate kinase	A	X(q13)
Phosphoglycerate mutase	M	7p12–7p13
	B	10
Lactate dehydrogenase	M(A)	11
	H(B)	12

limb-girdle dystrophy or polymyositis. A distinctive feature in approximately one-third of patients is early ventilatory insufficiency, which is out of proportion to limb weakness. Visceral organs are not affected.

The serum CK concentration is consistently increased in all forms. Electromyography (EMG) shows myopathic features associated with fibrillation potentials, positive waves, bizarre high-frequency discharges, and myotonic discharges. In adult patients, these EMG abnormalities may be more evident in paraspinal muscles. In infantile AMD, electrocardiography shows a short P-R interval, giant QRS complexes, and signs of left ventricular or biventricular hypertrophy. Chest radiography shows massive cardiomegaly in all infantile cases. Studies of pulmonary function show markedly decreased vital capacity, maximal breathing capacity, maximal expiratory and inspiratory static pressure, and early diaphragmatic fatigue.

Genetic and Biochemical Features

Inheritance of all three forms is autosomal recessive, consistent with the assignment to chromosome 17 of the gene encoding acid maltase. The striking difference in clinical expression between infantile and late-onset forms of AMD appears to be due to the presence of a small but crucial amount of residual acid maltase activity in childhood and adult cases but not in infantile AMD. The infantile and late-onset forms of AMD are allelic disorders. Allelic diversity with various combinations of homo-allelic and hetero-allelic mutant genotypes has been suggested as the basis for the clinical and biochemical heterogeneity of AMD and could explain a few families with apparent discrepancy between biochemical levels of acid maltase and clinical phenotype. Prenatal diagnosis can be accomplished by measuring acid maltase activity in cultured amniotic fluid fibroblasts or in chorionic villus samples.

Full-length cDNAs encoding human acid maltase have been reported. The coding region is 2,856 bp in length, encompassing 20 exons and corresponding to 952 amino acids. Genetic errors detected so far in patients with AMD include nonsense, missense, and frameshift mutations, and the majority of patients appear to be compound heterozygotes. Three mutations seem to be the most frequent: (1) deletion of exon 18 (del exon 18); (2) a single base pair deletion (525delT) in exon 2; and (3) a splice site mutation (IVS1-13T→G) in the consensus sequence of the acceptor splice site of intron 1 that results in the splicing out, in frame, of exon 2.

Treatment

In addition to conventional treatment of heart failure and respiratory infection, some experimental interventions have been tried in infantile AMD. Lysosome-labilizing agents, such as vitamin A, progesterone, or hyperbaric oxygen, were administered in the hope of releasing intralysosomal glycogen, and epinephrine was given to promote the glycogenolytic action of extralysosomal enzymes. Liver glycogen decreased without clinical improvement. Enzyme replacement appears to be promising, although the impermeability of the blood-brain barrier limits its application to childhood-onset and adult-onset AMD.

Debrancher Deficiency

Clinical Features

Debrancher deficiency (glycogenosis type III; Cori-Forbes disease) is usually a benign disease of childhood characterized by symptoms and signs of liver dysfunction: hepatomegaly, growth retardation, fasting hypoglycemia, and, sometimes, seizures. These tend to resolve spontaneously during puberty, and most patients live normal adult lives. Although the enzyme defect involves both liver and muscle, clinical myopathy is uncommon and often manifests in adult life, long after liver symptoms have remitted. Wasting of distal leg muscles and intrinsic hand muscles is common. The course is slowly progressive, and the myopathy is rarely incapacitating. EMG may show myopathic features alone or more commonly combined with fibrillations, positive sharp waves, and myotonic discharges. This "mixed" EMG pattern with abundant fibrillations in patients with distal wasting often suggests the diagnosis of motor neuron disease. Nerve conduction velocities are decreased in many patients.

Genetic and Biochemical Features

Inheritance is autosomal recessive, although a male predominance exists among patients with myopathy. The gene encoding the human debranching enzyme has been cloned, sequenced, and assigned to chromosome 1p21. Prenatal diagnosis is possible by immunoblot analysis of cultured amniocytes. The debranching enzyme is a single 160-kD polypeptide with two distinct and independent catalytic functions, oligo-1,4–1,4-glucantransferase and amylo-1,6-glucosidase. Most patients lack both transferase and glucosidase activities in both muscle and liver. A much smaller number of patients also lack both enzyme activities, but muscle and heart are spared. Six distinct mutations have been identified in these two groups.

Treatment

Infants and young children with debrancher deficiency should be protected from fasting hypoglycemia with frequent feedings and nocturnal gastric infusions of glucose and uncooked cornstarches. A 7-year-old boy with severe diffuse weakness and wasting showed remarkable clinical improvement after 6 months of high-protein nocturnal intragastric therapy. No benefit, however, was noted after 6 months of high-protein diet in an adult with myopathy and wasting of distal muscles.

Brancher Deficiency

Clinical Features

Brancher deficiency (glycogenosis type IV; Andersen's disease) is a rapidly progressive disease of infancy characterized by liver dysfunction with hepatosplenomegaly, progressive cirrhosis, and chronic hepatic failure. Death from hepatic failure or gastrointestinal bleeding usually occurs before 4 years of age. Although muscle wasting and hypotonia occur, they are usually overshadowed by liver disease. Isolated myopathy was reported in five patients, with ages of onset from infancy to middle age.

Genetic and Biochemical Features

Inheritance is autosomal recessive. Because, in the more typical presentation with liver disease, the enzyme defect is expressed in fibroblasts and amniocytes, prenatal diagnosis is feasible. Branching enzyme catalyzes the last step in glycogen biosynthesis by attaching short glucosyl chains to naked peripheral chains of glycogen; the newly added stubs are then elongated by glycogen synthetase. The gene for human branching enzyme has been cloned, sequenced, and assigned to chromosome 3. Three pathogenic point mutations were found in two patients with typical presentation, and two distinct point mutations in separate alleles were found in a patient with nonprogressive hepatopathy. A patient with myopathy and cardiopathy had slicing site mutation resulting in a 210-bp deletion and complete loss of branching activity in expression experiments.

Treatment

There is no specific therapy for brancher deficiency. Liver transplantation has been reported beneficial in 10 children and should be considered; however, this procedure does not protect patients from developing the disease in other organs.

Muscle Phosphorylase Deficiency

Clinical Features

Muscle phosphorylase deficiency (glycogenosis type V; McArdle's disease) causes exercise intolerance with premature fatigue, myalgia, and cramps in exercising muscles, relieved by rest. Onset of exercise intolerance occurs in childhood; cramps and myoglobinuria develop later. Symptoms may be caused by brief, intense isometric contractions or less intense but sustained dynamic exercise. If patients slow down or pause briefly at the first appearance of symptoms, they can soon resume exercising at the original pace without difficulty. Fixed weakness is seen in approximately one-third of older patients. The resting serum CK concentration is usually increased. Electrical activity is not recorded from maximally shortened muscles during cramps.

Genetic and Biochemical Features

Phosphorylase initiates glycogen breakdown by removing α-1,4-glucosyl residues phosphorylytically from the outer branches of glycogen with liberation of glucose-1-phosphate. Phosphorylase activity is undetectable in muscle biopsy specimens of most patients. Inheritance is autosomal recessive, and the gene for myophosphorylase has been localized on chromosome 11. The coding region of the human myophosphorylase gene is 2,523 bp long and consists of 20 exons separated by 19 introns. Mutations identified in patients with McArdle's disease include nonsense, missense, and frameshift mutations. The most common genetic error in white patients is a nonsense mutation at codon 49. No clear genotype-phenotype correlation has been identified.

Treatment

Attempts to bypass the metabolic block by providing glycolytic substrates to working muscle or to raise blood glucose indirectly by injections of glucagon have failed.

Phosphorylase b Kinase Deficiency

Clinical Features

Phosphorylase b kinase deficiency (glycogenosis type VIII) causes four main clinical syndromes:

1. A benign liver disease of infancy or childhood characterized by hepatomegaly, growth retardation, delayed motor development, and fasting hypoglycemia. Inheritance is X-linked recessive.
2. Liver and muscle disease, with hepatomegaly usually resolving with age, and apparently nonprogressive myopathy. Transmission is autosomal recessive in most cases.
3. Myopathy and exercise intolerance, probably inherited as an autosomal recessive trait.
4. Cardiomyopathy, apparently isolated and probably inherited as an autosomal recessive trait, causing death in infancy.

Genetic and Biochemical Features

Phosphorylase b kinase is a multimeric enzyme composed of four different subunits, α, β, γ, and δ. The γ-subunit is catalytic, and activity is regulated by the degree of phosphorylation of the α- and β-subunits. Four genes encoding different subunits of phosphorylase b kinase have been cloned and chromosomally mapped (see Table 16.1).

Treatment

No specific therapy is available.

Muscle Phosphofructokinase Deficiency

Clinical Features

Muscle phosphofructokinase deficiency (glycogenosis type VII; Tarui's disease) is indistinguishable from myophosphorylase deficiency. There is lifelong intolerance to vigorous exercise, often accompanied by cramps and nausea that are relieved by rest. Clinical heterogeneity is illustrated by two groups of patients: one with hemolytic anemia without myopathy, the other with fixed weakness of early or late onset.

Genetic and Biochemical Features

Inheritance is autosomal recessive, although there is an unexplained predominance of affected men. All patients in the United States for whom ethnic origin was known have been of Eastern European Ashkenazi Jewish descent. The site of the metabolic block has been documented in vitro by showing no lactate production by phosphofructokinase-deficient muscle extracts with glycogen, glucose-1-phosphate, glucose-6-phosphate, and fructose-6-phosphate but normal formation of lactate with fructose-1,6-diphosphate as substrate. The genes encoding subunits of the enzyme have been localized to chromosomes 1, 10, and 21. An in-frame deletion that removes exon 5 of the gene (D5) is the most common genetic error among the Ashkenazi Jewish patients, possibly related to a founder effect. Ten additional mutations, including deletions and missense point mutations, have been identified in patients of various ethnic origins.

Treatment

The problems in attempting to bypass the metabolic block are similar to those discussed for phosphorylase deficiency, with the added complication that glucose is not an alternative substrate for phosphofructokinase-deficient muscle.

Defects of Terminal Glycolysis

Phosphoglycerate mutase (PGAM) deficiency, phosphoglycerate kinase (PGK) deficiency, LDH deficiency, and aldolase deficiency are clinically and pathophysiologically similar and can be considered together.

Phosphoglycerate Kinase Deficiency

CLINICAL FEATURES. PGK deficiency can be clinically silent or cause hemolytic anemia, seizures, and mental retardation. Involvement of muscle alone has been reported in three patients: a 13-year-old boy, a 31-year-old man, and a 37-year-old man. All three had exercise intolerance, cramps, and myoglobinuria. In five other patients, myopathy was associated with hemolytic anemia, mental retardation, or both.

GENETIC AND MOLECULAR FEATURES. PGK is a single polypeptide controlled in all tissues except spermatogenic cells by a gene on the X chromosome. Studies of physical and kinetic characteristics of the mutant enzymes in eight patients with myopathy showed that the enzymes differed from each other, suggesting genetic heterogeneity. A full-length cDNA for the normal human X-linked gene has been obtained. Different molecular defects were identified in two patients with myopathy: a missense mutation and a splice junction mutation.

Phosphoglycerate Mutase Deficiency

CLINICAL FEATURES. PGAM deficiency occurs mainly in black Americans. It causes exercise intolerance, cramps, and myoglobinuria.

GENETIC AND CHEMICAL FEATURES. Glycogen concentration in muscle is normal or moderately increased. Studies of anaerobic glycolysis in all cases showed decreased lactate production with glycogen and with all hexose-phosphate intermediates, consistent with a partial block of terminal glycolysis. PGAM is a dimeric enzyme composed of a muscle-specific (M) and a brain-specific (B) subunit. The small residual activity found in muscle biopsy specimens of all patients was exclusively the BB isozyme. PGAM-M deficiency is transmitted by autosomal recessive inheritance. A full-length cDNA and the genomic clone containing the entire gene for PGAM-M have been isolated and sequenced, and the gene has been localized to chromosome 7. Three mutations in patients with PGAM deficiency have been identified, all of which were within a short segment of exon 1.

Lactate Dehydrogenase Deficiency

CLINICAL FEATURES. Hereditary deficiency of the muscle-specific subunit of LDH (LDH-A) causes exercise intolerance and myalgia after intense exercise, often followed by myoglobinuria. In addition to muscle symptoms, three affected women suffered from stiffness of the uterine muscle at the onset of delivery, necessitating cesarean section, and a few patients presented a dermatologic disorder characterized by follicular papules or erythematous patches.

Genetic and Biochemical Features. LDH is a tetrameric enzyme composed of two subunits: one (A) predominant in skeletal muscle, liver, smooth muscle, and skin; and the other (B) predominant in heart muscle. The relative abundance of the A subunit in different tissues explains the coexistence of myopathy, uterine dystocia, and skin problems as well as the lack of cardiopathy in patients with LDH-A deficiency. The gene encoding LDH-A has been localized to chromosome 11. Multiple molecular genetic defects have been identified in patients with LDH-A deficiency, including nonsense and missense point mutations, deletions, and in-frame splicing errors. The gene encoding LDH-B has been localized to chromosome 12.

Aldolase Deficiency

Clinical Features. Aldolase deficiency has been described in a 4-year-old boy with exercise intolerance, mild weakness, developmental delay, a hemolytic trait, and repeated episodes of rhabdomyolysis during febrile illnesses. The muscle biopsy specimen showed no glycogen storage by histochemistry, but biochemical analysis showed a severe isolated defect of aldolase activity, which was 3.8% of the normal mean.

Genetic Features. Intermediate aldolase levels were found in muscle specimens from the boy's asymptomatic parents and brother. A homozygous mutation was identified changing a negatively charged glutamic acid to a positively charged lysine at residue 206.

DISORDERS OF GALACTOSE METABOLISM

Galactosemia falls into three biochemically, clinically, and genetically distinct forms. The most common is due to galactose-1-phosphate uridyltransferase (GALT) deficiency (classic galactosemia; transferase-deficient galactosemia). The other forms of galactosemia are due to galactokinase (GALK) deficiency and uridine diphosphate galactose-4-epimerase (epimerase) deficiency. The end result of the three normal enzyme reactions is the conversion of galactose-1-phosphate to glucose-1-phosphate.

Classic Galactosemia (Galactose-1-Phosphate Uridyltransferase Deficiency)

Clinical Features

Infants with GALT deficiency present with jaundice, abdominal swelling, and failure to thrive. Sepsis is common, and many newborns die of overwhelming infection, often without the diagnosis of galactosemia. Some infants are born with cataracts; presumably, they have received enough galactose transplacentally from their heterozygous mothers for lens damage to occur. In others, cataracts develop during infancy if galactose intake is not restricted. Neurologic disturbances in the newborn are limited to increased intracranial pressure characterized by a bulging anterior fontanelle. Untreated galactosemia usually has a fatal outcome in infancy.

Two principal approaches have been used to screen for galactosemia. The first of these depends on measuring the activity of GALT, whereas the second depends on the use of microorganisms to determine the amount of galactose in the blood sample. Treatment of classic galactosemia with a galactose-free diet is effective, but intellectual development, although greatly improved over that of the untreated patient, is probably not entirely normal. Neurologic symptoms are common in older children and adults with galactosemia believed to be under satisfactory dietary control. These may include progressive cerebellar and extrapyramidal motor disturbances, developmental regression, and seizures.

Genetic and Biochemical Features

Several variants have been characterized biochemically. Some patients, mainly of African ancestry, have higher residual amounts of GALT than do patients with typical galactosemia. Of particular interest is the Duarte allele that expresses half of the normal GALT activity. One mutation, an A-to-G transition at nucleotide 591, leading to a substitution of arginine for glutamine at amino acid 188, accounts for 70% of cases. The mutation that produces the Duarte variant has also been identified.

Galactokinase Deficiency

Clinical Features

Affected newborns are not ill but develop cataracts early in infancy. Those heterozygous for GALK deficiency may have an increased incidence of cataracts early in life. Neurologic symptoms are not expected.

Genetic and Biochemical Features

Patients with GALK deficiency have so little residual enzyme in their red cells that nothing is known of the characteristics of the residual enzyme. A common allele (the Philadelphia variant) that lowers the enzyme activity has been found among patients of African ancestry. A cDNA encoding a human GALK has been cloned and localized to chromosome 15. Using somatic hybrids, however, a gene for GALK has been mapped to a different location, chromosome 17q23–25. The relationship between the disease and these two genes of GALK is not yet known.

Epimerase Deficiency

Clinical Features

Most patients with epimerase deficiency are asymptomatic. The mutation may affect only red blood cells. A more generalized deficiency of epimerase, however, may result in severe neurologic disease. Only two cases have been described. One patient had hypotonia, failure to thrive, and liver disease; the other showed severe mental retardation and profound sensorineural deafness in spite of early diagnosis and institution of a galactose-free diet.

Genetic and Biochemical Features

At least two types of mutations can cause this deficiency. Human epimerase has not yet been cloned.

MOLECULAR BIOLOGY OF ALCOHOL DEPENDENCE

Alcoholism is a chronic disease characterized by addiction to ethanol. Alcoholics crave alcoholic beverages, and with continued drinking, display tolerance to the intoxicating effects of ethanol. If alcoholics discontinue drinking, they develop neurologic signs of withdrawal, thereby demonstrating physical dependence on ethanol. Alcoholism has been distinguished from alcohol abuse, which is characterized by recurrent episodes of heavy alcohol consumption with adverse economic, social, or health consequences to the user. Alcohol abuse does not usually produce serious physical dependence.

Clinical Pharmacology

Ethanol Intoxication

Virtually all alcohol is metabolized in the liver, where alcohol dehydrogenase converts ethanol to acetaldehyde, which is, in turn, metabolized by aldehyde dehydrogenase to acetate. Excessive accumulation of acetaldehyde causes an alcohol-flush reaction. Asian people have a mutation in an aldehyde dehydrogenase isoenzyme, resulting in reduced acetaldehyde metabolism. Affected individuals experience hot sensations associated with vasodilatation and facial flushing, tachycardia, and nausea.

Ethanol readily crosses the blood-brain barrier, and brain and blood alcohol concentrations equilibrate rapidly after drinking. Intoxication develops in nonalcoholics at blood alcohol levels of 11–33 mmol/liter (50–150 mg/dl) and is more severe when blood levels are rising rather than falling. These concentrations usually cause euphoria, loss of social inhibitions, and garrulous behavior, but some intoxicated people are gloomy and belligerent. At higher blood ethanol levels, cerebellar and vestibular function deteriorates, and lethargy and stupor may supervene. In nonalcoholics, a blood alcohol concentration of 500 mg/dl can be fatal because of respiratory depression and hypotension. Alcoholics are more resistant to ethanol intoxication than nonalcoholics.

Alcoholic blackouts reported during heavy drinking are characterized by hours of amnesia while awake. New events are forgotten, but immediate recall and long-term memory are normal, as in patients with transient global amnesia. Alcoholic blackouts may be related to ethanol inhibition of *N*-methyl-D-aspartate receptor–stimulated calcium currents in the hippocampus.

Acute and Chronic Tolerance to Alcohol

Acute tolerance develops quickly, and after several hours of drinking, an individual can appear to be sober at the same blood ethanol levels initially associated with intoxication. Chronic tolerance occurs in all alcoholics after several days of heavy drinking. Acute and chronic tolerance are due to adaptive molecular changes in the central nervous system.

Alcohol Withdrawal Syndrome

People with ethanol dependence develop a hyperexcitable state if drinking is abruptly reduced or discontinued. The clinical features include tremulousness, disordered perceptions, convulsions, and delirium tremens. These arise from the persistence of adaptive neural mechanisms no longer opposed by the depressant effects of ethanol.

Tremor is the first and most common symptom, beginning 6–8 hours after the last drink. Sympathetic hyperactivity is also apparent. Disordered perceptions may parallel the development of tremor and sympathetic hyperactivity, becoming most pronounced at 24–36 hours and clearing in a few days. Generalized tonic-clonic convulsions can develop within 7–48 hours after reducing or stopping drinking. Delirium tremens develop abruptly several days later, characterized by agitation, global confusion, insomnia, frightening hallucinations, and sympathetic hyperactivity.

Genetic Studies of Alcoholism

Heritability of Alcoholism

Alcoholism is approximately seven times more frequent in first-degree relatives of alcoholics than in the general population. In addition, 16–26% of fathers and 2–6% of mothers of alcoholics also have alcoholism. Identical twins have a significantly higher concordance of alcoholism than fraternal twins. Among alcoholics with severe alcohol-related behavioral or medical complications, adoptees have a 2.5 times greater chance of developing alcoholism if at least one biological parent is an alcoholic. Alcoholism in the biologic father is a better predictor for alcoholism in the son than is the environment in which the boy is raised.

Linkage Analysis of Alcoholism

Genes responsible for genetic forms of alcoholism have not yet been identified. An initial report linking alcoholism with a minor allele of the dopamine D_2-receptor gene remains inconclusive because of supporting and conflicting studies. No structural abnormality in the D_2-receptor gene has been identified in alcoholism. Preliminary evidence indicates that treatment with bromocriptine, a dopaminergic agonist, may benefit alcoholics carrying this minor allele. Studies linking alcoholism with the chromosome 4q blood group marker MNS and the esterase D marker on chromosome 13q have also been reported, but these results are inconclusive for significant linkage.

Alcohol-Related Neurologic Disorders

Alcoholics often obtain as much as 50% of their calories from ethanol, and some develop serious nutritional deficiencies, particularly of protein, thiamine, folate, and niacin. On the other hand, the cases of well-nourished alcoholics with skeletal and cardiac myopathy suggest that a lifetime ethanol consumption threshold is exceeded before irreversible damage occurs. In addition, genetic factors may contribute to the diverse toxicity of ethanol.

Wernicke's Encephalopathy

Wernicke's encephalopathy is caused by thiamine deficiency. The typical triad is ataxia, oculomotor abnormalities, and global confusion (Korsakoff's psychosis), although most patients do not have the complete triad. Wernicke's encephalopathy should be suspected in any poorly nourished patient with altered mental status. In alcoholics, thiamine deficiency may result from an inadequate diet, impaired intestinal absorption, and decreased hepatic thiamine storage. Four enzymes involved in intermediary metabolism require thiamine pyrophosphate as a cofactor: pyruvate dehydrogenase, α-ketoglutarate dehydrogenase, transketolase, and branched-chain α-ketoacid dehydrogenase. The affinity of transketolase for thiamine is reduced in patients with Wernicke's encephalopathy. Such individuals would be at greater risk to develop functional thiamine deficiency when thiamine levels in the diet are marginal.

Alcoholic Cerebellar Degeneration

Some alcoholics develop a cerebellar syndrome characterized by gait ataxia, with lesser degrees of limb ataxia affecting the legs more than the arms. The syndrome occurs after several years of alcoholism and is usually gradual in onset. Some alcoholics may be more vulnerable to developing cerebellar damage because of genetic factors. Cerebellar dysfunction frequently improves or stabilizes with abstinence and improved nutrition.

Alcoholic Dementia

Several disorders may cause impaired cognitive function in alcoholics. These include thiamine deficiency, pellagra, hepatocerebral degeneration, recurrent head trauma, and Marchiafava-Bignami disease. In addition, some alcoholics have cognitive deficits attributed to a direct neurotoxic effect of ethanol for which no specific brain lesions have been described.

Central Pontine Myelinolysis

Central pontine myelinolysis (CPM) is an uncommon disorder found in alcoholics. Hyponatremia frequently precedes CPM, and aggressive correction of chronic hyponatremia appears to be the major precipitating factor. Typically, the disorder develops over several days to weeks in severely ill patients. Mental confusion is a prominent early feature. Demyelination of pontine corticobulbar fibers may lead to dysarthria or mutism, dysphagia, facial and neck weakness, conjugate gaze palsies, and impaired movement of the tongue. Corticospinal tract lesions in the pons produce paraparesis or quadriparesis. In severe cases, a locked-in syndrome may develop.

Alcoholic Neuropathy

Polyneuropathy is a common neurologic complication. Patients report paresthesias, pain, and weakness, especially in the feet. Dysesthesias can be so severe as to interfere with walking. On examination, there is often reduced pain and temperature sensation. Distal muscle weakness and atrophy are common and are more severe in the legs. Tendon reflexes are reduced, and ankle reflexes are usually absent, even in asymptomatic patients.

Alcoholic Myopathy

Acute alcoholic myopathy is a life-threatening disorder that can develop after several days of heavy binge drinking. Muscle pain, cramps, tenderness, and proximal weakness and swelling of the muscles are sometimes associated with cardiac arrhythmias. Blood creatine phosphokinase levels are elevated. Myoglobinuria is a frequent complication and may lead to hyperkalemia, renal failure, and death. Recovery usually occurs within days to weeks of abstinence, but a residual proximal muscle weakness may remain.

Chronic alcoholic myopathy is usually a painless syndrome of proximal muscle weakness and atrophy that is often not recognized. Nearly 50% of asymptomatic alcoholics probably have a skeletal myopathy. Alcoholic skeletal myopathy and alcoholic cardiomyopathy develop simultaneously, and a direct relationship exists between the amount of ethanol consumed and the severity of the myopathies.

For a more detailed discussion see DiMauro S, Servidei S, Tsujino S. Disorders of Carbohydrate Metabolism: Glycogen Storage Diseases (Chapter 62; pp. 1067–1097); Beutler E. Disorders of Galactose Metabolism (Chapter 63; pp. 1099–1108); Messing RO, Diamond I. Molecular Biology of Alcohol Dependence (Chapter 64; pp. 1109–1126), in RN Rosenberg, SB Prusiner, S DiMauro, RL Barchi (eds),* The Molecular and Genetic Basis of Neurological Disease *(2nd ed). Boston: Butterworth–Heinemann, 1997.

17

Amino Acid Disorders

INBORN ERRORS OF AMINO ACID METABOLISM AND TRANSPORT

Of the disorders of amino acid transport, only Hartnup disease is characterized by neurologic abnormality. It is discussed in Chapter 7.

CLASSIC ORGANIC ACIDEMIAS

The classic organic acidemias are propionic acidemia, methylmalonic acidemia, multiple carboxylase deficiency, isovaleric acidemia, and 3-oxothiolase deficiency.

Clinical Features

The clinical presentation in each of the organic acidemias is similar. After the initial symptom-free period, vomiting, anorexia, and lethargy are followed rapidly by life-threatening ketosis and acidosis. The latter lead to dehydration, coma, apnea, and, in the absence of successful intensive care, death—a picture similar to neonatal sepsis. True sepsis may coexist. In infants surviving the initial episodes, recurrent episodes of ketosis and acidosis occur after infection or dietary intake of ordinary amounts of protein.

Episodes are characterized by massive ketonuria, systemic acidosis, and, in infancy, hyperammonemia. Rare episodes are complicated by hypoglycemia. Large quantities of glycine are found in the blood and urine. Organic acidemia affects the marrow, causing anemia in the newborn and neutropenia and thrombocytopenia during infancy. Toxicity to T and B cells leads to impairment of immune function and attendant monilial infection.

Some specific findings occur in individual disorders. Both forms of multiple carboxylase deficiency are characterized by alopecia and a bright red, scaly dermal eruption. Biotinidase deficiency is associated with ataxia, optic and auditory nerve degeneration, and spastic paraplegia. In isovaleric acidemia, the smell of isovaleric acid is acrid and nothing like sweaty feet. Failure to thrive may occur in any of these conditions but is most prominent in methylmalonic acidemia. Renal tubular acidosis and chronic interstitial nephritis are also more common in methylmalonic acidemia.

Chronic neurologic disability, seizures, and developmental delay are more the consequences of hypovolemic shock, hypoglycemia, or neonatal hyperammonemia than of the disease itself. Patients diagnosed early and treated effectively may be neurologically normal. Hypotonia, seizures, myoclonus, and coma occur in most patients with propionic acidemia. The initial features of biotinidase deficiency may be seizures or ataxia. Methylmalonic and propionic acidemia may be complicated by a stroke involving the basal ganglia, associated with spasticity, dystonia, chorea, or death.

Definitive diagnosis is by organic acid analysis of the urine.

Biochemical and Genetic Features

The mode of inheritance in each of these conditions is autosomal recessive. The defect in propionic acidemia is in propionyl-CoA carboxylase, which catalyzes the conversion of propionyl CoA to methylmalonyl CoA. Propionyl-CoA carboxylase can be assayed in lymphocytes or cultured fibroblasts and is less than 2% of control. cDNA clones have been isolated that code for α- and β-subunits of the human enzyme. The gene for the α chain has been localized to chromosome 13 and that for the β chain to chromosome 3q13.3–22. Mutations have been identified, such as a deletion in an intron in the β gene, that causes a frameshift and exon skipping.

The defect in methylmalonic acidemia is in methyl-malonyl-CoA mutase, which catalyzes the conversion of methylmalonyl CoA to succinyl CoA. The mutase is a B_{12} coenzyme–requiring protein. Some defects are in the conversion of B_{12} to deoxyadenosylcobalamin; others are due to apoenzyme abnormalities. In general, the former patients are B_{12}-responsive, whereas the latter are not. The gene for the mutase enzyme has been cloned, and its locus mapped to chromosome 6p12–21.2. Mutations have been identified.

The gene for isovaleryl-CoA dehydrogenase, the site of the defect in isovaleric acidemia, has been cloned and localized to chromosome 15q12–15. One identified mutation results in a truncated precursor protein, which is inefficiently imported into mitochondria and prematurely degraded in the cytoplasm.

In multiple carboxylase deficiency, the activity in lymphocytes of all of the biotin-requiring carboxylases, propionyl-CoA carboxylase, 3-methylcrotonyl-CoA carboxylase, and pyruvate carboxylase, are defective. The primary defect in the most severe form, which usually presents in infancy, is in the enzyme holocarboxylase synthetase, which attaches biotin to newly synthesized carboxylase proteins conferring activity. In the other form of multiple carboxylase deficiency, the defect is in biotinidase, an enzyme that is easily measured in serum.

Treatment

Treatment depends on a specific diagnosis. In multiple carboxylase deficiency, 10 mg/day of oral biotin reverses all manifestations of the disease except for optic or auditory nerve damage. The B_{12}-responsive form of methylmalonic acidemia is easier to manage than the unresponsive forms. Dietary therapy is always required, however, as it is in propionic acidemia and isovaleric acidemia. The principle of dietary therapy is the restriction of protein containing the precursors to just those quantities required for anabolism and growth, along with adequate amounts of calories. The precursors of propionate and methylmalonate are isoleucine, valine, threonine, and methionine, whereas leucine is the precursor of isovalerate. Carnitine supplementation is useful to reverse the deficiency of free carnitine that regularly occurs, and to form carnitine esters of accumulated toxic organic acid CoA esters; these carnitine esters are readily excreted in the urine. In isovaleric acidemia, glycine supplementation accomplishes a further detoxification by the excretion of increased amounts of isovalerylglycine.

Glutaric Aciduria Type I

Clinical Features

Glutaric aciduria type I is a degenerative neurologic disorder characterized by spasticity, dystonia, intellectual impairment, and choreoathetosis. Macrocephaly may be present at birth or develop in early infancy, often accompanied by attacks of sweating or unexplained fever. Delayed motor development is usually severe. Facial grimacing and opisthotonos may be associated. Episodes of coma followed by dyskinesia and dystonic extensor and flexor spasms may occur, resulting in a picture of choreoathetoid cerebral palsy. Some patients develop normally for as long as 2 years, until neurologic manifestations occur acutely after an infection. Later infections are followed by coma, convulsions, and increased neurologic deterioration.

Magnetic resonance imaging (MRI) usually shows some cortical atrophy. Decreased attenuation in putamen and caudate nuclei with increased signal on T2-weighted images may be seen followed by caudate atrophy. Frontotemporal atrophy is typical and may be found before the onset of clinical symptoms. The key findings on organic acid analysis of the urine are large amounts of glutaric acid and 3-hydroxyglutaric acid as well as glutaconic acid.

Biochemical and Genetic Features

The basic defect is in the enzyme glutaryl-CoA dehydrogenase. Some patients have no activity, whereas others have some. The gene is located on the short arm of chromosome 19.

Treatment

Treatment with a diet low in protein to restrict the intake of lysine and tryptophan rapidly decreases the excretion of glutaric acid and other metabolites. A combination of L-carnitine and riboflavin, 100–300 mg/day, may yield clinical and biochemical improvement along with increased levels of gamma-aminobutyric acid (GABA) in the cerebrospinal fluid (CSF). The GABA agonist baclofen may be a useful adjunct.

Gamma Hydroxybutyric Aciduria

4-Hydroxybutyric aciduria is an unusual inborn error in the metabolic pathway for 4-aminobutyrate (GABA) in which the compound that accumulates has neuropharmacologic activity.

Clinical Features

Most patients are hypotonic in infancy and have developmental delays in language and motor function. This is followed by mild to severe mental retardation, hyperactivity or somnolence, spastic diplegia, and seizures. Some have ocular apraxia. MRI may be normal or show generalized cerebral atrophy.

Biochemical and Genetic Features

Inheritance is autosomal recessive. The molecular defect is in the enzyme succinic semialdehyde dehydrogenase, an enzyme that is predominantly active in the brain. It can be assayed in normal lymphocytes and cultured human lymphoblasts.

Treatment

The only available treatment is anticonvulsant control of seizures.

Phenylketonuria and Disorders of Biopterin Metabolism

Clinical Features

Mental retardation is virtually uniform (IQ less than 30) in untreated phenylketonuria (PKU). Other features are fair skin, blonde hair, and blue eyes. Itching or an eczematoid rash may occur. Spastic paraplegia, seizures, and extrapyramidal signs occur in some patients. Hyperkinetic behavior is a regular feature of untreated PKU.

Not all newborns with hyperphenylalaninemia do not have classic PKU. Some with phenylalanine levels not exceeding 20 mg/dl have a mild variant in which phenylalanine hydroxylase is only partially deficient. Others have defects in biopterin metabolism that do not respond to dietary therapy. Affected patients have marked hypotonia as well as spasticity and dystonic posturing. Some have seizures, myoclonus, and electroencephalogram (EEG) abnormalities. Drooling is common. The delay in psychomotor development is usually profound.

Biochemical and Genetic Features

The defective enzyme in PKU is phenylalanine hydroxylase. It converts phenylalanine to tyrosine. In its absence, phenylalanine accumulates and is converted to phenylpyruvic acid, phenyllactic acid, phenylacetic acid, and phenylacetylglutamine. Tetrahydrobiopterin is an essential cofactor for the phenylalanine hydroxylase enzyme. In the course of the reaction, tetrahydrobiopterin is oxidized to dihydrobiopterin, and it must be reduced with nicotinamide-adenine dinucleotide in a reaction catalyzed by dihydropteridine reductase to regain cofactor activity. Biopterin is synthesized from guanosine triphosphate. Defects in the synthesis of tetrahydrobiopterin or in the enzyme dihydropteridine reductase prevent the conversion of phenylalanine to tyrosine. Tetrahydrobiopterin is also the cofactor for the hydroxylation of tryptophan and tyrosine, and its deficiency interferes with the synthesis of serotonin, dihydroxyphenylalanine, and norepinephrine. Severe neurologic disease may occur in the presence of only mild hyperphenylalaninemia, suggesting that tetrahydrobiopterin levels may be relatively more adequate for phenylalanine hydroxylation than for that of tryptophan or tyrosine.

The gene for phenylalanine hydroxylase has been cloned and localized to chromosome 12q. Several restriction fragment length polymorphism haplotypes have been identified. In Northern Europeans, as many as 90% of the mutant alleles for phenylalanine hydroxylase are accounted for by only four haplotypes. At least 31 different mutations in the hydroxylase gene have been identified.

Treatment

The clinical manifestations of PKU may be successfully prevented by restriction of the dietary intake of phenylalanine. Phenylalanine blood concentrations are maintained at less than 300 mmol/liter. Early diagnosis and consistent treatment prevent mental retardation. Newborns with biopterin abnormalities are treated with tetrahydrobiopterin, dopamine, and 5-hydroxytryptophan, along with carbidopa, to inhibit peripheral decarboxylases that would prevent these compounds from entering the central nervous system.

Nonketotic Hyperglycinemia (Glycine Encephalopathy)

Nonketotic hyperglycinemia (NKH) is a primary disorder of glycine metabolism in which large amounts of glycine are found in body fluids and in which accumulation of glycine in the CSF is particularly prominent.

Clinical Features

The disorder usually presents as neonatal seizures. Frequent hiccups is a unique feature. Progression to coma and respiratory arrest is common. Ventilatory assistance must be provided or death will ensue. Most patients die in the neonatal period, many probably without diagnosis. In those who survive the early crisis, spontaneous respiration begins, and apneic episodes do not usually occur. Developmental delay is severe, however, and intractable seizures are the rule. Those surviving the early neonatal crisis usually die in infancy. Neonates are hypotonic but eventually become spastic and often opisthotonic. Most are microcephalic. The prognosis in classic NKH is so bad that continued ventilator support seldom seems justifiable. This issue has been complicated by a transitory form of NKH. Two neonates presented with hypotonia, intractable seizures, and high concentrations of glycine in the CSF. In one patient, CSF levels became normal by 7 days. A small number of patients have milder clinical presentations. In one family, three girls were mildly retarded, only one seriously enough to warrant admission to an institution.

EEG shows a burst suppression pattern and MRI shows cerebral atrophy. The corpus callosum is abnormally thin, but no patient has had complete agenesis. Abnormalities in MRI do not correlate with levels of glycine in plasma or CSF.

Biochemical and Genetic Features

Concentrations of glycine in the plasma are 6–12 times control levels. The excretion of glycine in the urine is often greater than 1 g/day, and levels in the CSF are always elevated. The ratio of glycine in the CSF to that of the plasma is generally used to make the diagnosis. In control individuals, the ratio is less than 0.04; in NKH, the ratio is greater than 0.10.

The fundamental defect is a deficient activity of the glycine cleavage system. The glycine cleavage system is composed of four proteins now designated *P, H, T,* and *L*. The P protein contains pyridoxal phosphate and catalyzes the decarboxylation of glycine. The H protein is a lipoic acid–containing protein, which is the aminomethyl carrier protein. The T protein is a tetrahydrofolate-requiring flavoprotein that transfers carbon 2 of glycine to tetrahydrofolate. The L protein is a dihydrolipoyl dehydrogenase that catalyzes the oxidation of the lipoic acid of the H protein to its disulfide.

Defects in the P protein are most common, followed by defects in the T protein and in the H protein. Classic neonatal NKH is usually associated with virtual absence of the P protein. T protein abnormalities may have classic or milder phenotypes, and an H protein defect was associated with a progressive degenerative disease presentation. The genes for the P protein and the H protein cDNA have been cloned.

Treatment

There is no satisfactory treatment for NKH. Intractable seizures can be reduced or eliminated by the administration of sodium benzoate in doses sufficient to decrease CSF levels of glycine. The rationale is to conjugate benzoate with glycine to form hippuric acid, which is excreted, thus lowering plasma levels of glycine first and, by diffusion, those of the CSF. In the acute management of the neonatal crisis, benzoate usually improves the patient's condition enough to allow discontinuation of the ventilator; exchange transfusion or dialysis may accomplish the same thing.

Urea Cycle

Clinical Features

The initial features of urea cycle disorders are usually life-threatening hyperammonemia and coma in the neonatal period. If untreated, these disorders are uniformly fatal. The blood concentrations of ammonia are greater than 500 mmol/liter and often greater than 1,000 mmol/liter. Most infants are flaccid and unresponsive; others are tremulous and have seizures. Tendon reflexes may be brisk early in the course but are absent in deep coma. Shallow respirations or respiratory alkalosis may be followed by respiratory arrest and death unless the infant is intubated and given assisted ventilation.

The four diseases that produce this clinical picture are carbamyl phosphate synthetase (CPS) deficiency, ornithine transcarbamylase (OTC) deficiency, argininosuccinate synthetase deficiency (citrullinemia), and argininosuccinase (ASA) deficiency.

The differential diagnosis includes secondary hyperammonemia caused by organic acidemia. This can be excluded by defining the acid-base status. Patients with organic acidemia are acidotic and usually ketotic, whereas those with urea cycle defects have a normal pH and occasionally a respiratory alkalosis.

Arginase deficiency, the other urea cycle enzyme, causes a different clinical syndrome characterized by progressive spastic tetraplegia, opisthotonos, convulsions, and microcephaly. Some patients with urea cycle defects have a later onset and a more indolent course. Episodes of hyperammonemia begin any time from late infancy to adulthood. Some patients may have a history of recurrent vomiting. Others have episodes of ataxia, headache, or slurring of speech. Nonspecific mental retardation and behavioral abnormalities are rare presentations.

OTC deficiency is transmitted as an X-linked trait. Expression in females is variable depending on how many cells contain the inactivated normal X chromosome. Some female infants are as fully affected as males, others are clinically normal, and some have intermediate phenotypes. A small number of males have milder OTC phenotypes similar to those found in females. Similarly, milder variants of citrullinemia and ASA deficiency occur, and a late-onset form of citrullinemia is common in Japan. Older patients with ASA deficiency may have apparent alopecia because of friable hair.

Newborns with hyperammonemia, lacking diagnostic excretion of amino acid and orotic acid, either have CPS deficiency or a self-limited condition called *transient hyperammonemia of the newborn* (THN). Newborns with THN get well if they live until approximately the fifth day. Their blood ammonia concentrations and risk of dying are as great as for patients with the urea cycle defects, but they have an excellent prognosis if they can be successfully treated for just a few days. THN can sometimes be distinguished from CPS deficiency by the presence of modest levels of citrulline and arginine in plasma. These are zero in severe CPS deficiency. If the distinction cannot be made, all such infants should be given vigorous treatment and support for 5 days, when the distinction should become apparent.

Biochemical and Genetic Features

OTC and CPS are normally expressed only in the liver, and liver biopsy is required for definitive diagnosis of the deficiency state. Citrullinemia and ASA deficiency may be diagnosed by assay of the enzymes in cultured fibroblasts, and arginase deficiency by determining the activity of the enzyme in erythrocytes.

The gene for OTC has been cloned, and in families in whom the proband has been defined by study of the DNA, prenatal diagnosis and carrier detection may be accomplished by molecular biologic methods. The gene has been localized to Xp21.1, a site just proximal to the Duchenne muscular dystrophy locus. It is also adjacent to genes for glycerol kinase and for adrenal insufficiency, and large deletions have been observed that include two or even four of these loci with their attendant disease phenotypes. Deletions have been detected in approximately 10% of hemizygous males with OTC deficiency.

CPS is also expressed only in the liver. The gene is located on chromosome 2p, and cDNAs have been cloned. Large deletions have not been identified by examination of genomic DNA with the cDNA probe.

The gene for citrullinemia is located on chromosome 9q34. The cDNA for human argininosuccinate synthetase has been cloned and several sequences used as probes. Several mutations of this gene have been discovered, and many patients are compound heterozygotes for different mutations. Most of these lead to no immunoreactive enzyme.

ASA has been studied at the protein molecular level. The gene is located on chromosome 7cen-q11.2. Several mutations have been defined.

A cDNA clone for arginase is available, and the gene has been mapped to chromosome 6q23. Two mutations associated with arginase deficiency have been described.

Treatment

The treatment of choice for neonatal hyperammonemic coma is hemodialysis. Later episodes should be recognized early, and intervention should be prompt. Measures to promote alternate routes of waste nitrogen excretion are effective. These include intravenous arginine, sodium benzoate, and sodium phenylacetate. Continuing therapy for OTC or CPS deficiency requires dietary restrictions of nitrogen intake and use of oral benzoate and phenylacetate. Oral citrulline may be used in place of arginine. Patients with ASA deficiency or citrullinemia may be managed with supplemental arginine alone. Oral benzoate and phenylacetate appear to be useful adjuncts to dietary therapy in arginase deficiency.

Maple Syrup Urine Disease

Maple syrup urine disease (MSUD) is caused by deficiency of the branched-chain α-keto acid dehydrogenase (BCKAD) complex. It is transmitted as an autosomal recessive trait.

Clinical Features

The classic presentation of MSUD is early neonatal hypertonicity and opisthotonos. Tendon reflexes are increased, and there may be clonus. Generalized seizures are common. Lethargy progresses rapidly to coma, apnea, and death unless intensive care, including intubation and artificial ventilation, is initiated promptly. At this stage, the patient is flaccid, and reflexes may be absent. Serum concentrations of branched-chain amino acids (BCAAs) and branched-chain keto-acids (BCKAs) are markedly elevated.

Three variant forms are recognized: intermediate, intermittent, and thiamine responsive. In the intermediate form, BCAA and BCKA levels are moderately elevated without obvious ketoacidosis. Psychomotor delay is present, but the diagnosis is not usually established until the first or second year of life. These patients come to attention medically because of the psychomotor retardation. Institution of dietary therapy often results in some improvement.

The intermittent form, also discussed in Chapter 7, presents with episodic ketoacidosis precipitated by infections or excess protein intake. Between episodes, these children are asymptomatic with normal psychomotor development. The BCAA and BCKA levels are also normal between exacerbations but rise during ketoacidotic episodes. Patients with the intermittent and intermediate forms of MSUD have residual decarboxylation activity greater than 2% and as high as 25–40% of normal. The residual decarboxylation activity in fibroblasts from variant MSUD patients is not directly related to the phenotype, although it correlates with tolerance for dietary protein.

The thiamine-responsive type was first shown in an 11-month-old girl who had excessive BCAAs and BCKAs in the urine and exhibited developmental retardation. The patient was placed on a low protein diet and 10 mg/day of thiamine hydrochloride. The BCAA levels in her plasma fell within several days. Withdrawal of thiamine resulted in a prompt rise of plasma BCAA levels to pre–thiamine treatment levels, which was again rapidly reversed by restarting thiamine. Thiamine responsiveness has been reported in other MSUD patients, but biochemical improvement required several weeks of therapy. Thiamine may stabilize the enzyme complex and delay its degradation. All patients are managed on a combination of thiamine and dietary therapy.

All forms of MSUD can be detected in newborn screening programs by the elevation of leucine in spots of blood. Confirmation is by quantitative analysis of the BCAAs in plasma. Heterozygotes can be detected and prenatal diagnosis accomplished by assay of cultured amniocytes or chorionic villus samples.

Biochemical and Molecular Features

BCKAD is an enzyme complex composed of three major subunits. Defects have been localized in a small number of patients to the E1, E2, or E3 proteins. E3 deficiency also causes lactic acidemia. The cofactor for the E1 is thiamine pyrophosphate, which is involved in the decarboxylation reaction. E2 contains covalently bound lipoic acid to which the acyl group is transferred. This is then transferred to coenzyme A to form the acyl-coenzyme A product E3, which contains flavin adenine dinucleotide and uses nicotinamide adenine dinucleotide to reoxidize dihydrolipoate in E2 to the disulfide. E3 is also a component of pyruvate dehydrogenase and 2-oxoglutarate dehydrogenase. BCKAD activity is regulated by phosphorylation/dephosphorylation. A kinase phosphorylates the E1 component, causing inactivation, whereas activity is restored by a phosphatase. The liver enzyme is primarily in the active form, whereas the muscle enzyme is primarily in the phosphorylated inactive form.

The E1α gene is located on chromosome 19q13.1–13.2, and the E1β gene is found at 6p21–22. At least seven mutations in the E1α gene have been identified, but only one in E1β, a deletion in Japanese patients. Eleven mutations have been reported in E2 and two missense mutations in E3. The E2 gene has been localized to chromosome 1.

Treatment

Some patients respond to treatment with large doses of thiamine. The mechanism of the response may involve decreased affinity of the mutant enzyme for thiamine pyrophosphate or increased stabilization of the enzyme by thiamine pyrophosphate. All newly diagnosed patients should be tested for thiamine responsiveness. Doses range between 10 and 300 mg/day. All thiamine-responsive patients have residual BCKAD activity.

The treatment of MSUD consists of a diet low in BCAAs. Optimal treatment, initiated before the onset of damaging ketoacidotic episodes, can lead to normal development. Newborns with lethargy or coma should be treated aggressively. Peritoneal dialysis has been used, but leucine is not readily removed in this way. BCAA-free parenteral nutrition has been used for the management of acutely ill patients. Once the acute episode is controlled, protein and BCAA intake is limited to provide the minimum quantity of BCAAs necessary for growth. Patients must be carefully observed by monitoring plasma amino acid concentrations repeatedly.

Homocystinuria

Several metabolic defects result in homocystinuria. The most common defect is a deficiency of cystathionine β-synthase (homocystinuria I). Two other causes are defects of methylcobalamin synthesis (homocystinuria II) and defects in tetrahydrofolate metabolism (homocystinuria III).

Clinical Features

Homocystinuria I is a recessively inherited disorder of methionine metabolism. A subset of patients with this cystathionine β-synthase deficiency respond to pyridoxine. The unresponsive form has a more severe phenotype.

The most common feature is subluxation of the lens (ectopia lentis). Other eye complications are myopia, glaucoma, and, rarely, optic atrophy. Median IQ is 64 (range, 10–138) and seizures occur in 20%. Psychiatric abnormalities include episodic depression, chronic behavioral problems, obsessive-compulsive behaviors, and personality disorders. One-third of patients have stroke, 10% have myocardial infarction, 11% have peripheral arterial occlusion, and 51% have peripheral venous occlusion, including pulmonary emboli. Homocystinuria is one of the most common causes of stroke in childhood. Skeletal changes include osteoporosis, leading to collapse of vertebrae and scoliosis.

Infants with homocystinuria I may be identified through neonatal screening for methionine. The cyanide nitroprusside test detects homocystine in urine. The diagnosis is confirmed by quantification of the amino acids of plasma and urine. Prenatal diagnosis for homocystinuria can be accomplished by assay of the enzyme in cultured amniocytes.

Homocystinuria II can be caused by three different blocks in cobalamine metabolism. All three are characterized by megaloblastic anemia and homocystinuria.

Homocystinuria III is also transmitted as an autosomal recessive disorder. Central nervous system manifestations tend to be more striking than in homocystinuria I. A boy died at 7½ years with severe mental retardation, spasticity, and intractable seizures after a rapid deterioration in the previous 6 months. Low CSF folate levels are usually found, along with normal concentrations of methionine in plasma. Some patients are folate responsive.

Biochemical and Genetic Features

Synthase deficiency is characterized by homocystinuria, homocystinemia, and methioninuria. Deficiencies in the methylation of homocysteine to methionine cause normal or low levels of methionine in plasma and elevated levels of homocystine in plasma and urine. This results from defects in cobalamin metabolism, which cause homocystinuria and methylmalonic aciduria, or defects in methylcobalamin metabolism, which cause homocystinuria without methylmalonic aciduria. Deficiency of methylene tetrahydrofolate reductase leads to homocystinuria and normal or low levels of methionine in plasma.

The genetic defect in synthase deficiency is heterogeneous but constant within sibships. Most patients who are responsive to pyridoxine have residual cystathionine β-synthase activity in fibroblasts ranging from 0% to 10% of normal. Decreased activity has also been documented in the liver and brain. The cDNA for cystathionine β-synthase has been cloned. The gene is located on chromosome 21q22.3. At least 14 mutations have been identified. Phenotype does not appear to correlate with genotype. Heterozygosity for cystathionine β-synthase is associated with an increased risk of arteriosclerosis.

Treatment

The therapeutic approach to homocystinuria is to reduce methionine and homocystine levels by restricting methionine intake and raising the cystine levels by increasing that of cystine. Betaine has been used to increase the methylation of homocysteine to methionine and lower plasma homocystine levels in an alternate pathway catalyzed by betaine-homocysteine methyltransferase.

Pyridoxal phosphate is a cofactor for cystathionine synthase, and 500–1,000 mg/day of pyridoxine are effective in lowering homocysteine levels in more than one-third of patients. Most pyridoxine nonresponsive patients have no detectable synthase activity, whereas most responders have residual activity. Excessive pyridoxine can produce a sensory neuropathy.

DISORDERS OF GLUTATHIONE METABOLISM

Glutathione (GSH) occurs in all regions of the brain and may be a neuromodulator or neurotransmitter. All the enzymes of the γ-glutamyl cycle—glutathione disulfide reductase, GSH peroxidases, thiol transferases, and GSH *S*-transferases—are present in the brain. Several inborn errors of the γ-glutamyl cycle are known. The fact that many patients with such defects have neurologic symptoms attests to the importance of this cycle in brain function.

Severe Glutathione Synthetase Deficiency (5-Oxoprolinuria)

Clinical Features

In severe GSH synthetase deficiency, life-threatening acidosis may occur soon after birth. Survivors are mentally retarded and have spastic tetraparesis, signs of cerebellar damage, an ataxic gait, and pronounced tremor. Metabolic acidosis recurs with stress. An increased rate of hemolysis may be present. Some affected individuals may be neurologically normal at birth and then show neurologic deterioration.

Biochemical and Genetic Features

The disorder is transmitted as an autosomal recessive trait. GSH synthetase deficiency is generalized. The levels of 5-oxoproline in the plasma, CSF, and urine are markedly elevated. In the absence of GSH, feedback inhibition of γ-glutamylcysteine synthetase is markedly decreased, leading to increased formation of γ-glutamylcysteine, which is efficiently converted to 5-oxoproline. Patients have low or undetectable levels of GSH in erythrocytes, diminished plasma GSH, and 10–20% of normal levels of GSH in leukocytes.

Treatment

Vitamin E improves granulocyte and erythrocyte function in some cases. The brain lesions on postmortem examination resemble those seen after mercury poisoning. Treatment of severe GSH synthetase deficiency with antioxidants may be beneficial.

Glutathione Synthetase Deficiency without 5-Oxoprolinuria

Clinical Features

All patients with GSH synthetase deficiency without 5-oxoprolinuria have well-compensated hemolytic anemia. Three-fourths have enlarged spleens. There are no reports of neonatal jaundice or neurologic impairment.

Biochemical and Genetic Features

In the less severe form, the deficiency appears to be confined to the erythrocytes, and oxoprolinuria does not occur. The genetic lesion apparently leads to synthesis of a catalytically competent but unstable GSH synthetase.

Treatment

Patients with severe and mild forms of GSH deficiency exhibit increased rates of hemolysis, and in this respect they resemble patients with glucose-6-phosphate dehydrogenase (G6PD) deficiency. It has been recommended that such patients avoid certain drugs and foods known to precipitate hemolytic crises in patients with G6PD deficiency.

γ-Glutamylcysteine Synthetase Deficiency

Clinical Features

γ-Glutamylcysteine synthetase deficiency is an inborn error that has been reported only in two siblings who had a syndrome of hemolytic anemia, spinocerebellar degeneration, peripheral neuropathy, myopathy, and amino aciduria associated with GSH deficiency.

Biochemical Features

The disease is probably inherited as an autosomal recessive trait. In both patients, GSH levels in erythrocytes, peripheral leukocytes, and muscle were less than 3%, less than 50%, and approximately 25% of normal, respectively. γ-Glutamylcysteine synthetase activity is markedly reduced in erythrocytes, and generalized amino aciduria is present. In contrast to the patients with severe GSH synthetase deficiency, patients with γ-glutamylcysteine synthetase deficiency have a severely impaired ability to synthesize γ-glutamyl compounds.

γ-Glutamyl Transpeptidase Deficiency

Clinical Features

Two definite and three probable cases of γ-glutamyl transpeptidase deficiency have been reported. The disease is inherited in an autosomal recessive fashion. The syndrome is one of moderate mental retardation associated with glutathionuria and glutathionemia.

Biochemical Features

Cultured skin fibroblasts show little to no γ-glutamyl transpeptidase activity. The percentage of excretion of glutamine (plus asparagine) is higher than the corresponding values for serine, alanine, tyrosine, and methionine, consistent with a deficiency of glutamine transport in the kidney.

5-Oxoprolinase Deficiency

Clinical Features

Five individuals with 5-oxoprolinase deficiency have been described. Two brothers, 16 and 11 years old, had periods of enterocolitis and urolithiasis. They had normal erythrocyte GSH levels and did not exhibit acidosis, neurologic symptoms, or hemolysis. The cultured skin fibroblasts of both individuals showed low levels of 5-oxoprolinase. The activity in the patients' fibroblasts was 2% of normal, whereas the activity in the cells from their parents was intermediate between those of the patients and those of controls, suggesting recessive inheritance.

A third case of 5-oxoprolinuria was discovered in a woman who had given birth to three children with birth defects. The third and only surviving child had prolinuria before surgical correction of a heart defect. Both parents were mentally retarded. The mother had 5-oxoprolinemia and 5-oxoprolinuria. The mother's blood GSH level was normal, and the erythrocyte GSH synthetase activities of the mother and child were normal. Two brothers were discovered to have 5-oxoprolinase deficiency and excreted large amounts of 5-oxoproline. Both appeared normal at ages 4 and 8.

Biochemical Features

In 5-oxoprolinase deficiency, the GSH synthetase activities of erythrocytes, leukocytes, and cultured skin fibroblasts are normal, as are the γ-glutamylcyclotransferase and γ-glutamylcysteine synthetase levels of erythrocytes. Evidently, urinary excretion of 5-oxoproline in individuals with 5-oxoprolinase deficiency is less than in those with GSH synthetase deficiency.

For a more detailed discussion see Nyhan WL, Haas R. Inborn Errors of Amino Acid Metabolism and Transport (Chapter 65; pp. 1129–1150); Mize CE, Waber LJ. Urea Cycle Disorders (Chapter 66; pp. 1151–1174); Cox RP, Chuang JL, Chuang DT. Maple Syrup Urine Disease: Clinical and Molecular Genetic Considerations (Chapter 67; pp. 1175–1193); Cooper AJL. Glutathione in the Brain: Disorders of Glutathione Metabolism (Chapter 68; pp. 1195–1230), in RN Rosenberg, SB Prusiner, S DiMauro, RL Barchi (eds),* The Molecular and Genetic Basis of Neurological Disease *(2nd ed). Boston: Butterworth–Heinemann, 1997.

18

Purines

LESCH-NYHAN DISEASE

Clinical Features

Infants with Lesch-Nyhan disease typically develop normally for the first 4–6 months. The first sign of disease is usually crystalluria, often described as orange sand in the diapers. Delayed neurologic development is apparent within the first year, and affected children cannot sit unassisted, or lose the ability if achieved. They never stand unassisted or walk. Choreoathetosis and dystonia develop in the first year. Severe spasticity and opisthotonic spasms are regularly present. Dysarthria and dysphagia are common features. Most patients eat poorly and vomit frequently. IQ is usually in the 40–70 range. Aggressive, self-injurious behavior is one of the most distinctive features and is always present in the fully developed disease. Patients typically bite their lips and fingers, with resulting loss of soft tissue and sometimes phalanges of the fingers. Lesch-Nyhan patients are not insensitive to pain and are usually relieved when restrained to prevent self-injury. The abnormal behavior appears to be compulsive, and physical restraint and extraction of teeth are the only effective preventive methods. The types of movements seen in Lesch-Nyhan disease closely resemble the adult form of Huntington chorea, but the self-injurious behavior is a unique feature. Megaloblastic anemia is sometimes present; in some cases, it is severe enough to require regular blood transfusions. Megaloblastic changes may occur in the bone marrow in the absence of clinical anemia.

Hyperuricemia and hyperuricuria is present in all patients. Hyperuricemia is invariably associated with hypoxanthine-guanine phosphoribosyltransferase (HPRT) deficiency. It is explained by an accelerated rate of purine biosynthesis de novo, reaching levels 10 times greater than normal. The main mechanism underlying this increase in purine biosynthesis is probably the underuse, and thereby elevated level, of 5-phosphoribosyl-1-pyrophosphate (PRPP) that occurs with HPRT deficiency.

Partial Deficiency of Hypoxanthine-Guanine Phosphoribosyltransferase

HPRT activity in classic Lesch-Nyhan disease is less than 1.4% of normal. HPRT activity ranging from 1.6% to 8% of normal can be associated with all the features of Lesch-Nyhan disease, or with a partial syndrome in which intelligence is normal. HPRT activity between 8% and 60% of normal is associated with hyperuricemia without neurologic disease.

Serum levels of uric acid, as well as the amount excreted in urine, are similar to those found in the classic Lesch-Nyhan patient. Urate crystalluria is the rule, and the initial feature is nephrolithiasis or adult-onset gout.

Biochemical and Molecular Features

HPRT is a cytoplasmic purine salvage enzyme that catalyzes the reaction of hypoxanthine or guanine with PRPP to form their respective nucleotides, inosinic and guanylic acid (Figure 18.1). In HPRT deficiency, the underusage of hypoxanthine and guanine leads to increased excretion of their degradation product, uric acid, and the accompanying underusage of PRPP gives rise to an increased activity in the de novo pathway, further enhancing uric acid production. The plasma concentration of uric acid in Lesch-Nyhan disease is 5–10 mg/dl, as compared with less than 4 mg/dl in normal children.

The gene for HPRT is coded on the X chromosome and has been mapped to the distal part of the long arm at position Xq2.6–Xq2.7. In addition, autosomal nonfunctional HPRT-like sequences, probably pseudogenes, have been identified at four locations in the human genome. Two of these have been mapped to chromosome 11, one to chromosome 3, and one to chromosome 5. Because HPRT is coded on the X chromosome, Lesch-Nyhan disease usually occurs in males. A Japanese female exhibited all features of the disease and had normal cytogenetic analysis. The abnormal HPRT gene was shown to be the result of a de novo microdeletion in the maternal gamete involving the entire HPRT gene. No HPRT mRNA was made by her cells. It was further shown that the paternally derived X chromosome was subjected to nonrandom inactivation, making this patient completely deficient in HPRT activity. At least two other Lesch-Nyhan females have been identified, in one of whom there

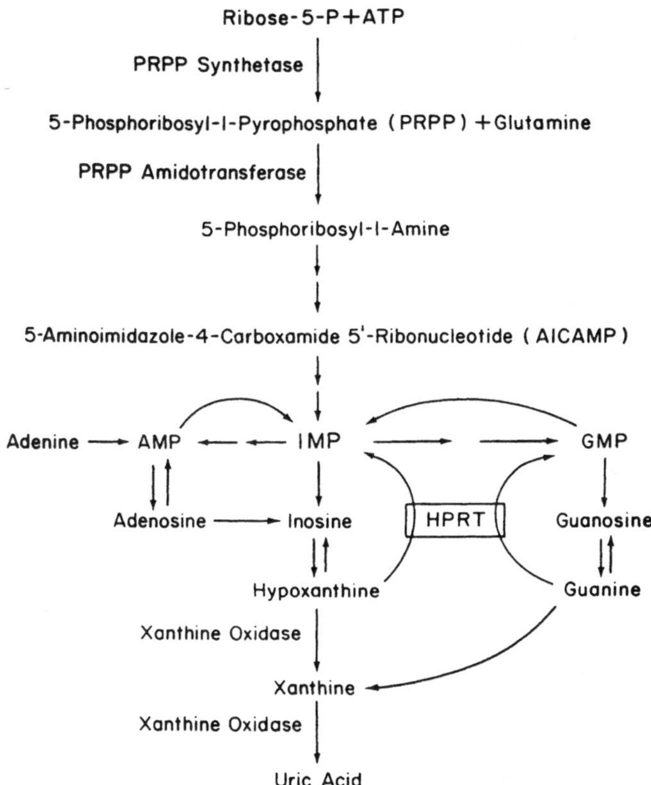

Figure 18.1 Diagram of purine metabolic pathways.

was evidence of nonrandom inactivation of a normal maternally derived X chromosome.

Diagnosis

A preliminary diagnosis of classic Lesch-Nyhan disease can usually be made on the basis of the phenotype. Choreoathetosis and spasticity in combination with the typical self-injurious behavior is almost diagnostic. In the case of partial HPRT deficiency, the clinical phenotype is less distinct. In virtually all instances of HPRT deficiency, hyperuricemia and increased excretion of uric acid are present. A serum concentration in a child of more than 4–5 mg uric acid/dl and a urine uric acid to creatinine ratio of 3 to 4 or greater are highly suggestive of HPRT deficiency, especially in combination with neurologic symptoms. A definitive diagnosis requires analysis of HPRT enzyme activity.

The technique most commonly used for carrier detection is the hair root assay. Embryonic development of hair follicles is mainly clonal, and most follicles express only one of the two X chromosomes. HPRT activity is assayed in a number of individual hair roots, and most of the time a clear pattern of mosaicism is seen in the heterozygous individual. Prenatal diagnosis can be performed on amniocytes and chorionic villus cells.

Treatment

The excessive uric acid production is best treated with daily administration of allopurinol. A dose of 20 mg/kg/day promptly leads to normal plasma concentrations of uric acid and prevention of symptoms related to hyperuricemia. The reduction of uric acid increases the urinary levels of hypoxanthine and xanthine, raising the possible risk of xanthine stone formation. Allopurinol administration does not affect the neurologic or behavioral manifestations. The most effective management of the self-injurious behavior remains physical restraint and in some cases extraction of teeth to prevent self-biting.

For a more detailed discussion see Sege-Peterson K, Nyhan WL. Lesch-Nyhan Disease and Hypoxanthine-Guanine Phosphoribosyltransferase Deficiency (Chapter 69; pp. 1233–1252), in RN Rosenberg, SB Prusiner, S DiMauro, RL Barchi (eds),* The Molecular and Genetic Basis of Neurological Disease *(2nd ed). Boston: Butterworth–Heinemann, 1997.

19

The Porphyrias

HEME AND PORPHYRIN METABOLISM

The porphyrias are a group of disturbances in which intermediates or by-products in the pathway of heme synthesis are produced in excess. The building blocks of heme are succinyl CoA and glycine, which combine to form δ-aminolevulinic acid (ALA). In subsequent reactions, two molecules of ALA combine to form porphobilinogen (PBG). Four PBGs are linked, yielding an intermediate linear tetrapyrrole—hydroxymethylbilane—that is cyclized to the initial porphyrin of the pathway, uroporphyrinogen. Uroporphyrinogen is converted to coproporphyrinogen and protoporphyrinogen. The biosynthetic sequence involves intermediates of progressively decreasing water solubility. ALA, PBG, and uroporphyrin appear in urine, coproporphyrin in both urine and feces, and protoporphyrin entirely in feces. The true porphyrin intermediates are the porphyrinogens and protoporphyrin. Uroporphyrin and coproporphyrin are irreversibly oxidized by-products destined for excretion. Normally, they represent a minute fraction of the total flow of intermediates through the pathway. Their appearance in excess in urine or feces indicates a defect in the pathway.

The effect of a partial enzyme deficiency is amplified by the fact that the pathway as a whole is regulated by its end product, heme. ALA synthase, the enzyme mediating the initial step of the pathway, limits the rate of heme synthesis; its activity is subject to end-product (heme) regulation, such that the rate of heme synthesis is appropriate to the needs of the organism. With induction of heme-requiring proteins (such as hepatic cytochrome P-450 after the administration of barbiturates), heme use is increased. This results in up-regulation of ALA synthase and an increase in the flow of precursors along the pathway until the demand for heme is met. If heme synthesis is reduced by a defective enzyme at a distal step (as in the hereditary porphyrias), a prolonged, exaggerated increase in ALA synthase results, with marked overproduction of intermediates before the blocked step.

Table 19.1
Classification of hereditary porphyrias.

	Acute ("Neurologic")	*Cutaneous*
Hepatic		
Acute intermittent	+++	0
Coproporphyria	++	+
Variegate	++	++
Cutanea tarda	0	++
ALA uria	+	0
Erythropoietic		
Congenital (Gunther's)	0	+++
Protoporphyria	0	++

ALA = δ-aminolevulinic acid; 0 = symptom complex absent; + = mild symptoms present; ++ = moderate symptoms present; +++ = severe symptoms present.

PORPHYRIA: CLINICAL ASPECTS

The porphyrias fall into two groups: those that mainly cause neurologic or cutaneous features, and those in which the porphyrin overproduction is most evident in liver or bone marrow (Table 19.1).

This discussion focuses on neurologic manifestations of the acute attack porphyrias, a group of disorders comprising acute intermittent porphyria (AIP), hereditary coproporphyria, variegate porphyria, and δ-aminolevulinic aciduria. Although these are genetically and biochemically distinct disorders, they all cause abdominal or back pain, which is aching more often than colicky but can suggest inflammation of a hollow viscus. An important differentiating point in porphyric pain is the lack of fever, leukocytosis, or rebound tenderness. Neurologic evaluation may be sought for psychosis or seizures, which occur early in the course of an attack. The history of abdominal pain in the preceding days should suggest the possibility of porphyria rather than a primary neuropsychiatric disorder. Mental abnormalities accompany attacks in 50–75% of cases and range from depression to delusions; psychosis is unusual. Patients are often judged "hysterical" or, because the demand for pain relief seems inconsistent with the physical findings, drug-seeking.

When generalized seizures are an initial feature of porphyria, they represent a particular challenge because many anticonvulsants are contraindicated in porphyria (Table 19.2). A history of preceding abdominal pain or dark urine is the clue to diagnosis. Treatment other than measures to suppress acutely the seizures should be withheld pending

Table 19.2
Use of medications in porphyria.

	Unsafe	*Believed To Be Safe*
Anticonvulsants	Barbiturates	Bromides
	Carbamazepine	Diazepam
	Clonazepam	Magnesium sulfate
	Ethosuximide	
	Phenytoin	
	Primidone	
	Valproic acid	
Hypnotics/sedatives	Barbiturates	Chloral hydrate
	Chlordiazepoxide	Chlorpromazine
	Ethchlorvynol	Diphenhydramine
	Glutethimide	Lithium
	Meprobamate	Lorazepam
	Methyprylon	Meclizine
		Trifluoperazine
Other	α-Methyldopa	Adrenocorticotropic hormone
	Danazol	Allopurinol
	Ergot preparations	Aminoglycoside
	Estrogens	Antibiotics
	Griseofulvin	Aspirin
	Imipramine	Codeine
	Pentazocine	Colchicine
	Pyrazinamide	Furosemide
	Sulfonamides	Ibuprofen
		Insulin
		Meperidine
		Morphine
		Naproxen
		Warfarin

the results of a rapid urine test for PBG (the Watson-Schwartz test). Neuropathy occurs in 40% of acute attacks, usually 1–4 weeks after onset. Proximal, symmetric weakness can involve the arms, legs, or all four limbs. The rate of progression is variable but can mimic Guillain-Barré syndrome. Mild paresthesias and numbness occur in half of the patients.

The first attack is rarely recognized as caused by porphyria. Laboratory tests are always required for establishing the diagnosis and characterizing the type of porphyria in an individual case. Marked elevation of PBG in urine is a hallmark of all acute porphyrias except δ-aminolevulinic aciduria. This can be established rapidly with the Watson-Schwartz test.

All positive Watson-Schwartz test results should be confirmed and quantitated with a column assay.

Typing of the porphyria requires quantitative assay of ALA, PBG, and porphyrins in urine and feces, because a specific pattern of excretion is associated with each type of acute porphyria. The defective enzyme in AIP, PBG deaminase (PBG-D), is present in erythrocytes. Because PBG-D does not fluctuate with disease activity, it is a useful adjunct to urine studies in screening for genetic carriers among the first-degree relatives of an index case. On average, affected individuals have 50% of normal activity. By combining urine studies, PBG-D activity, and pedigree analysis, 80–90% of carriers of AIP can be identified.

INDUCERS OF ACUTE PORPHYRIA

Most acute attacks of porphyria are associated with a known precipitating condition, although apparently spontaneous attacks do occur. Most often, the precipitating factor is a pharmaceutical (see Table 19.2). The most hazardous pharmaceuticals are those that stimulate hepatic heme synthesis. The most widely encountered inducers, if not the most potent, are barbiturates and related compounds.

Fasting predisposes to acute porphyria by sensitizing the heme synthetic pathway to the effects of an inducing drug. The involvement of female sex steroids in acute exacerbations is suggested by the fact that attacks are more common in women than in men (despite an even distribution of the genetic defect) and have a peak incidence in the third and fourth decades. Attacks before puberty are rare, and cyclic exacerbations occur in some women, just before menstruation.

BIOCHEMICAL AND MOLECULAR FEATURES

The enzymatic defect for each of the acute porphyrias has been identified. Each protein has been purified, most of the corresponding genes cloned, and mutational analysis performed. The enzyme affected in AIP is PBG-D. The gene of AIP is located on chromosome 11. The complete genomic sequence for PBG-D has been identified, and analysis of defects in individual families with AIP has revealed 10 polymorphisms and 58 different mutations. The enzymes affected in hereditary coproporphyria and variegate porphyria are coproporphyrinogen oxidase (chromosome 3q12) and protoporphyrinogen oxidase (chromosome 1q). The fourth type of acute porphyria, δ-aminolevulinic aciduria, is clinically silent except in individuals who are homozygous for defective PBG synthase (chromosome 9q34).

TREATMENT

Initial management is directed at pain relief, metabolic support for conditions such as hyponatremia, and elimination of factors that may have precipitated the attack. Chlorpromazine is suggested for pain relief, although excessive sedation can be troublesome. Propranolol counters the tachycardia and may also relieve pain. Propranolol should be started at a low dose; hypotensive reactions have occurred in some patients. Adequate analgesia sometimes requires meperidine or morphine. All nonessential medications, in addition to those implicated as a cause of acute attacks, should be discontinued. For reversing a fasting state (present in most patients because of pain and nausea), carbohydrate is given with the goal of providing approximately 400 g of dextrose daily.

Administration of hematin constitutes definitive therapy. In patients without neurologic signs, conservative care may be pursued for 2–3 days, supplemented by hematin if the clinical picture is unchanged or deteriorating. In patients presenting with neurologic signs, hematin is started as early as possible, together with carbohydrates and supportive care. Freshly prepared hematin is given at a dose of 1.5–2.0 mg/kg of body weight by slow intravenous infusion (over 10 minutes) every 24 hours. Adverse effects of hematin are minor and infrequent, provided that the recommended dose is not exceeded.

For a more detailed discussion see Bissell DM. The Porphyrias (Chapter 70; pp. 1255–1269), in RN Rosenberg, SB Prusiner, S DiMauro, RL Barchi (eds),* The Molecular and Genetic Basis of Neurological Disease *(2nd ed). Boston: Butterworth–Heinemann, 1997.

20

Metal Metabolism

DISORDERS OF COPPER METABOLISM

Copper is an essential trace element that functions as cofactor for several enzymes. The mean copper intake in American diets is approximately 1 mg/day. Healthy adults absorb 40–70% of dietary copper. The absorption site is probably in the proximal portion of the gastrointestinal tract. The metallothioneins (MTs), a family of metal-binding proteins, are involved in regulating the absorption, intestinal transport, and initial hepatic uptake of copper. Three major isoforms are identified: MT-1, MT-2, and MT-3. All MT genes have been mapped to the long arm of chromosome 16. MT-3 is expressed only in the brain.

After its intestinal uptake, copper enters plasma, where it is bound to albumin in the form of cupric ion. Within 2 hours, the absorbed copper is incorporated by a two-stage process into a liver protein. First, it is dissociated from its transport protein, and then probably taken up by MT, which transports it across the cell membrane. In the liver, copper either is stored in liver lysosomes in a polymeric form of MT or combined with apoceruloplasmin in hepatocytes to form ceruloplasmin, which is then secreted into plasma. At least 95% of serum copper is in the form of ceruloplasmin. Ceruloplasmin is believed to be the major vehicle for the transport of the metal from the liver and functions as a copper donor in the formation of copper-containing enzymes, notably cytochrome *c* oxidase and superoxide dismutase.

The normal plasma concentration of ceruloplasmin is 20–40 mg/dl. It is elevated in pregnancy and other conditions with high estrogen concentrations, infections, cirrhosis, malignancies, hyperthyroidism, and myocardial infarction. Dietary intake of copper far exceeds the daily trace amounts required by the body. Its intracellular content must be regulated within narrow limits because in its free form it is extremely toxic to cells.

Table 20.1
Initial neurologic signs in 31 patients with Wilson's disease.

Sign	*Percentage of Patients*
Dysarthria	97
Dystonia	65
Dysdiadochokinesia	58
Rigidity	52
Abnormal posture	42
Abnormal gait	42
Abnormal facial expression	39
Tremor	32
Abnormal eye movements	32
Drooling	23
Bradykinesia	19
Motor impersistence	19
Frontal release signs	19
Athetosis	10

Source: Adapted from GJ Brewer, V Yuzbasiyan-Gurkan. Wilson disease. Medicine 1992;71:139.

Wilson's Disease (Hepatolenticular Degeneration)

Clinical Features

Wilson's disease (WD) is transmitted as an autosomal recessive trait. It occurs mainly in groups with a high rate of inbreeding. Onset is usually between the ages of 11 and 25 years. Overt or subclinical liver disease is the initial feature in 40% of patients. In young children, initial symptoms may be jaundice or portal hypertension, leading quickly to death without neurologic abnormalities. More commonly, the initial acute hepatitis is self-limited. Psychiatric symptoms or a slowly progressive dementia is the initial presentation in 10–25% of patients; neurological dysfunction is the initial feature in 40% of patients (Table 20.1).

Most untreated patients develop tremor, rigidity, and contractures. The tremor is often bizarre, localized to the arms and described as *wing beating*. It is usually absent at rest and develops after a short latent period when the arms are extended. The arms are thrown up and down in a wide arc and the movements increase in severity. Many patients have a fixed, open-mouth smile. Rigidity and muscle spasms are often present. Dystonia of the laryngeal and pharyngeal muscles can lead to dysarthria and dysphagia. Drooping of the lower jaw and excess salivation are common. Tendon reflexes are increased, but extensor plantar responses are exceptional. Many patients with WD have behavioral and psychiatric manifestations that antedate by years the appearance of a movement disorder. Some have dementia whereas others have emotional lability. Without treatment, death ensues within 1–3 years of the onset of dystonia and is usually due to hepatic insufficiency.

An intracorneal, ring-shaped pigmentation, the Kayser-Fleischer (KF) ring, is best seen with slit-lamp examination. The ring is present in 75% of patients with hepatic symptoms and in all patients with cerebral symptoms. Its absence in a patient with neurologic symptoms essentially rules out the diagnosis of WD; its presence may antedate overt symptoms of the disease. The important features of WD are progressive extrapyramidal symptoms starting during the second or third decade, coupled with abnormal liver function and absent or decreased ceruloplasmin. Magnetic resonance imaging studies show abnormal signals (hypointense on T1-weighted images and hyperintense on T2-weighted images) in the lenticular, caudate, and dentate nuclei and thalamus.

Approximately 5% of patients with WD have normal plasma concentrations of ceruloplasmin. In affected families, the identification of presymptomatic homozygotes is important because they should be given preventative treatments. Low ceruloplasmin concentrations in an asymptomatic family member suggest the presymptomatic stage of the disease; however, 5% of heterozygotes have ceruloplasmin levels of less than 15 mg/dl. When low ceruloplasmin levels are found on routine screening and are unaccompanied by abnormal hepatic function, the subject is most likely a heterozygote for WD. If the diagnosis remains unresolved, a liver biopsy must be performed to measure hepatic copper content. Copper levels exceeding 250 μg/g dry weight are diagnostic of WD. Liver biopsy may also be required in patients who present with hepatic disease exclusively. WD hepatitis can raise serum ceruloplasmin levels. In many such patients, KF rings are absent. The measurement of urinary copper is a less satisfactory diagnostic procedure because, in some asymptomatic homozygotes, cupriuria is not significantly increased.

The presence of numerous mutations in the WD gene and the necessity of finding two mutant alleles to establish a diagnosis preclude the use of DNA analysis for the diagnosis of a subject without affected family members. Haplotype analysis, however, does predict the presence of the disease in family members with nearly 100% accuracy.

Several variants of WD exist. One is probably caused by a failure in copper absorption from the lower gut. It begins in adolescence and is marked by progressive tremor, dysarthria, disturbed eye movements, and dementia. Plasma copper and ceruloplasmin concentrations are low, as are liver copper concentrations, and KF rings are absent. Another type of WD is characterized by extrapyramidal movements without an associated KF ring or liver disease. Blood copper concentrations are low, but cytoplasmic hepatic copper concentrations are elevated.

Molecular Genetics and Biochemical Pathology

WD was first thought to represent a simple ceruloplasmin deficiency. The gene for WD localizes to 13q14.3, however, whereas the gene that encodes ceruloplasmin is located on chromosome 3. The gene for WD encodes a copper-transport protein with up to 76% amino acid homology to that encoded by the gene for kinky hair disease (KHD). The WD gene encodes a protein of 1,411 amino acids that functions as a P-type adenosine triphosphatase (ATPase). The P-type ATPases are a large family of enzymes so named because of a phospho-aspartate intermediate in the ATP-driven cation transport cycle.

Several mutations in this gene may occur in WD. The most common are a point mutation and a frameshift mutation, seen in approximately 30% of American patients. The remainder of patients have mutations scattered throughout the gene. Most homozygotes for WD are actually compound heterozygotes. The 5% of WD patients with normal ceruloplasmin concentrations probably have mutations that allow normal transport of copper into ceruloplasmin but prevent copper excretion.

Treatment

The aim of treatment is twofold: (1) removal of the excessive and toxic amounts of copper deposited in tissue, and (2) lifelong prevention of copper reaccumulation. D-Penicillamine is the drug of choice for forming a soluble complex with tissue copper. It is administered orally in divided doses, at least 0.5 g twice daily or 0.25 g in four divided doses for adults or 0.02 g/kg/day for children younger than 10 years. The exact dosage depends on the clinical response and rate of copper excretion. The dosage of penicillamine is adjusted to allow losses of copper of more than 2 mg/day at the start of therapy. Later, the excretion rate returns to normal; raising the dosage can again cause a transitory excretion. Penicillamine has an antipyridoxine effect, and pyridoxine supplementation, 25 mg/day, is needed. Adverse effects of penicillamine are fever, rash, adenopathy, pyridoxine-responsive optic neuritis, nephrotic syndrome, pyridoxine deficiency, and infrequently, thrombocytopenia and leukopenia. In addition, penicillamine-induced myasthenia has been observed on several occasions. These effects improve with temporary interruption of therapy. The neurologic symptoms of many patients may worsen during the first few weeks of penicillamine therapy.

Alternate drugs for the initial treatment of patients with neurologic symptoms are triethylene tetramine (Trientine), 1.0 to 1.5 g/day, and tetrathiomolybdate, 100–220 mg/day. Zinc acetate, 50 mg three times per day, is used during the maintenance phase of treatment and in the management of presymptomatic patients. It induces intestinal MT synthesis, which binds copper and produces a significant negative copper balance.

These regimens produce a gradual neurologic improvement. The KF ring begins to fade within 6–10 weeks and disappears completely in 2 years. Serial computed tomography scans show progressive reduction in the hypodense areas in the basal ganglia. Total serum copper and ceruloplasmin concentrations fall, and the aminoaciduria and phosphaturia diminish. A low-copper diet and penicillamine or zinc acetate are recommended for presymptomatic children. Discontinuation of chelation therapy causes rapid deterioration.

Kinky Hair Disease (Menkes' Disease)

Kinky hair disease (KHD) is a multifocal degenerative disease of gray matter caused by a primary defect in copper metabolism. It is transmitted as an X-linked trait.

Clinical Features

The severity of clinical expression is variable. The most common phenotype has its onset in the newborn with hypothermia, hypoglycemia, poor feeding, and impaired weight gain. Hypotonia, seizures, and progressive deterioration of neurologic function follow. The facies are "cherubic" in appearance with a depressed nasal bridge, ptosis, and reduced facial movements. Ocular findings include optic disc pallor and microcysts of the pigment epithelium and iris. Hydronephrosis, hydroureter, and bladder diverticuli are common. The most striking feature is the colorless and friable appearance of the hair, most often manifesting as pili torti (twisted hair), monilethrix (varying diameter of hair shafts), and trichorrhexis nodosa (fractures of the hair shaft at regular intervals).

Radiographs of long bones show osteoporosis, metaphyseal spurring, a diaphyseal periosteal reaction, and scalloping of the posterior aspects of the vertebral bodies. On arteriography and magnetic resonance angiography, the cerebral vessels are markedly elongated and tortuous. Similar changes are seen in the systemic vasculature. The mean age at death is 19 months, but survival to 13 years has been recorded.

Several variants of the disorder exist that probably reflect the multiplicity of gene defects. In these variants, symptoms are less severe, and development is normal until sometime in infancy. Initial symptoms may be ataxia, mild mental retardation, and an extrapyramidal movement disorder.

The clinical features should suggest the diagnosis that is then confirmed by ^{64}Cu uptake studies in cultured fibroblasts. Prenatal diagnosis is based on the increased copper content of cultured amniocytes and chorionic villus samples. Mutation analysis is possible in families in which the gene defect has been identified. In heterozygotes, areas of pili torti constitute 30–50% of the hair.

Molecular and Biochemical Pathology

The gene for KHD is located at Xq13. Like the defective gene in WD, the gene for KHD codes for a copper-transporting P-type ATPase. The gene is expressed in all tissue except liver. Its predicted gene product is a protein located on the membrane of an intracellular organelle, possibly the endoplasmic reticulum, where it is involved in copper uptake into the lumen. Partial gene deletions are seen in approximately 15–20% of patients. Other mutations result in an abnormal splicing process and exon skipping. All mutations are unique to each family, and almost all have been associated with a decreased level of mRNA for copper transport.

The characteristic copper metabolism abnormality is a maldistribution of body copper such that copper accumulates to abnormal levels in a form or location that is inaccessible for the synthesis of copper enzymes. Copper is not absorbed orally, but intravenous administration causes a prompt rise in serum copper and ceruloplasmin. The activities of several copper enzymes are significantly reduced in cells or tissue derived from patients with KHD (Table 20.2).

Treatment

Oral or parenteral therapy with copper salts is not effective in arresting the progressive cerebral degeneration, although parenterally administered copper can correct the hepatic copper deficiency and restore serum copper and ceruloplasmin levels to normal.

NEUROAXONAL DYSTROPHY

Neuroaxonal dystrophy (ND), previously known as *Hallervorden-Spatz disease*, is a rare heredodegenerative disorder of childhood and adolescence. It is an autosomal recessive trait.

Table 20.2
Cuproenzymes affected in kinky hair disease.

Affected Enzyme	*Clinical Manifestation*
Tyrosinase	Depigmentation of hair, skin pallor
Lysyl oxidase	Defective elastin and collagen cross-linking, frayed and split arterial intima
Cytochrome *c* oxidase	Hypothermia, impaired myelination, hypotonia, mitochondrial abnormalities
Ascorbate oxidase	Skeletal demineralization
Monoamine oxidase	Unknown
Superoxide dismutase	Diminished protection against free radicals, cytotoxic effects
Dopamine-β-hydroxylase	Unknown
Peptidylglycine α-amidating monooxygenase	Reduced activity of many neuroendocrine peptides, notably melanocyte-stimulating hormone

Clinical Features

Affected children are normal for the first 5 years. The typical childhood form is characterized by a motor disorder affecting the extrapyramidal system and includes rigidity, dysarthria, dystonia, choreoathetosis, tremors, and progressive intellectual impairment. The patients develop progressive difficulty with gait due to stiffness of the legs and foot deformities such as equinovarus or pes cavus. The adult-onset form looks like parkinsonism. Cerebellar ataxia occurs in some cases, but seizures and sensory findings are uncommon. Other unusual associated features are distal muscle atrophy and behavioral and affective changes.

Ocular findings are common and include optic atrophy, pigmentary degeneration of the retina, macular cherry-red spots, and a bull's-eye maculopathy. Patients with pigmentary degeneration of the retina form a distinct group in which the disease starts early and has a more rapid course, with death occurring in late childhood. The diagnosis of ND is difficult to make during life. Definitive diagnosis is based on the unique pathologic findings.

Biochemical Changes

The characteristic pathologic feature in ND is a rust-brown discoloration of the medial segment of both globi pallidi, with a less striking discoloration in the zona reticularis of the substantia nigra. These changes are associated with slight to marked atrophy and enlarged ventricles. Histologic examination reveals accumulation of iron and possibly of zinc and copper in the globus pallidus and substantia nigra. Iron-positive pigments are located in macrophages, neurons, and hyperplastic astrocytes or may be free in the tissue.

Marked elevations of cystine and cysteine concentrations in the globus pallidus may be caused by reduced activity of the enzyme cysteine dioxygenase, which converts cysteine to taurine. Accumulated cysteine in the globus pallidus might chelate iron and other trace metals. Iron plays a role in dopamine binding and may contribute to peroxidation. The combination of cysteine and ferrous iron increases lipid peroxidation, which may result in generation of free radicals. The free radicals in turn have extensive destructive effects throughout the globus pallidus by causing damage to neuronal membranes, with neuronal death and subsequent gliosis and a dysmyelinative state in the globus pallidus.

Another pathologic hallmark of ND is widely disseminated neuraxonal swelling or axonal spheroids, similar to those seen in neuraxonal dystrophy. These can be found at all levels of the central nervous system but are most prominent in the globus pallidus. They can also be found in other brain stem nuclei, neurons of the posterior column, spinal gray matter, cortex, and cerebellum. Both the infantile and late infantile forms of ND may show evidence of pallidonigral spheroids.

Therapy

No effective treatment for ND is available. Treatment with iron-chelating agents is not effective. An interdisciplinary team approach to rehabilitation and family support is reasonable but does not change the course of the disease.

For a more detailed discussion see Menkes JH. Disorders of Copper Metabolism (Chapter 71; pp. 1273–1290); Paulson GW, Reider C, Dadmehr N. Hallervorden-Spatz Disease (Chapter 72; pp. 1291–1297), in RN Rosenberg, SB Prusiner, S DiMauro, RL Barchi (eds),* The Molecular and Genetic Basis of Neurological Disease *(2nd ed). Boston: Butterworth–Heinemann, 1997.

21

Vitamins

INHERITED DISORDERS OF COBALAMIN AND FOLATE TRANSPORT AND METABOLISM

Inherited Disorders of Cobalamin Metabolism

Cobalamin (vitamin B_{12}, Cbl) is a water-soluble vitamin derived almost exclusively from animal tissues. Cbl deficiency is best known as the cause of pernicious anemia. In addition, several inherited disorders of Cbl transport and metabolism have been identified.

Absorption

Absorption of dietary Cbl depends on the combined action of gastric, pancreatic, and ileal elements. Ingested Cbl is released from dietary protein in the stomach. Free Cbl initially binds to a group of glycoproteins known as *R binders* (transcobalamin (TC) O, TC I, TC III, cobalophyllin, hepatocorrin). Pancreatic trypsin digests the R binders in the upper small intestine, and the free Cbl binds to another specific glycoprotein known as *intrinsic factor* (IF). IF is secreted by gastric parietal cells, and the IF-Cbl complex binds to specific ileal receptors located on the brush border of enterocytes. Calcium-dependent transport from brush border to portal vein is followed by release of Cbl from IF, and binding to TC II. All newly absorbed Cbl is bound to TC II, which is required for its intestinal uptake. R binders (TC I and TC II) in plasma contain 75% of total endogenous Cbl. R binders also bind several biologically inactive Cbl analogues, and may remove potentially noxious Cbl analogues.

Cellular Uptake and Metabolism

Specific cell surface receptors recognize the circulating TC II-Cbl, and the complex is internalized. Lysosomal processing of the TC II-Cbl complex results in the release of free Cbl. Cbl is an essential cofactor in two intracellular reactions catalyzed by methionine synthase and methylmalonyl-

CoA mutase. Lysosomal processing of the TC II-Cbl complex results in degradation of TC II and release of Cbl from the complex. The Cbl is transported across the lysosomal membrane and released into the cytosol as trivalent Cbl. The divalent Cbl [Cob(II)alamin] may remain in the cytosol and proceed to methylcobalamin (MeCbl) synthesis or enter the mitochondria and proceed to adenosylcobalamin (AdoCbl) synthesis.

Inherited Disorders of Cobalamin Absorption and Transport

R Binder Deficiency

Only six patients with R binder (TC I) deficiency have been reported, and it is not clear if any neurologic dysfunction is attributable to lack of Cbl-binding proteins.

Defective Intrinsic Factor

Defective IF is the juvenile form of pernicious anemia. Onset is usually between 1 and 5 years of age. The main features are megaloblastic anemia, global developmental delay, and myelopathy. Serum Cbl levels are low, gastric function and morphology are normal, and autoantibodies to IF are absent. The absorption of Cbl can be corrected by mixing with normal gastric juice as a source of IF. Defective IF can be caused by failure to secrete IF, reduced affinity for IF receptor sites, or enhanced degradation by proteolytic enzymes. IF cDNA has been cloned, and the gene localized to chromosome 11.

Defective Cobalamin Transport by Enterocytes (Imerslund-Gräsbeck Syndrome)

Defective cobalamin transport by enterocytes is a disorder caused by a selective specific malabsorption of Cbl. Onset is after infancy with megaloblastic anemia, failure to thrive, global developmental delay, and myelopathy, often with associated proteinuria. Serum Cbl concentrations are decreased, and IF and TC II concentrations are normal.

Transcobalamin II Deficiency

The onset of TC II deficiency is in early infancy. The features are megaloblastic anemia, failure to thrive, and global developmental delay. When treated only with folic acid and not Cbl, mental retardation and myelopathic features resembling subacute combined degeneration develop in some patients who survive infancy. Serum Cbl concentrations are normal or moderately decreased, with normal IF and absent TC II. Symptoms develop once maternally derived Cbl stores are depleted. The TC II gene is located on chromosome 22, and the cDNA has been cloned.

Treatment

Treatment of the disorders of Cbl absorption requires only the injection of adequate Cbl. Folic acid supplementation is effective in improving the hematologic abnormality. Complete reversal of neurologic deficits depends on the duration of symptoms before instituting proper treatment.

Cobalamin Use Defects

In these disorders, target cells fail to use Cbl. Cbl use defects cause more severe disease than the transport defects.

Impaired Methylcobalamin and Adenosylcobalamin Synthesis

Impaired methylcobalamin and adenosylcobalamin synthesis is a group of disorders that includes three distinct complementation classes: CblC, CblD, and CblF. The block is at sites common to the intracellular biosynthetic pathways of both MeCbl and AdoCbl. Patients are suspected to have both methylmalonic aciduria and homocystinuria. Most cases are caused by CblC defects. Usually presenting in infancy, the initial features are feeding difficulty, lethargy, failure to thrive, megaloblastic anemia, and global developmental delay. Seizures and microcephaly are common. Multiorgan failure with thrombotic microangiopathy is an early feature. The remaining CblC patients have a later onset and are characterized by delirium, psychosis, and spasticity.

Only two brothers with CblD defects are known. The elder boy presented in early adolescence with behavioral problems and was found to be mildly mentally retarded. Thrombotic stroke occurred at age 18 years. His younger brother, although biochemically affected, was asymptomatic. Of five known patients with CblF defects, failure to thrive was noted in most, confusion in one, hypotonia in three, abnormal movements in two, and seizure in one. CblC and CblF defects are presumed to be transmitted as autosomal recessive traits.

Patients with impaired synthesis of MeCbl and AdoCbl have normal serum Cbl and TC II concentrations and usually have megaloblastic anemia, homocystinuria, and methylmalonic aciduria.

Treatment of CblC disease consists of administration of OHCbl (up to 1 mg intramuscularly daily) titrated to control the patient's homocystinuria and methylmalonic aciduria. Adjunctive therapies include moderate protein restriction, carnitine supplementation (to enhance organic acid excretion), folic acid supplementation, and betaine administration (250 mg/kg/day). Despite apparent good metabolic control, surviving patients have shown signs of moderate to severe mental retardation, and many early-onset patients died despite therapy. The CblF patients responded to therapy with OHCbl, although one infant in good metabolic control died suddenly.

Impaired Methylcobalamin Synthesis Only

The term *impaired methylcobalamin synthesis only* refers to a group of disorders that includes two distinct complementation classes: CblE and CblG. These patients have homocystinuria and megaloblastic anemia without methylmalonic aciduria, suggesting a block at a site unique to methyl-Cbl synthesis or activity. Clinically and biochemically, these patients are similar, but they can be differentiated by complementation analysis. Vomiting, lethargy, and poor feeding usually begin before 3 months of age. Neurologic features include psychomotor delay, hypotonia, and frequent seizures. Other features are megaloblastic anemia, homocystinuria, and hypomethioninemia without methylmalonic aciduria.

Treatment consists of OHCbl (1 mg/day to 1 mg/week) titrated to control metabolic parameters. The value of adjunctive therapy with combinations of folic acid, methionine, betaine, pyridoxine, and carnitine supplementation is not established.

Impaired Adenosylcobalamin Synthesis Only

The term *impaired adenosylcobalamin synthesis only* refers to a group of disorders that includes two distinct complementation classes: CblA and CblB. These patients have methylmalonic aciduria without homocystinuria, or megaloblastic anemia with secondary ketosis, acidosis, hypoglycemia, and hyperammonemia. Each class has an early-onset and late-onset presentation. The infantile onset variant consists of failure to thrive, lethargy, recurrent vomiting, dehydration, and hypotonia. Late-onset cases begin in childhood and may present acutely with coma or, in a more indolent fashion, with developmental retardation. Inheritance is presumed to be autosomal recessive.

Therapy involves both dietary protein restriction and OHCbl supplementation. Almost all CblA patients (90%) respond biochemically to therapy, whereas only 40% of CblB patients respond.

Defective Methylmalonyl-CoA Mutase

Methylmalonyl-CoA mutase deficiency is not a disorder of Cbl processing but is considered here because of its biochemical and clinical similarity to CblA and CblB mutations.

Clinical Features

The typical presentation is one of acute neonatal ketoacidosis, with vomiting, lethargy, dehydration, and profound hypotonia. A benign phenotype exists in which the infant is asymptomatic despite methylmalonic aciduria. Several intermediate phenotypes involve growth and psychomotor delay in the absence of acidosis, childhood ketoacidosis, stroke-like episodes with prominent extrapyramidal symptoms, and interstitial nephritis.

Biochemical and Molecular Features

Inheritance of methylmalonyl-CoA mutase deficiency is autosomal recessive. The gene for the disorder has been localized to chromosome 6p12–21.2.

Treatment

Dietary restriction of protein is recommended. Carnitine supplementation may also be useful to replenish depleted stores and to enhance organic acid excretion.

Inherited Disorders of Folate Metabolism

Folate (pteroylglutamate) refers generically to a group of compounds that are conjugates of pterin, para-aminobenzoate, and glutamate. Folates are essential cofactors in several critical single carbon transfer reactions involved in the synthesis of purines, pyrimidines, and methionine, as well as in the degradation of serine, glycine, and histidine.

Methylenetetrahydrofolate Reductase Deficiency

The cDNA for methylenetetrahydrofolate dehydrogenase has been isolated and the gene localized to chromosome 14q24. Age of onset of methylenetetrahydrofolate reductase (MTHFR) deficiency ranges from the newborn to adult life. Presentation within a family varies from biochemically affected but clinically asymptomatic to severely impaired. Most patients present in infancy with global developmental delay, frequently associated with recurrent apneic episodes, seizures, microcephaly, and progressive neurologic deterioration. Childhood onset is characterized by psychomotor delay and myelopathy, and adult onset by recurrent cerebrovascular disease.

The metabolic block is at the level of the reduction of MTHFR to methyltetrahydrofolate. MTHFR activity is low in lymphocytes, leukocytes, hepatic samples, and confluent cultured fibroblasts.

Clinical severity is only roughly correlated with residual enzyme activity. The recommended therapeutic protocol consists of oral betaine combined with folic acid, pyridoxine, and Cbl. The prognosis is poor once neurologic involvement is evident. The best result was in a patient diagnosed prenatally and treated with betaine from birth.

Glutamate Formiminotransferase Deficiency

Age of onset of glutamate formiminotransferase deficiency is between 3 months and 42 years, and two clinical phenotypes are identified. The severe phenotype is characterized by mental retardation and seizures with cortical atrophy. The other phenotype may consist of speech delay or may be represented by an asymptomatic biochemically affected sibling of a symptomatic index case. The metabolic block is in the catabolism of histidine and involves a failure to form 5,10-methylenetetrahydrofolate. The severe phenotype is attributed to cyclodeaminase deficiency and the mild phenotype to a defect in formiminotransferase.

Hereditary Folate Malabsorption

Hereditary folate malabsorption is also called *congenital malabsorption of folate*. Onset is early in infancy with severe megaloblastic anemia combined with oral ulcers, diarrhea, and failure to thrive. Although most patients have seizures and progressive neurologic deterioration, some are asymptomatic. Some patients have intracranial calcification and others a propensity to recurrent infections, which are attributed to low immunoglobulin and partial deficiency of both humoral and cellular immunity. All have a severe abnormality in the intestinal absorption of orally administered folic acid or reduced folates. Severely reduced serum and red blood cell folate combined with severe megaloblastic anemia are the laboratory diagnostic clues.

Inheritance is presumed to be autosomal recessive. Therapy is directed at maintaining serum, red blood cell, and cerebrospinal fluid folate levels above those seen in folate deficiency (4, 150, and 15 ng/ml, respectively). This may be accomplished by oral administration of large doses of folic acid, folinic acid, or methyltetrahydrofolate (up to 100 mg daily). If oral treatment is inadequate, parenteral administration may be necessary. Therapy invariably results in hematologic correction and often in neurologic improvement, especially with respect to seizure control.

DISORDERS OF BIOTIN METABOLISM

Biotin Holocarboxylase Synthetase Deficiency

Clinical Features

Onset of biotin holocarboxylase synthetase deficiency is at birth, with the initial symptom of vomiting. Skin rash develops at 1 month and tachypnea and coma at 5 months. Coma is associated with metabolic ketoacidosis and excretion of large quantities of β-methylcrotonic acid and β-methylcrotonylglycine in the urine. Some patients become symptomatic later in infancy. Abnormal urine odor from hyperammonemia may be noted.

Biochemical and Molecular Features

Holocarboxylase synthetase deficiency is inherited as an autosomal recessive trait. Holocarboxylase synthetase deficiency is usually suspected when high concentrations of the metabolites β-hydroxyisovalerate, β-methylcrotonylglycine, β-hydroxypropionate, methylcitrate, or lactate are found in the urine. Definitive diagnosis requires the demonstration of deficient activity of holocarboxylase synthetase in peripheral blood leukocytes or skin fibroblasts. The cDNA for the enzyme has been isolated and sequenced, and the gene has been localized to chromosome 21q22.1.

Treatment

Most patients with holocarboxylase synthetase deficiency improve markedly after the oral administration of 10 mg biotin per day. Biochemical abnormalities correct quickly with improvement of many of the clinical symptoms. If treatment is delayed, many of the neurologic abnormalities fail to improve. Prenatal diagnosis of holocarboxylase synthetase deficiency can be accomplished, and prenatal treatment is possible by treating the mothers with 10 mg biotin orally.

Biotinidase Deficiency

Clinical Features

In biotinidase deficiency, age of onset of symptoms varies from 1 week to 10 years of age, with a mean age between 3 and 6 months. The most common neurologic features of this disorder are seizures and hypotonia. Several children exhibit hyperventilation, stridor, and apnea. Later they show ataxia, developmental delay, neurosensory hearing loss, and ophthalmologic abnormalities (infections, optic neuropathies, motility disturbances, and retinal pigment changes). Other features are skin rash, varying degrees of alopecia, and cellular immunologic abnormalities. Most enzyme-deficient individuals show metabolic ketolactic acidosis and organic aciduria similar to that seen in holocarboxylase synthetase deficiency. The most commonly elevated urinary organic acid is β-hydroxyisovalerate.

Biochemical and Molecular Features

Biotinidase deficiency is inherited as an autosomal recessive trait. The cDNA that encodes for biotinidase has been cloned and sequenced. The gene is on chromosome 3p25. The primary biochemical defect in most patients with late-onset multiple carboxylase has been shown to be deficient activity of biotinidase in serum. Patients with profound biotinidase activity have less than 10% mean normal activity, and their parents usually have serum enzyme activities intermediate between the children and normal.

In addition to patients with profound biotinidase deficiency, newborns with 10–30% of mean normal activity have been identified by screening. Clinical consequences of partial deficiency were not known until one such child, who was not treated with biotin, exhibited hypotonia, skin rash, and hair loss during a bout of gastroenteritis at 6 months of age. Biotin rapidly resolved the symptoms.

Treatment

All symptomatic children with biotinidase deficiency have improved after treatment with 5–10 mg biotin per day. Biotin must be in the free form. Biochemical abnormalities and seizures rapidly resolve after biotin treatment, followed by improvement of the cutaneous manifestations. Hair growth returns over a period of weeks to months in the alopecic children. Optic atrophy and hearing loss are the most resistant to therapy. Some treated children have rapidly achieved developmental milestones, whereas others have continued to show deficits.

For a more detailed discussion see Shevell MI, Cooper BA, Rosenblatt DS. Inherited Disorders of Cobalamin and Folate Transport and Metabolism (Chapter 73; pp. 1301–1321); Wolf B. Disorders of Biotin Metabolism: Treatable Neurologic Syndromes (Chapter 74; pp. 1323–1339), in RN Rosenberg, SB Prusiner, S DiMauro, RL Barchi (eds),* The Molecular and Genetic Basis of Neurological Disease *(2nd ed). Boston: Butterworth–Heinemann, 1997.

22

The Genetics of Bipolar Disorder and Schizophrenia

BIPOLAR DISORDER

Bipolar Phenotype

Bipolar disorder (BP) consists of episodes of elevated mood state, or mania, and lowered mood state, or major depression. These episodes typically include disturbances in sleep, appetite, energy, concentration, sexual activity, and self-esteem. Impaired judgment and loss of perspective are characteristic of mania as well as depression. Either state may include periods of psychosis. BP type I consists of at least one episode each of mania and major depression, whereas BP type II requires at least one full episode of major depression and at least one episode of elevated mood (hypomania) without full mania. Cyclothymia consists of episodic elevations and depressions of mood that fail to meet either the duration or the severity requirements of major depression or mania.

Family Studies

Family studies are designed to show patterns of aggregation for a particular disorder. The principal findings of these studies are as follows: (1) Although major depression aggregates in the adult relatives of probands with major depressive disorder (MDD) or BP illness, BP aggregates only in the families of BP probands; (2) Rates of major depression are higher among female relatives, whereas rates of BP show a roughly equal gender ratio, and proband gender does not affect the degree of familial aggregation; (3) Early-onset MDD (age <30 years) is related to increased risk of MDD in adult relatives and children; and (4) Onset of major depression in probands younger than 20 years is associated with increased risk of early-onset depression in offspring, beginning at puberty. Family studies have not resolved several issues that are important in attempting to identify specific disease-promoting genes. The most important questions are: (1) What is the extent of genetic heterogeneity? (2) How can one distinguish genetically related phenotypes from genetically unrelated ones? and (3) What is the mode of genetic transmission?

Genetic Heterogeneity

Linkage studies of BP suggest the possibility of extensive genetic heterogeneity—that is, several independent BP susceptibility mutations, each accounting for similar behavioral phenotypes. Currently, heterogeneity can only be inferred; conclusive proof requires the identification of at least two independent disease-promoting genes.

Mode of Transmission

Linkage studies of BP hypothesize autosomal dominant or X-linked dominant transmission involving action of a single major gene. Although the size and structure of the pedigrees are consistent with this assumption, it has not been strongly supported by segregation analyses.

Linkage Studies of Bipolar Disorder

Several linkage studies of BP used the highly polymorphic human leukocyte antigen (HLA) markers on chromosome 6 and phenotypic markers on the X chromosome. These studies were not conclusively positive, and others have excluded linkage between HLA and mood disorders. Other studies suggest segregation with color blindness and with the glucose-6-phosphate dehydrogenase site on the X chromosome. Although Xq26–q27 represents the only positive linkage between BP and markers on the X chromosome, cytogenetic abnormalities in the 11q21–q22 region have been found in several families. As part of an ongoing study of Old Order Amish, restriction fragment length polymorphism markers were used to analyze 81 members of a single, multigenerational pedigree heavily loaded for BP. Linkage to two markers previously localized to chromosome 11, the insulin gene and the H-*ras* oncogene, was identified. These findings could not be replicated in independent pedigrees.

SCHIZOPHRENIA

Schizophrenic Phenotype

Schizophrenia (SC) is a clinical syndrome marked by a combination of negative (e.g., deterioration of social, work, or self-care functioning) and positive symptoms (e.g., auditory or visual hallucinations and delusions), with onset after childhood. Although several lines of evidence point to a heritable predisposition to SC, the search for genetic loci is difficult because SC is hard to define. Relatively few families with SC are compatible with mendelian transmission; 81% of SC patients have no first-degree relatives with the disorder, and 63% have no family history of SC.

Biochemistry

The advent of antipsychotic medications that diminish positive symptoms in many affected individuals has indicated that irregularities of the dopaminergic system are fundamental to the pathology of SC. Neuroimaging studies have implicated regions of the brain known to have dopaminergic neurons. Neurotransmitters other than dopamine may have a role in at least a subgroup of schizophrenics. The distinctive efficacy/clinical profile of different types of antipsychotic medications suggest the possibility of further subtyping of SC, but family and genetic studies have not yet been done to show whether drug responsiveness defines genetically distinct types of SC. For example, haloperidol binds predominantly to D_2 receptors and is effective in treating positive symptoms, whereas clozapine binds preferentially to D_4 dopamine receptors and treats both positive and negative symptoms.

Family and Twin Studies

Family studies have shown an approximately 10-fold increase in risk for SC among first-degree relatives of index cases as compared with relatives of controls. Adoption studies indicate that increased familial aggregation is not simply the result of environmental factors. Using probands and controls identified from adoption records, a greater concentration of SC and SC-spectrum disorders is found in biological relatives of adoptees who were later diagnosed with SC than in their adoptive relatives. Twin studies comparing concordance rates in monozygotic and dizygotic twins show a concordance of approximately 40–50% for monozygotic twins versus 9–10% for dizygotic twins. This ratio is higher than would be expected with a single dominant locus but is compatible with either a recessively acting locus or polygenic model. Family risk data show a higher risk to offspring of affected individuals than to their siblings, implying that a recessive mode of inheritance is unlikely.

Linkage and Association Studies of Schizophrenia

Linkage and association studies in SC have not produced a replicable linkage finding. Considering the typically small size of SC families, progress in SC genetics has been particularly dependent on the identification of highly polymorphic DNA markers. The coexistence of a trisomy (of the 5q11–q13 chromosomal region) and SC in a young adult proband and his maternal uncle was reported. The mother of the proband, who was phenotypically normal, carried a balanced translocation of this region and part of chromosome 1. The report of linkage between SC or other psychiatric disorders and DNA markers on chromosome 5 in other families further increased interest in chromosome 5. Subsequently, several reports excluding linkage between chromosome 5 markers and SC in independently collected families have concluded that, if the finding remains after more markers are tested, the chromosome accounts for only a small percentage of familial cases.

A second site of expected linkage is on chromosome 6p22. After an initial screen of 35 markers showed a lod score of 1.4 at a marker on the 6p22 region in one of the models, six additional markers in that region were tested. Using the broad diagnostic model and an intermediate mode of transmission, four of the additional markers in this region provided positive lod scores, with one marker peaking at a lod score of between 3.2 and 3.5 (under homogeneity and heterogeneity models, respectively). Multipoint analyses of these markers (analyzing results with pairs of markers instead of single markers) showed conflicting results. Further analysis showed the lod score results on the border of a significance value of $P = .05$.

A third site of possible linkage with SC is a locus on chromosome 22q. Peak lod scores greater than 2.0 have been reported in a large series of pedigrees, indicating a possible locus, but results are preliminary as many of the markers responsible for the positive scores are not highly informative. The chromosome 5 trisomy and the chromosome 6p and chromosome 22 linkage have received the most attention; however, SC has also been described in conjunction with abnormalities on several other chromosomes, including 2, 3, 8, 18, and 19. The apparent clinical heterogeneity of chronic psychotic syndromes suggests that alternative phenotypes be considered.

For a more detailed discussion see Escamilla MA, Freimer NB, Reus VI. The Genetics of Bipolar Disorder and Schizophrenia (Chapter 75; pp. 1343–1362), in RN Rosenberg, SB Prusiner, S DiMauro, RL Barchi (eds),* The Molecular and Genetic Basis of Neurological Disease *(2nd ed). Boston: Butterworth–Heinemann, 1997.

23

Gene Therapy and the Human Genome

PRACTICAL ASPECTS OF GENE THERAPY

Gene or Gene Product to Be Introduced

For most recessive genetic diseases resulting from the loss of a specific genetic function, it is necessary to identify the mutant gene, clone its normal homologue, and introduce a functional copy into the diseased cells. This approach is not likely to work for dominant genetic diseases resulting from gain of function mutations. In these, it may be necessary to correct the mutant gene directly, to prevent expression of the mutant gene, or to introduce another gene that masks the functional consequences of the dominant mutation. Expression of a dominant mutation might be masked by inserting sequences that direct the production of dominant negative alleles, antisense mRNA molecules, or ribozymes that recognize and inactivate the mutant sense mRNA transcripts produced in affected cells.

Gene transfer methods may be applicable to certain neurologic diseases of nongenetic origin. In Parkinson's disease, it may be possible to provide symptomatic control by introducing genes or cells expressing tyrosine hydroxylase or aromatic amino acid decarboxylase to restore dopamine levels.

Strategy for Gene Transfer

The two general strategies for developing gene therapy are the in vivo approach and the ex vivo approach. The in vivo approach involves the introduction of genetic material directly into the tissues of an affected individual. The ex vivo approach is technically more demanding. First, a suitable cell type is harvested from a donor and grown in tissue culture. Next, the gene is introduced into the cells in vitro, and cells expressing the transgene are amplified. The genetically altered cells are then harvested and reimplanted into an affected host. This approach requires the growth of suitable cells in vitro and their subsequent survival after implantation. The advantage of this approach is that it does not require an efficient method for gene transfer because the genetically altered cells may be amplified in vitro before implantation.

Method for Introduction of Transgenes

The simplest approach to the introduction of foreign genetic material is the direct injection of DNA or RNA into an affected area. This requires that naked genetic material be taken up by cells and expressed. This procedure is rarely efficient. A more efficient approach is to introduce transgenes that have been incorporated into a viral vector. These vectors take advantage of the mechanisms viruses have evolved to mediate efficient introduction, replication, and expression of their genetic cargo. The retroviruses have been used extensively for this process. These viruses are capable of efficiently infecting many cell types of different animal species. One disadvantage is that they require active cell replication for stable integration of their genetic cargo, so they are not useful for introducing genes into postmitotic cells such as neurons or glia of the adult nervous system. The herpes simplex virus type 1 may be suitable for that purpose because it is neurotropic and capable of infecting nondividing cells. The adenoviruses can infect postmitotic neurons and glia and do not integrate into the host genome. However, they tend to induce an immune response that may be responsible for the eventual disappearance of gene expression and resistance to reinfection.

Cell Type and Region Affected

In metabolic disorders, it may be necessary to introduce genetic material into all cells throughout the nervous system. In other disorders, only a restricted subpopulation of neurons in a particular brain subregion may need to be targeted. Genetic modification of glial cells or myocytes may be required for the correction of diseases of myelin and muscle, respectively. The treatment of diseases affecting specific subclasses of cells in anatomically defined areas seems the easier task because gene transfer vectors or genetically modified cells can be delivered to one or a few brain regions by microsurgical injection.

Amount of Transgene Expression Required

Many inherited metabolic diseases do not require complete restoration of gene function to correct important aspects of the disease phenotype.

In phenylketonuria, restitution of less than 10% of normal phenylalanine hydroxylase activity is sufficient.

Age of the Affected Host

In many diseases affecting the nervous system, irreversible developmental or neurodegenerative processes occur during infancy. These must be corrected at birth or before.

CONSEQUENCES OF MAPPING AND SEQUENCING THE HUMAN GENOME FOR NEUROLOGIC DISEASES

Human Genome Project

The human genome consists of approximately 3 billion base pairs (bp) of DNA arranged into 24 different chromosomes. This DNA is believed to contain the information necessary to code for 50,000–100,000 genes. Half of these genes are believed to direct the synthesis of proteins that are present in significant quantities only in the central nervous system. The major challenge for human geneticists is to find all the genes in the human genome and set the stage for determining their functions. Conventional human disease gene searches start from a phenotype, such as an inherited neurologic disorder, and use the pattern of inheritance of this phenotype, in combination with other inherited markers, to determine the approximate chromosomal position of the gene responsible for the disorder. This approach to gene identification has been called *reverse genetics* or *positional cloning*.

Applications of the Human Genome Project

The current human genetic map has an average resolution of approximately 1 Mb. Thus, genetic data can potentially locate a typical gene of interest within a 1- to 5-Mb interval. Sometimes data indicate roughly where the gene lies within that interval. In an average 5-Mb genomic region, there are likely to be 150 genes. If a large number of human families segregating disease alleles of the gene are available, it is possible to use this finer genetic map and eventually localize the desired gene to within approximately 1 Mb. For rare disease genes, this may not be possible, because the number of informative families may be inadequate.

When completed, the Human Genome Project will show the DNA sequence of tens of thousands of previously uncharted genes. Initially, there will be few clues about the function of most of these genes, but some should correspond to the several thousand known genetic diseases. Others will be close relatives of genes already studied in other organisms, and many will have no connection with anything previously studied. Most of these uncharted genes are likely to function only in the central nervous system.

For a more detailed discussion see Jinnah HA, Friedmann T. Gene Therapy and Neurologic Disease (Chapter 76; pp. 1365–1373); Smith CL, Cantor CR. Consequences of Mapping and Sequencing the Human Genome for Neurologic Diseases (Chapter 77; pp. 1375–1388), in RN Rosenberg, SB Prusiner, S DiMauro, RL Barchi (eds),* The Molecular and Genetic Basis of Neurological Disease *(2nd ed). Boston: Butterworth–Heinemann, 1997.

Index

In this index, page numbers followed by "t" and "f" indicate tables and figures, respectively.